Metabolic and Bariatric Surgery

Editor

ADRIAN G. DAN

SURGICAL CLINICS
OF NORTH AMERICA

www.surgical.theclinics.com

Consulting Editor
RONALD F. MARTIN

August 2016 • Volume 96 • Number 4

ELSEVIER

1600 John F. Kennedy Boulevard • Suite 1800 • Philadelphia, Pennsylvania, 19103-2899

http://www.surgical.theclinics.com

SURGICAL CLINICS OF NORTH AMERICA Volume 96, Number 4

August 2016 ISSN 0039–6109, ISBN-13: 978-0-323-45989-1

Editor: John Vassallo, j.vassallo@elsevier.com

Developmental Editor: Colleen Viola

Surgical Clinics of North America (ISSN 0039–6109) is published bimonthly by Elsevier Inc., 360 Park Avenue South, New York, NY 10010-1710. Months of publication are February, April, June, August, October, and December. Business and Editorial Offices: 1600 John F. Kennedy Blvd., Suite 1800, Philadelphia, PA 19103-2899. Periodicals postage paid at New York, NY and additional mailing offices. Subscription prices are $375.00 per year for US individuals, $707.00 per year for US institutions, $100.00 per year for US students and residents, $455.00 per year for Canadian individuals, $895.00 per year for Canadian institutions, $510.00 for international individuals, $895.00 per year for international institutions and $250.00 per year for Canadian and foreign students/residents. To receive student/resident rate, orders must be accompanied by name of affiliated institution, date of term, and the *signature* of program/residency coordinator on institution letterhead. Orders will be billed at individual rate until proof of status is received. Foreign air speed delivery is included in all *Clinics* subscription prices. All prices are subject to change without notice. POSTMASTER: Send address changes to *Surgical Clinics*, Elsevier Health Sciences Division, Subscription Customer Service, 3251 Riverport Lane, Maryland Heights, MO 63043. **Customer Service (orders, claims, online, change of address): Telephone: 1-800-654-2452 (U.S. and Canada); 314-447-8871 (outside U.S. and Canada). Fax: 314-447-8029. E-mail: journalscustomerservice-usa@elsevier.com (for print support); journalsonline support-usa@elsevier.com (for online support).**

Reprints. For copies of 100 or more, of articles in this publication, please contact the Commercial Reprints Department, Elsevier Inc., 360 Park Avenue South, New York, New York 10010-1710. Tel. 212-633-3874, Fax: 212-633-3820, E-mail: reprints@elsevier.com.

The *Surgical Clinics of North America* is also published in Spanish by McGraw-Hill Interamericana Editores S.A., P.O. Box 5-237 06500 Mexico D.F. Mexico; and in Portuguese by Interlivros Edicoes Ltda., Rua Comandante Coelho 1085, CEP 21250, Rio de Janeiro, Brazil; and in Greek by Paschalidis Medical Publications, Athens Greece.

The *Surgical Clinics of North America* is covered in *MEDLINE/PubMed (Index Medicus)*, *EMBASE/Excerpta Medica*, *Current Contents/Clinical Medicine*, *Current Contents/Life Sciences*, *Science Citation Index*, and *ISI/BIOMED*.

Contributors

CONSULTING EDITOR

RONALD F. MARTIN, MD, FACS
Colonel (ret.), United States Army Reserve York Hospital, York, Maine

EDITOR

ADRIAN G. DAN, MD, FACS, FASMBS
Director, Advanced Gastrointestinal Minimally Invasive and Bariatric Surgery Fellowship Program; Chief, Division of Robotic General Surgery; Co-Director, Bariatric Care Center, Akron City Hospital–Summa Health System, Akron, Ohio; Assistant Professor of Surgery, Northeast Ohio Medical University, Rootstown, Ohio

AUTHORS

OMODELE AYENI, MD, FRCSC
Southlake Regional Health Centre, Newmarket, Ontario, Canada

DAN E. AZAGURY, MD
Assistant Professor of Surgery, Section of Bariatric and Minimally Invasive Surgery, Stanford University School of Medicine, Stanford University, Stanford, California

LINDSAY BERBIGLIA, DO
Minimally Invasive and Bariatric Surgery Fellow, Akron, Ohio

LAURENT BIERTHO, MD
Department of Metabolic and Bariatric Surgery, Institut Universitaire de cardiologie et pneumologie de Québec – Université Laval, Quebec City, Quebec, Canada

SIMON BIRON, MD, MSc
Department of Metabolic and Bariatric Surgery, Institut Universitaire de cardiologie et pneumologie de Québec – Université Laval, Quebec City, Quebec, Canada

STACY BRETHAUER, MD
Staff Surgeon, Bariatric and Metabolic Institute, Associate Professor of Surgery, Cleveland Clinic Lerner College of Medicine, Cleveland Clinic, Cleveland, Ohio

JAMES ROSSARIO CASELLA MARIOLO, MD
Bariatric and Metabolic Surgery, Division of Diabetes and Nutritional Sciences, King's College London and King's College Hospital, London, United Kingdom

LIDIA CASTAGNETO-GISSEY, MD
Bariatric and Metabolic Surgery, Division of Diabetes and Nutritional Sciences, King's College London and King's College Hospital, London, United Kingdom

ADAM C. CELIO, MD
Bariatric Surgery Research Fellow and General Surgery Resident, Department of Surgery, Brody School of Medicine, East Carolina University, Greenville, North Carolina

BIPAN CHAND, MD
Associate Professor of Surgery, Director, Loyola Center for Metabolic Surgery and Bariatric Care, Stritch School of Medicine, Loyola University Medical Center, Maywood, Illinois

JESSE CLANTON, MD
Assistant Professor, Department of Surgery, West Virginia University Charleston Division, Charleston, West Virginia

ADRIAN G. DAN, MD, FACS, FASMBS
Director, Advanced Gastrointestinal Minimally Invasive and Bariatric Surgery Fellowship Program; Chief, Division of Robotic General Surgery; Co-Director, Bariatric Care Center, Akron City Hospital–Summa Health System, Akron, Ohio; Assistant Professor of Surgery, Northeast Ohio Medical University, Rootstown, Ohio

A. DANIEL GUERRON, MD
Department of General Surgery, Duke University Health System, Durham, North Carolina

MATTHEW DAVIS, MD
Section of Surgical Endoscopy, Department of General Surgery, Digestive Disease Institute, Cleveland Clinic Lerner College of Medicine, Cleveland, Ohio

GEORGE EID, MD, FACS
System Director, Bariatric and Metabolic Institute, Allegheny Health Network, Pittsburgh, Pennsylvania; Adjunct Professor, Biomedical Engineering, Carnegie Mellon University, Pittsburgh, Pennsylvania; Clinical Professor of Surgery, Temple University, Philadelphia, Pennsylvania

TAMMY FOUSE, DO
Advanced Laparoscopic and Bariatric Fellow, Cleveland Clinic, Cleveland, Ohio

LAURENT GENSER, MD
Bariatric and Metabolic Surgery, Division of Diabetes and Nutritional Sciences, King's College London and King's College Hospital, London, United Kingdom

RICHDEEP S. GILL, MD, PhD, FRCSC
Minimally Invasive Upper Gastrointestinal and Bariatric Surgeon; Assistant Professor, Department of Surgery, Peter Lougheed Hospital, University of Calgary, Calgary, Alberta, Canada

KELLEN HAYES, MD
Bariatric and Metabolic Institute, Allegheny Health Network, Pittsburgh, Pennsylvania

FRÉDÉRIC-SIMON HOULD, MD
Department of Metabolic and Bariatric Surgery, Institut Universitaire de cardiologie et pneumologie de Québec – Université Laval, Quebec City, Quebec, Canada

DENNIS J. HURWITZ, MD
Director of the Hurwitz Centre For Plastic Surgery, Clinical Professor of Plastic Surgery, University of Pittsburgh Medical School, Pittsburgh, Pennsylvania

FRANÇOIS JULIEN, MD
Department of Metabolic and Bariatric Surgery, Institut Universitaire de cardiologie et pneumologie de Québec – Université Laval, Quebec City, Quebec, Canada

SHAHZEER KARMALI, BSc, MD, MPH, FRCSC, FACS
Surgical Director Weight Wise Bariatric Clinic; Associate Professor, Department of
Surgery, Minimally Invasive Gastrointestinal and Bariatric Surgery, University of Alberta,
Edmonton, Alberta, Canada

MATTHEW KROH, MD
Director, Section of Surgical Endoscopy, Department of General Surgery, Digestive
Disease Institute, Associate Professor of Surgery, Cleveland Clinic Lerner College of
Medicine, Cleveland, Ohio

STÉFANE LEBEL, MD
Department of Metabolic and Bariatric Surgery, Institut Universitaire de cardiologie
et pneumologie de Québec – Université Laval, Quebec City, Quebec, Canada

EMANUELE LO MENZO, MD, PhD, FACS, FASMBS
Director of Center for Research, The Bariatric and Metabolic Institute, Cleveland Clinic
Florida, Weston, Florida

SIMON MARCEAU, MD
Department of Metabolic and Bariatric Surgery, Institut Universitaire de cardiologie et
pneumologie de Québec – Université Laval, Quebec City, Quebec, Canada

ERIC MARCOTTE, MD, MS
Assistant Professor of Surgery, Stritch School of Medicine, Loyola University Medical
Center, Maywood, Illinois

JOHN MAGAÑA MORTON, MD, MPH, FACS, FASMBS
Chief, Section of Bariatric and Minimally Invasive Surgery, Stanford University School of
Medicine, Stanford University, Stanford, California

SPYROS PANAGIOTOPOULOS, MD, PhD
Bariatric and Metabolic Surgery, Division of Diabetes and Nutritional Sciences, King's
College London and King's College Hospital, London, United Kingdom

WALTER J. PORIES, MD, FACS
Professor of Surgery, Biochemistry, and Kinesiology, Department of Surgery, Brody
School of Medicine, East Carolina University, Greenville, North Carolina

DANA D. PORTENIER, MD
Department of General Surgery, Duke University Health System, Durham, North Carolina

RAUL ROSENTHAL, MD, FACS, FASMBS
Chairman, Department of General Surgery; Director, The Bariatric and Metabolic Institute
Co-Director Fellowship Training Advanced GI Surgery; Cleveland Clinic Florida, Weston,
Florida

FRANCESCO RUBINO, MD
Chair of Bariatric and Metabolic Surgery, Bariatric and Metabolic Surgery, Division of
Diabetes and Nutritional Sciences, James Black Centre, Consultant Bariatric Surgeon,
King's College London and King's College Hospital, London, United Kingdom

PHILIP SCHAUER, MD
Director, Bariatric and Metabolic Institute, Professor of Surgery, Cleveland Clinic Lerner
College of Medicine, Cleveland Clinic, Cleveland, Ohio

VADIM SHERMAN, MD, FRCSC, FACS
Assistant Professor of Surgery, Weill Cornell Medical College, Medical Director, Bariatric
and Metabolic Surgery Center, Houston Methodist Hospital, Houston, Texas

MICHAEL SUBICHIN, MD
Department of Surgery, Summa Health System, Akron, Ohio

NOAH J. SWITZER, MD
CAMIS Research Fellow, Department of Surgery, University of Alberta, Edmonton, Alberta, Canada

SAMUEL SZOMSTEIN, MD, FACS, FASMBS
Director, Fellowship Training Advanced GI Surgery; Associate-Director, The Bariatric and Metabolic Institute, Cleveland Clinic Florida, Weston, Florida

JOHN G. ZOGRAFAKIS, MD, FACS, FASMBS
Director, Advanced Laparoscopic Surgical Services, Director, Bariatric Care Center, Co-Director Minimally Invasive and Bariatric Surgery Fellowship, Associate Professor of Surgery, Northeast Ohio Medical University, Rootstown, Ohio

Contents

This article examines the progression of bariatric surgery since its creation more than 60 years ago with a focus on the effect of surgery on weight loss, comorbidity reduction, and safety. The success has been remarkable. It is possible to cure severe obesity, type 2 diabetes, and hyperlipidemia in addition to the many other manifestations of the metabolic syndrome with remarkable safety. Equally important are the opportunities for research afforded by the surgery and its outcomes. Until better treatments become available, bariatric surgery is the therapy of choice for patients with morbid obesity for weight control and comorbidity improvement.

Bariatric surgery has been shown in many studies to be the most effective long-term treatment for severe obesity and obesity-related comorbidities. Economic analysis has demonstrated cost-effectiveness as well as cost-savings in select subgroups of patients. Despite the health and economic benefits of bariatric surgery, relatively few eligible patients receive this treatment. This disparity in access to care must be addressed by health policy decision-makers.

Several gastrointestinal (GI) operations originally developed for the treatment of severe obesity (bariatric surgery) promote sustained weight loss as well as dramatic, durable improvements of insulin-resistant states, most notably type 2 diabetes mellitus (T2DM). Experimental evidence shows that some rearrangements of GI anatomy can directly affect glucose homeostasis, insulin sensitivity, and inflammation, supporting the idea that the GI tract is a biologically rational target for interventions aimed at correcting pathophysiologic aspects of cardiometabolic disorders. This article reviews the pathophysiology of metabolic disease and

Nonalcoholic fatty liver disease (NAFLD) is an under-recognized but increasingly important manifestation of the metabolic syndrome. Bariatric surgery, both through direct weight loss and more indirect effects on insulin resistance and improvements in inflammatory proteins, can have a profound effect on NAFLD, resulting in improvement or resolution of even high-grade liver disease.

Bariatric surgery is the most effective and durable treatment of severe obesity. In addition to weight loss, these operations result in significant improvement or resolution of many obesity-related comorbid diseases. There are now numerous studies demonstrating that bariatric surgery decreases all-cause mortality long-term compared with cohorts of patients who did not undergo surgery. Decreases in cancer, diabetes, and cardiovascular-related mortality are major contributors to this overall effect on life expectancy after bariatric surgery.

Patient safety and quality improvement have been part of bariatric surgery since its inception, and there have been significant improvements in outcomes of bariatric surgery over the past two decades. A strong accreditation program exists. This program defines two tiers of accredited centers: low-acuity and comprehensive centers similar to the trauma systems. Accreditation has been shown to have a favorable impact on outcomes of bariatric surgery. Bariatric surgery lends itself well to improvements in processes and use of perioperative protocols, such as ulcer and thromboembolic prophylaxis prevention or gallstone prevention and management.

Bariatric surgery is the most effective way to improve comorbidities related to obesity. Since the introduction of minimally invasive laparoscopic surgery in the bariatric surgery techniques, the number of procedures has increased substantially; advances in techniques and the transition from open to minimally invasive procedures have decreased morbidity and mortality. Multidisciplinary teams in charge of the operative planning, surgical act, and postoperative recovery are determinant in the success of the management of high-risk bariatric patients; careful identification and preoperative management of these higher-risk patients is crucial in decreasing complications after weight loss surgery.

with duodenal switch. The standard follow-up requirements, including vitamin supplementation and long-term risks associated with metabolic surgery, are also discussed. Most of the data reported here are based on the authors' experience with 4000 biliopancreatic diversions with duodenal switch performed in their institution since 1990.

Revisional bariatric procedures are increasingly common. With more primary procedures being performed to manage severe obesity and its complications, 5% to 8% of these procedures will fail, requiring revisional operation. Reasons for revisional bariatric surgery are either primary inadequate weight loss, defined as less than 25% excess body weight loss, or weight recidivism, defined as a gain of more than 10 kg based on the nadir weight; however, each procedure also has inherit specific complications that can also be indications for revision. This article reviews the history of each primary bariatric procedure, indications for revision, surgical options, and subsequent outcomes.

Bariatric surgery is well-recognized for its effects on health, beyond weight-loss. It underwent a revolution recently with the growing performance of laparoscopic procedures, leading to enhanced recovery and a reduction in procedural risk. However, surgical complications, although rare, do develop. It is important to recognize the complications, and ideally prevent them from happening. This article reviews the risks of the four most commonly performed bariatric procedures, with an emphasis on technique and management in the intraoperative and postoperative period. The nutritional aspect of bariatric surgery is of the utmost importance, because catastrophic consequences have been linked to malnutrition and vitamin deficiencies.

The burden of obesity and weight-related comorbid disease is significant. Existing laparoscopic techniques show excellent efficacy and safety. New endoscopic and laparoscopic procedures offer different approaches, as primary and revisional techniques, to treat obesity and associated metabolic disease.

Plastic surgeons subspecializing in body contouring are meeting the challenge of postbariatric surgery massive weight loss patients. With an appreciation of the magnitude of the surface deformity, and altered metabolism, nutrition, and psychological makeup of these patients, innovative plastic surgeons have forged an organized approach to preparation, operative technique, and postoperative care. Patients at greatest risk for complications are identified, appraised, and either their condition improved or they are counselled to reduce expectations. Beyond the removal of excess skin and adipose tissue, advanced gender-specific techniques have improved aesthetics.

SURGICAL CLINICS
OF NORTH AMERICA

ISSUE OF RELATED INTEREST

Endocrinology and Metabolism Clinics, June 2016 (Vol. 45, Issue 2)
Pediatric Endocrinology
Robert Rapaport, *Editor*
Available at: www.endo.theclinics.com

THE CLINICS ARE AVAILABLE ONLINE!
Access your subscription at:
www.theclinics.com

Foreword

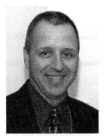

Ronald F. Martin, MD, FACS
Consulting Editor

This issue of the *Surgical Clinics of North America* is the third issue that we have dedicated entirely to bariatric surgery and/or metabolic surgery since my time as Consulting Editor. I would like to tell our readership that we have made tremendous advances in this disease epidemic of obesity, but unfortunately, I cannot. Not to be misunderstood, we have made great strides in the operative management of uncontrolled excess weight and of the metabolic complications that are associated with it, as Dr Dan and his colleagues reveal through their collective contributions. That acknowledged, we collectively have fallen far short in the management of the disease itself.

For many years, a main focus of surgical inquiry was how to keep people from starving. The development of enteral nutrition and subsequent parenteral nutrition built careers and some industries. Gut transplant has remained challenging but possible after years of refinement of understanding of fundamental biology and technical and supportive care. Now the most rapidly growing threat to our collective health may be the consequences of increased caloric ingestion.

We are increasing our ability to alter "normal anatomy" to prohibit the consequences to attempting to consume more than one can physiologically manage. Yet, the underlying disease begins well before the excess weight goes on. And while the disease strikes all social strata, it is unevenly divided to most significantly affect the poorer segments of more affluent cultures. It remains a disease of the unhinging of our consumption from our needs.

We have to ask our selves, why? What is it that has brought us to this place over the last several decades? If there were a simple answer, I suppose we would all know it. Clearly, we have shifted our economy from one that is mainly agrarian to manufacturing to service to information, each representing a potential for decreased caloric expenditure to make a living. We have retreated to vehicles for transportation rather than walking. We don't even let our children walk. In short, we have decreased the number of calories needed to keep ourselves employed and productive. At the same time, we have massively increased the amount of calories that we consume in total and per meal. Not only has caloric content gone up but also a shift to less complex carbohydrates leads the way, adding its own nutritional dimension. Even our socialization has become more digital and less physical in the aggregate.

Surg Clin N Am 96 (2016) xiii–xiv
http://dx.doi.org/10.1016/j.suc.2016.06.004
0039-6109/16/$ – see front matter © 2016 Published by Elsevier Inc.

surgical.theclinics.com

We live in a culture of increased consumerism and short-term expectations. More instant gratification and less personal responsibility abound in our culture. And this does not solely apply to the United States; this is a worldwide issue affecting all nations with the resources to create this dilemma.

It is truly impressive what our colleagues in the metabolic and bariatric surgical disciplines have been able to learn and refine to help manage this problem for individual patients. On the larger scale, we need a different approach. Perhaps we should look more to our colleagues in the trauma world. They too developed systems and techniques to care for traumatized patients that were and are very impressive. Yet, they also developed collaborations and partnerships that allowed for safer transportation using safer vehicles and better roads. We still have a ways to go with gun violence, but one battle at a time. The point being, they worked on prevention as much as treatment. In all likelihood, the yield on prevention was probably a better return on investment.

So why can't we do that with food? It's hard to say. Maybe, we can charge and will pay more for a safer car. Maybe, it's easier for people to be horrified by the carnage caused by a car wreck in which a couple of teenagers die tragically and suddenly so we collectively will do what we can to solve the problem—put in a stop light, make seatbelts mandatory, enforce drunk-driving laws. I can't say what the analogous situation is for obesity. Charging more for better food isn't working because the less nutritious foods are cheaper. People don't generally like to pay more for what they perceive to be less. Also, let's face it, getting sick by eating, short of choking, is a slow process: as much the opposite of a car crash or fire as it could be. It is a lot easier to ignore getting obese or to believe that one can turn the situation around—tomorrow.

If we were improving our trauma care while letting trauma rates quintuple or if we were improving our ability to revascularize our hearts while ignoring the use of statins and other preventive measures, there would be riotous indignation looking for prevention, both on the public and on governmental levels. That is not so with obesity.

For the meantime, it appears to be what it is. Dr Dan and his colleagues have assembled an excellent collection of articles to address this disease. I am indebted to them. As a group of professionals, we need to seek to reduce the demand for these services, not by restricting them for those in need, but by reducing the number of people who need them in the first place. This may be the defining medical issue of the industrialized world at this time.

Ronald F. Martin, MD, FACS
Colonel (ret.), United States Army Reserve York Hospital
16 Hospital Drive, Suite A
York, ME 03909, USA

E-mail address:
rmartin@yorkhospital.com

Preface

Obesity—The Epidemic Crisis of Our Time

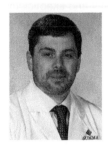

Adrian G. Dan, MD, FACS, FASMBS
Editor

Seldom does a specific disease entity become a "plague" to humanity and thereby define that period of time in the history of mankind. Today, one such phenomenon is the obesity epidemic, which spares no socioeconomic subset or geographic region of the world. The problem has reached a critical point becoming profoundly ubiquitous in the general population. A drastic change has occurred in the past few decades, unlike any other seen in the evolution of the human species. Rates of morbid obesity are skyrocketing to unprecedented levels, particularly in more affluent regions of the world. The simultaneous advances in agriculture, industry, and technology are testing our species in novel ways. In fact, more individuals now suffer from obesity and its health ravages than endure hunger and malnutrition.

For the first time in the *Surgical Clinics of North America* series, Metabolic Surgery has taken precedence in the title of an issue, emphasizing the metabolic capabilities of surgical procedures that have been refined over the span of six decades. These operations have been developed into some of the most effective and well-studied therapies in modern medicine. The myth that "weight loss is the sole objective of bariatric surgery" has dissipated and given way to the avalanche of scientific evidence validating the metabolic benefits made possible with surgical alterations of the gastrointestinal tract. Every single organ system is impacted by morbid obesity and may be positively affected by the metabolic changes conferred with bariatric procedures. The potential to prevent and resolve associated conditions, significantly reduce the incidence of malignancies, and increase longevity makes bariatric surgery the ultimate weapon in the era of population health management. Obesity reaches far beyond the issues limited to the patient-physician relationship, and the psychologic, social, cultural, and economic ramifications penetrate all facets of our life. This issue is designed to cover a wide range of such topics pertinent to contemporary bariatric practice. It is intended to serve as a current and robust reference for surgical residents, bariatric fellows, practicing surgeons, collaborating physicians, and health care policymakers.

Surg Clin N Am 96 (2016) xv–xvi
http://dx.doi.org/10.1016/j.suc.2016.06.001
0039-6109/16/$ – see front matter © 2016 Published by Elsevier Inc.

surgical.theclinics.com

It has been a privilege to gather some of the brightest and most prolific surgical minds of our time in an effort to comprehensively review the major topics of our specialty. The opportunity to organize this issue and to serve as guest editor is the single greatest honor of my academic career. I extend my deepest gratitude to the authors whose immense efforts have collectively culminated in this compilation. Finally, I would like to dedicate this issue to those visionaries and pioneers of bariatric surgery whose efforts and contributions, often in the face of adversity and skepticism, have paved the way to the current state of Metabolic and Bariatric Surgery.

Adrian G. Dan, MD, FACS, FASMBS
Bariatric Care Center–Summa Health System
95 Arch Street, Suite 260
Akron, OH 44304, USA

Northeast Ohio Medical University
Rootstown, OH, USA

E-mail address:
dana@summahealth.org

A History of Bariatric Surgery

The Maturation of a Medical Discipline

Adam C. Celio, MD, Walter J. Pories, MD*

KEYWORDS

- Bariatric • Obesity • Metabolic surgery • Intestinal bypass • Gastric bypass
- Gastric sleeve • Gastric band • Gastric balloon

KEY POINTS

- The history of bariatric surgery, one of the great medical advances of the last century, again documents that science progresses not as a single idea by one person, but rather in small collaborative steps that take decades to accept.
- Bariatric surgery, now renamed "metabolic surgery," has, for the first time, provided cure for some of the most deadly diseases, including type 2 diabetes, hypertension, severe obesity, NASH, and hyperlipidemias, among others, that were previously considered incurable and for which there were no effective therapies.
- With organization, a common database, and certification of centers of excellence, bariatric surgery, once one of the most dangerous operations, is now performed throughout the United States with the same safety as a routine cholecystectomy.

RECOGNITION

Obesity is now a worldwide public health problem, an epidemic, with increasing incidence and prevalence, high costs, and associated comorbidities.[1] Although the genes from our ancestors were helpful in times of potential famine, now in times of plenty, they have contributed to obesity.[1–4] The history of obesity is related to the history of food; the human diet has changed considerably over the last 700,000 years. Our ancestors at one time were hunter-gatherers, consuming large and small game along with nuts and berries. Their diets were high in protein and their way of life was strenuous; they were well suited for times of famine. Those able to store energy for long periods of time survived and passed on those genes.[2] About 8000 years ago, the development of farming allowed people to consume diets that were mainly complex

Disclosure Statement: The authors have nothing to disclose.
Department of Surgery, Brody School of Medicine, East Carolina University, 600 Moye Boulevard, Greenville, NC 27834, USA
* Corresponding author.
E-mail address: poriesw@ecu.edu

carbohydrates (wheat and barley).[3] More recently, sedentary lifestyles and the development of high-calorie fast foods with high levels of carbohydrates, saturated fat, and salt have contributed to the rise in obesity.[3]

Obesity became much more common and apparent in the 1900s as society progressed. Initially, medical means were used to attempt to help patients lose weight, dating back as far as the 1920s.[4] The results from the earliest attempts were largely unsuccessful and the patients that did achieve weight loss had great difficulty in maintaining their weight.[4,5] Medical modalities for treatment of obesity, namely a low-calorie balanced diet, anorectic drugs, behavioral therapy, and exercise, had little or nothing to offer most morbidly obese patients.[5]

The most important breakthrough in the history of bariatric surgery, that is, that surgery should be considered as a treatment of obesity, is too often forgotten. Although there are a few cultures, such as Hawaiian royalty, in which obesity was considered a sign of power, much of the world, especially in the United States, equates severe obesity with a lack of control. That bias is reflected in the difficulty millions of obese people have in finding such basic things as employment and acceptance in society.[6] Even today, there is great reluctance in admitting that medical therapy (ie, diets, behavioral modification, exercise, and drugs) fails, almost universally, in patients who are severely obese.

DEVELOPMENT OF PROCEDURES

The failure of medical therapy for severe obesity and the success of surgery has, over the last six decades, produced a remarkable series of new techniques and procedures for the treatment of obesity and its comorbidities. Bariatric operations have traditionally been divided into three groups based on their mechanism of weight loss production. Malabsorptive procedures induce weight loss totally by interference with digestion and absorption. Restrictive procedures produce weight loss solely by limiting intake. Mixed malabsorptive and restrictive procedures limit intake and produce malabsorption.[7] **Fig. 1** provides a diagrammatic overview of the operations currently in use and others for historical consideration. The following discussion of bariatric operations provides an overview. Multiple variations of each of the operations have been performed and discarded during the last 60 years with variations in, for example, the size of gastric pouches, length of limbs, type and size of anastomoses, and the use of vagotomy.

Malabsorptive Procedures: Intestinal Bypass

Surgeons have long known that shortened gut could lead to substantial weight loss.[8] The first application of these observations, the surgical treatment of obesity for the purpose of improving comorbidities, was in 1952 by a Swedish surgeon, Dr Viktor Henrickson. He noticed that small bowel resections performed for other disease processes usually produced no change in the patient's general status but, in some cases, resulted in significant weight loss.[9] Based on his observations, he resected 105 cm of small intestine from a 32-year-old obese female who could not complete a weight loss program. Interestingly, the patient lost only a small amount of weight but was noted to have an improved quality of life.[9] Although this was the first reported operation for obesity, it was not adopted for treatment in other patients because of its irreversibility. It would take the development of a reversible procedure for widespread adoption.

Surgeons in the United States were also investigating ways to shorten the intestines as a treatment of obesity and developed the intestinal bypass. Dr Varco, at the University of Minnesota, performed the first jejunoileal bypass (JIB) in 1953.[8] Kremen and

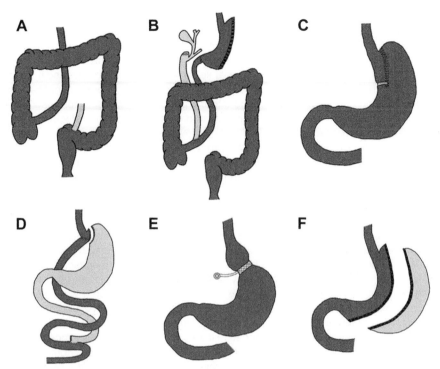

Fig. 1. Overview of bariatric surgical operations. (*A*) Jejunal-ileal bypass: end-to-end jejunoi-leostomy with ileosigmoidostomy. (*B*) Biliopancreatic diversion with a duodenal switch. (*C*) Vertical banded gastroplasty. (*D*) Roux-en-Y gastric bypass. (*E*) Adjustable gastric band. (*F*) Sleeve gastrectomy.

coworkers,[10] also at the University of Minnesota, published a report in 1954 describing the effects of small intestinal bypass on dogs. He bypassed various portions of the small bowel and found removing 50% of distal small bowel from the intestinal stream was associated with weight loss. This was done by diverting the proximal small intestine to the terminal ileum. They postulated that a bypass of much of the small intestine to the ileum could be used to produce weight loss in the severely obese and referenced the one human patient that had recently undergone the procedure.[10] Their procedure consisted of an end-to-end jejunoileostomy and an ileocecostomy.

Other surgeons began developing variations of intestinal bypasses of much of the small bowel. One of these was a diversion of the proximal small bowel to the colon. In 1963, Payne and colleagues[11] published a series of 10 patients that had jejunocolonic shunts performed. The bypassed intestine included some of the jejunum, the ileum, and the right colon with an end-to-side jejunotransverse colostomy. At the time, this was the largest series recorded of patients undergoing an operation to treat obesity. Initial results showed patients were able to lose weight and had some improvement in comorbidities. The operation was performed as a temporary measure, allowing a time for weight loss then reversal. However, after reversal, patients experienced significant weight gain so the procedure started to be performed with the intention of a long-term bypass with an option of reversal, if needed.[11]

In the following years, after the initial success of Payne, the JIB procedures increased in popularity. Subsequent follow-up over the next decade showed that although there was significant weight loss, the patients suffered from severe diarrhea, electrolyte disturbances, and nutritional deficits. More importantly, there was a reported death rate of up to 10%.[12] These complications led to a modification by Payne to preserve the ileocecal valve.[13] This consisted of anastomosing the first 14 inches of proximal jejunum to the side of the terminal ileum 4 inches from the ileocecal valve. This procedure became very popular. But despite the modifications, complications continued. Scott and coworkers[14] found that the proximal jejunal segment had elongated in several patients to almost 20 inches and on radiograph, there was reflux of barium into the bypassed ileum. This reflux allowed reabsorption of the contents and weight gain. He concluded that the procedure was still experimental and not ready for widespread therapeutic application.[14] New variations of the JIB were developed to reduce the small intestine's absorptive capability. These included an end-to-end anastomosis of jejunum to ileum and the transected ileum was anastomosed to the transverse colon for drainage of the bypassed segment.[15]

The JIB and its variations were popular in the 1960s and early 1970s, but despite some patient happiness with the results, the procedure had significant postoperative ramifications. Bypass enteritis, an overgrowth of the enteric bacteria in the bypassed small intestine, produced gas-filled blebs. Without any food or bile passage through this limb, there was no peristaltic activity. This created an environment favorable for bacterial overgrowth. Some patients presenting with abdominal pain were found to have pneumatosis of the small intestine on radiograph. This was from a functional ileus with passage of the gas through the bowel wall. Unfortunately, this led some patients to undergo an unneeded operation because it was later found that this process could be treated with antibiotics if diagnosed correctly.[16] Among the most serious complications of the JIB were liver disease from protein deficiency, which often progressed to liver failure and death.[17] Other complications included malabsorption of vitamins and nutrients, electrolyte imbalance, renal calculi, arthritis, significant diarrhea, cholelithiasis, colonic pseudo-obstruction, and osteomalacia.[18] These patients required very close surveillance, diet modifications, and antibiotics to avoid complications. Many patients underwent reversal of the procedure or modifications.[19] For these reasons, the surgeons were not well received, many advocated for its end, and the procedure was abandoned and replaced by other less morbid operations.[20,21] It is one of the darker periods in the history of surgery because more than 30,000 intestinal bypass operations were performed before it was recognized that the complications were unacceptable.[7]

Mixed Malabsorptive and Restrictive Procedures

Gastric bypass

Because the results of the JIB were proving to be unfavorable, other surgeons searched for safer bariatric operations. There was a major breakthrough in 1967, when Mason developed the first gastric bypass, which was the first restrictive and malabsorptive procedure. His team observed that weight loss was common in patients who underwent a gastrectomy for ulcer disease. They studied this using a gastroenterostomy on dogs and concluded that a subtotal gastric bypass could be used for obesity treatment in humans.[22] They reported a series of 24 obese patients in 1969. The procedure was essentially a modification of a Billroth II resection with a different goal.

Because surgeons were already comfortable with the gastric resection for the treatment of ulcer disease, the procedure was able to grow in popularity more quickly as opposed to a novel operation. This loop gastric bypass offered the possibility of reversal with use of the excluded stomach. Despite its' familiarity, the operation proved difficult with operating times in excess of 5 hours.

A series by Alden[23] published in 1977 compared patients that underwent JIB with the gastric bypass and concluded that the gastric bypass has fewer comorbidities, was equally safe, and resulted in equal weight loss. Griffen and coworkers[24] at the University of Kentucky noted that the largest technical difficulty of the Mason loop gastric bypass was obtaining the correct positioning of the stomach and small bowel loop. Several of his early patients had postoperative bilious emesis prompting the change from a loop to a Roux-en-Y type anastomosis in 1977.

The Greenville Gastric Bypass developed at East Carolina University was reported in 1983. Our study included 837 consecutive patients, all treated with an identical operation (30-mL gastric pouch, 10-mm handsewn gastroenterostomy, 60-cm alimentary jejunal segment) with a 95% follow-up from 1980 to 1986 with a mean duration of 9.2 years. This study documented that the procedure could be done safely, achieved a long-term mean weight loss of 102 lb, and most importantly produced long-term remission of type 2 diabetes in 83% of the patients with diabetes.[7,25] From the same series, MacDonald[26] was also the first to document the reduction in the mortality of diabetics by 78%. The study highlighted that patients lost to follow-up were treatment failures and that any new operative procedure requires thorough evaluation before widespread use.[27] The development of the Roux-en-Y was important because it eliminated bile reflux and provided less tension on the gastroenteric anastomosis.

In the 1980s and 1990s, there was additional experimentation and modifications made to improve the operation.[28] Although the gastric bypass had good results compared with the other available options, it also had its own set of new complications. Patients suffered from dumping syndrome if too high of a carbohydrate load was eaten; but some argued that this was beneficial for weight loss as a deterrence to overindulgence. More importantly, marginal ulcers were now a potential serious complication. As seen in other procedures, iron, vitamin B_{12}, and calcium supplements were necessary. In 1994, Wittgrove and coworkers[29] described the technique of the laparoscopic Roux-en-Y gastric bypass. This was a major advancement in bariatric surgery; one of the most difficult abdominal operations could be performed with laparoscopy safely. This approach offered the patients a shorter hospital stay and earlier return to activity among other benefits, and over time replaced the open technique.[7]

Biliopancreatic diversion and biliopancreatic diversion with duodenal switch

In 1979, after success on animal models, Scopinaro and coworkers[30] published a report of 18 patients that underwent a biliopancreatic diversion (BPD) with 1-year follow-up. The operation consisted of a partial gastrectomy with closure of the duodenal stump, transection of the jejunum 20 cm distal to the ligament of Treitz, and a gastrojejunostomy performed with the distal part of the transected jejunum for a limb about 250 cm long. The proximal part of the transected jejunum was anastomosed to the distal ileum forming a common channel of 50 cm with a preserved terminal ileum. This arrangement was created to keep the bypassed bowel from developing stasis and blind loop syndrome seen after older operations. The results from the initial case series showed that the procedure was a safe alternate to the JIB.[30]

The BPD proved to be safe and very successful. Scopinaro and coworkers[31] reported their experiences with the BPD over a 21-year period in 1998. The results of more than 2000 patients showed that the BPD was the most effective procedure in terms of initial weight loss and maintenance of weight. The procedure also had excellent reduction in comorbidities. However, potentially dangerous side effects were identified. The complications included diarrhea, foul-smelling stools, increased flatulence, anemia from poor iron absorption, stoma ulceration, protein malabsorption, dumping syndrome, peripheral neuropathy, Wernicke encephalopathy, and bone demineralization from poor calcium and vitamin D uptake. Among these, protein malnutrition was the most serious complication of BPD and the most common reason for late mortality after the operation. Surgeons recognized that careful lifetime follow-up was needed for surveillance and prevention of these complications.[32]

Although the BPD produced excellent weight loss, the long-term morbidity inspired others to attempt to improve on it. In 1998, Hess and Hess[33] described the BPD combined with a duodenal switch (DS). The procedure was essentially a hybrid of the BPD and an experimental operation initially used for duodenogastric reflux. The BPD with DS preserved the pylorus with a gastrectomy performed along the greater curvature. After 9 years follow-up, reported weight loss and comorbidity resolution was similar to the BPD data. The advantages of the BPD with DS over the BPD alone were that with the longer common channel there was incidence of less liver failure, renal failure, and electrolyte abnormalities. Additionally, with the preserved pylorus, marginal ulcers and dumping syndrome were not present. The BPD and the BPD with DS are difficult and long operations open and laparoscopically. The most serious complication, however, is the internal hernia, a problem that may need immediate attention to avoid bowel incarceration and necrosis. The complication was rare in the days of open surgery, but has become more common since the advent of laparoscopic surgery, an approach that produces fewer adhesions.[34] This, combined with the potential morbidity if not followed properly, has hindered the popularity of the operations despite the excellent weight loss results.

Restrictive Procedures

Vertical banded gastroplasty

Many surgeons sought other means to provide an operation for obesity that did not involve an enteric or gastric bypass. Gastroplasty was first reported in 1973, working off of the observation that extensive gastric resection with a Billroth II anastomosis produces weight loss, Printen[35] wanted to find a simpler procedure than the loop bypass that would not have the risk associated with bowel anastomoses, and proposed a partial horizontal transection of the stomach leaving a small upper gastric remnant with a narrow channel between the upper and lower gastric pouches. This entailed stapling across the stomach to provide a functional gastric transection with a greater curvature conduit of 1.0 to 1.5 cm between the upper and lower pouches. The gastroplasty resulted in less weight gain compared with gastric bypass, but the common channel could be stretched with excessive eating and become widened. Overtime, partition was modified and breakdown of the staple line remained a problem. To keep the gastric pouch the same size, Laws[36] added a silastic ring around the newly created gastric outlet after a vertical gastric partition in 1981.

One year later, Mason[37] published a series of 42 patients who underwent what he called a vertical banded gastroplasty (VBG). The procedure consisted of creating a vertical partition to create a small, less than 50-mL pouch, and banding of the lesser curvature pouch outlet with polypropylene mesh to keep the outlet diameter consistent over time. He noted that with horizontal stapling, the retaining sutures and staples often failed over time resulting in a larger stoma. The small gastric pouch put the patient at risk for reflux esophagitis. But with a vertical partition, the incidence was less as the angle between the stomach and the esophagus was maintained.[38] The long-term data showed that the silastic ring created stenosis of the gastric outlet in some patients and contributed to food intolerance and reflux esophagitis and had high rates of reoperation. Other surgeons began using marlex mesh to reinforce the gastric outlet created and this proved to be the superior material for the VBG procedure.[37]

The VBG had advantages compared with the other available weight loss operations available in the 1980s and early 1990s. First, it was not as technically challenging as the bypass procedures. Additionally, it avoided the potential complications of dumping and marginal ulcers. The VBG also was easier to reverse, if needed. However, over several years, patients began to regain their weight. Studies comparing VBG with the gastric bypass with long-term results began to surface in the mid-1990s. The Roux-en-Y bypass proved to be a better weight loss operation. The reports pointed out that the stapled partition began to breakdown over time and weight is regained.[38] Many patients underwent revisions to other bariatric operations. The VBG slowly fell out of favor and was rarely performed once the laparoscopic adjustable gastric band was widely available.

Adjustable gastric bands
In the mid-1970s, Wilkinson at the University of New Mexico began to search for other possible ways to surgically achieve early satiety and reduced caloric intake. He wanted to develop a more physiologic operation without disturbing the continuity of the gastrointestinal tract. He conducted canine experiments in which he tied prolene suture around the greater curvature of the stomach with a 1-cm bougie in the stomach. The dogs lost weight but after 3 to 4 months the stomach dilated back to normal size, so he changed to polypropylene mesh to prevent dilation. His first human patient underwent a similar operation with a polypropylene mesh wrap around the stomach in 1976.[39] The patient was pleased with their weight loss in the first 6 months but became discouraged at 1 year and underwent a gastric bypass.[39] Later, he published a series of 100 patients that underwent a Nissen fundoplication and gastric wrapping with polypropylene mesh. The fundoplication was performed to prevent postoperative reflux. His findings were that the procedure had satisfactory weight loss and gave the patients early satiety without any metabolic or physiologic changes.[40]

As the operation gained popularity and success, different sizes and materials of mesh were used to decrease inflammation and the potential for erosion. Fewer surgeons began wrapping the entire stomach as Wilkinson did initially and began using 1- to 2.5-cm bands placed across the stomach to create a small upper pouch and narrow channel to the remaining stomach. Among the most used materials was the Marlex mesh. In a series with 7 to 12 years follow-up from Sweden, the Marlex gastric band was not successful at long-term weight loss. Half of the patients underwent revision because of severe vomiting, esophagitis, and weight gain.[41] Other surgeons used silicone bands with better results. Despite this, the nonadjustable banding procedures were difficult in creating the correct stoma size and reoperations were at a high rate because of obstruction. Additionally, the gastric pouch could dilate over time contributing to reflux esophagitis.[42]

With further development of the procedure, the band was made adjustable. The adjustable bands were originally developed in Austria by work on rabbits. The goal was to develop a reversible gastric band that could be adjusted to the individual needs of the patient. A liquid-filled silastic cuff that is placed around the stomach adjacent to the cardia was used. The cuff diameter was adjusted by filling or draining fluid from a subcutaneous valve accessed by percutaneous needle puncture.[43]

The adjustable band provided patients with a variable size stoma that could be altered based on their symptoms. The procedure proved to be better at weight loss than the nonadjustable band and had fewer complications.[42] The adjustable bands easily displaced the nonadjustable in popularity. Around this time in the early 1990s, laparoscopy was starting to offer alternative ways of traditionally open procedures and in 1993, Belachew and coworkers[44] described laparoscopic adjustable silicone band placement. The laparoscopic gastric band became the most common bariatric operation in Europe and later the United States. Laparoscopic adjustable gastric banding was able to provide a significant loss of excess weight with few complications and a reduction in comorbidities. The procedure provided a less invasive and reversible operation than a gastric bypass with similar short-term weight loss, but with long-term potential risks of band slippage, erosion, and foreign body infection.[45] Although the operation has fallen out of favor in recent years, the adjustable gastric band remains a current option for obese patients.

Sleeve gastrectomy

The sleeve gastrectomy (SG) was originally described as a staging procedure for super obese patients to bridge them to a more definitive operation. After observing a high morbidity and mortality rate after BPD with DS in the super obese, Regan and Gagner developed the two-stage operative approach. The patients underwent an initial SG over a 60F catheter bougie, then in 6 to 12 months after plateau of weight loss, the patients would undergo a second stage BPD with DS or gastric bypass.[46] The SG separates the greater curvature from the lesser curvature and the antrum. The first laparoscopic SG (LSG) was reported in 1999 and the first report of SG as a standalone operation was in 2003.[47]

Many patients that underwent SG as a bridge operation lost enough weight with the SG that the secondary procedure was no longer necessary or wanted by the patient. Gagner and coworkers[47] published a comparison of LSG patients with laparoscopic adjustable gastric band patients. They found that the LSG was comparable in short-term 1-year weight loss and had the benefits of a decreased need for reoperation, no foreign material in the body, and decrease in ghrelin production.

The standalone LSG has increased in popularity in the last several years and now is the most common bariatric operation performed in the United States.[48] The SG has many advantages over other current operations. The SG is less technically demanding than the gastric bypass or BPD; has minimal morbidity; has no foreign material; and is without marginal ulcers, dumping syndrome, internal hernias, or nutritional deficiencies. Complications seen with the LSG are staple line leaks and strictures. Over time, the leak rate has decreased with improved surgical techniques. The LSG's favorable weight loss results, significant remission of comorbidities, and very low rates of postoperative mortality and morbidity have contributed to its rise in popularity.[49] The LSG is still a relatively new procedure without much long-term data; it has to be seen what the future holds for this operation.

Gastric balloon

Despite their knowledge of comorbidities associated with morbid obesity, some patients are reluctant to undergo bariatric surgery. Intragastric balloon placement offers an alternative to these patients. The intragastric balloon provides a temporary, reversible, and repeatable treatment. The balloon is placed endoscopically and typically the balloon is filled with 500 mL of saline and removed after 6 months.[50] Newer balloons with two intragastric chambers are available to help prevent migration. The therapy has been found to have only a temporary effect up to 3 years, despite repeat balloons.[51] The weight loss experienced does improve obesity-related comorbidities, but typically the weight is regained and the positive effect lost.[50] The balloon, along with diet and exercise, has shown better weight loss results against diet and exercise alone in a prospective randomized trial.[52] The balloon does not solve obesity and only with multiple placements can it control obesity in the long term, but in patients who decline surgery, it should be strongly considered.[50] However, up to 32% of patients who undergo gastric balloon placement eventually go on to have bariatric surgery.[50,51]

MEASUREMENT OF OUTCOMES

An innovation that advanced bariatric and metabolic surgery was quality control and documentation that operations could be done with minimal mortality and morbidity. Our studies, the Swedish Obese Subjects (SOS) study, and the National Institutes of Health/National Institute of Diabetes and Digestive and Kidney Diseases Longitudinal Assessment of Bariatric Surgery (LABS) all demonstrated the importance of long-term studies. The SOS study was a prospective controlled trial of 4047 obese patients, with 2010 undergoing bariatric surgery including gastric bypass, banding, and VBG; and 2037 in a matched control group undergoing conventional treatment. The patients were followed over a period of up to 15 years, with average 10.9 years of follow-up for 99.9% of patients. The results from SOS showed that compared with conventional treatment, the surgery group was associated with a long-term reduction in overall mortality and decreased incidence of diabetes, myocardial infarction, stroke, and cancer.[53] The LABS study was established to analyze the risks and benefits of bariatric surgery and its impact on the well-being of patients with obesity.[54] The consortium collected data starting in 2005. LABS first evaluated the 30-day outcomes after bariatric surgery, with data from 4776 bariatric surgery patients, with an overall 30-day mortality rate of 0.3% and low rate of adverse outcomes, comparable with a laparoscopic cholecystectomy.[55] LABS also evaluates long-term safety and efficacy of bariatric surgery and its data have led to multiple publications and newfound knowledge in bariatric surgery.

A FOCUS ON SAFETY

Another aspect of the quality control innovation was the development of Centers of Excellence (CoE). Confronted with reports of disastrous clinical outcomes in hospitals with limited experience, an increase of malpractice suits, and unaffordable insurance premiums, the leadership of the American Society of Bariatric and Metabolic Surgery created a program for the certification of CoE in 2003.[7] The certification required standardization of care paths, training of hospital personnel, well-equipped hospitals capable of managing very obese patients, and registering all patients and their outcomes. In addition, all sites were inspected at least once every 3 years, often with unannounced visits.[56]

Outcomes were recorded with the Bariatric Outcomes Longitudinal Database (BOLD) in the program that eventually included 425 hospitals in the United States and other centers in 22 countries. BOLD collected patient demographics and surgical outcomes for up to 2 years after their operation. BOLD provides information for providers to learn and provide better patient care. In 2006, the Centers for Medicare and Medicaid Services (CMS) restricted procedures coverage for bariatric procedures for Medicare patients to CoE.[57] In 2012, the program was absorbed by the American College of Surgeons, which had developed its own CoE program to ensure there would only be one set of standards for bariatric surgery. In an interesting development, centers that were not certified were forced to produce the same excellent outcomes to continue reimbursement by carriers. This "the tide lifts all boats" phenomenon then led the CMS to stop requiring center certification for reimbursement in 2013, the price of success.[57,58] Despite the CMS decision, private insurers continue to support accreditation and restrict coverage to high-volume centers.

SUMMARY

Currently in the United States there is a failure for the medical community as a whole to take full advantage of this breakthrough. More than one-third of Americans are obese and approximately 20% have a body mass index greater than 35.[59] Furthermore, there are 29.1 million Americans with type 2 diabetes, with close to 2 million newly diagnosed cases annually.[60] Despite this, there were only 179,000 bariatric operations performed in 2013.[61] Less than 1% of possible patients underwent a treatment that could cure them of diabetes, not to mention improvement in their other comorbidities. There are several prospective randomized studies that show superiority of the bariatric operations to intensive medical therapy.[62–65] There are also retrospective studies that show patients that underwent bariatric surgery compared with a matched control group without surgery have lower all-cause mortality and decreased deaths from diabetes, heart disease, and cancer.[66,67] Despite the benefits and the supporting data, patients remain afraid of surgery and many physicians are not convinced that traditional treatments are not effective.

This delay in acceptance of a revolutionary treatment has been seen many times throughout medicine. For example, Alexis Carrel developed the basic principles of vascular surgery in 1894 but the first vascular procedure did not occur until 1962.[68] Additionally, laparoscopy was used in 1901 by Georg Keiling on dogs[69] but it was not until 1981 that Kurt Semm performed a laparoscopic appendectomy.[70] Along those same lines, in the 1940s, Gerhard Kuntscher developed and used the first intramedullary nail in Europe during World War II. The procedure was described in Time magazine in a 1945 article "Amazing Thighbone," but American surgeons remained skeptical of his methods. It was not until the 1970s that the closed nailing technique was revisited and is now the standard of care for femoral shaft and tibial fractures requiring operative stabilization.[71]

With the obesity epidemic and the increasing prevalence of associated comorbidities, more work needs to be done to educate patients and physicians of the lifesaving ability of bariatric surgery.

REFERENCES

1. Eknoyan G. A history of obesity, or how what was good became ugly and then bad. Adv Chronic Kidney Dis 2006;13(4):421–7.
2. Deitel M. The obesity epidemic. Obes Surg 2006;16(4):377–8.
3. Deitel M. A brief history of the surgery for obesity to the present, with an overview of nutritional implications. J Am Coll Nutr 2013;32(2):136–42.
4. Rodger DE, McFetridge JG, Price TE. The management of obesity. Can Med Assoc J 1950;63(3):265–9.
5. Van Itallie TB. Morbid obesity: a hazardous disorder that resists conservative treatment. Am J Clin Nutr 1980;33:358–63.
6. Wolfe BM. Presidential address—obesity discrimination: what can we do? Surg Obes Relat Dis 2012;8(5):495–500.
7. Pories WJ. Bariatric surgery: risks and rewards. J Clin Endocrinol Metab 2008;93(11 Suppl 1):S89–96.
8. Buchwald H, Buchwald JN. Evolution of operative procedures for the management of morbid obesity 1950-2000. Obes Surg 2002;12(5):705–17.
9. Henrikson V. Can small bowel resection be defended as therapy for obesity? Obes Surg 1994;4(1):54.
10. Kremen AJ, Linner JH, Nelson CH. An experimental evaluation of the nutritional importance of proximal and distal small intestine. Ann Surg 1954;140(3):439.

11. Payne J, Dewind LT, Commons RR. Metabolic observations in patients with jeju-nocolic shunts. Am J Surg 1963;106(2):273–89.
12. Dewind LT, Payne JH. Intestinal bypass surgery for morbid obesity: long-term re-sults. JAMA 2014;312(9):966.
13. Payne J, Dewind LT. Surgical treatment of obesity. Am J Surg 1969;118(2):141–7.
14. Scott HW, Law DH, Sandstead HH, et al. Jejunoileal shunt in surgical treatment of morbid obesity. Ann Surg 1970;171(5):770–82.
15. Scott HW, Sandstead HH, Bill AB, et al. Experience with a new technic of intes-tinal bypass in the treatment of morbid obesity. Ann Surg 1971;174(4):560–72.
16. Passaro E, Drenick E, Wilson SE. Bypass enteritis. Am J Surg 1976;131(2): 169–74.
17. Brown RG, O'leary J, Woodward ER. Hepatic effects of jejunoileal bypass for morbid obesity. Am J Surg 1974;127(1):53–8.
18. Ravitch MM, Brolin RE. The price of weight loss by jejunoileal shunt. Ann Surg 1979;190(3):382–91.
19. Deitel M, Shahi B, Anand PK, et al. Long-term outcome in a series of jejunoileal bypass patients. Obes Surg 1993;3(3):247–52.
20. Bondar GF. Complications of small intestinal short-circuiting for obesity. Arch Surg 1967;94(5):707.
21. Herbert C. Intestinal bypass for obesity. Can Fam Physician 1975;21(7):56–9.
22. Ito C, Mason EE, Besten LD. Experimental studies on gastric bypass versus stan-dard ulcer operations. Tohoku J Exp Med 1969;97(3):269–77.
23. Alden JF. Gastric and jejunoileal bypass. Arch Surg 1977;112(7):799.
24. Griffen WO, Young VL, Stevenson CC. A prospective comparison of gastric and jejunoileal bypass procedures for morbid obesity. Ann Surg 1977;186(4):500–9.
25. Pories WJ, Swanson MS, Macdonald KG, et al. Who would have thought it? An operation proves to be the most effective therapy for adult-onset diabetes melli-tus. Ann Surg 1995;222(3):339–52.
26. Macdonald K. The gastric bypass operation reduces the progression and mortal-ity of non-insulin-dependent diabetes mellitus. J Gastrointest Surg 1997;1(3): 213–20.
27. Flickinger EG, Pories WJ, Meelheim HD, et al. The Greenville Gastric Bypass. Ann Surg 1984;199(5):555–62.
28. Brolin RE, Kenler HA, Gorman JH, et al. Long-limb gastric bypass in the super-obese. Ann Surg 1992;215(4):387.
29. Wittgrove AC, Clark GW, Tremblay LJ. Laparoscopic gastric bypass, Roux-en-Y: preliminary report of five cases. Obes Surg 1994;4(4):353–7.
30. Scopinaro N, Gianetta E, Civalleri D, et al. Bilio-pancreatic bypass for obesity: II. Initial experience in man. Br J Surg 1979;66(9):618–20.
31. Scopinaro N, Adami GF, Marinari GM, et al. Biliopancreatic diversion. World J Surg 1998;22(9):936–46.
32. Scopinaro N, Gianetta E, Adami GF, et al. Biliopancreatic diversion for obesity at eighteen years. Surgery 1996;119(3):261–8.
33. Hess DS, Hess DW. Biliopancreatic diversion with a duodenal switch. Obes Surg 1998;8(3):267–82.
34. Dowson HM, Bong JJ, Lovell DP, et al. Reduced adhesion formation following laparoscopic versus open colorectal surgery. Br J Surg 2008;95(7):909–14.
35. Printen KJ. Gastric surgery for relief of morbid obesity. Arch Surg 1973; 106(4):428.
36. Laws HL. Standardized gastroplasty orifice. Am J Surg 1981;141(3):393–4.
37. Mason EE. Vertical banded gastroplasty for obesity. Arch Surg 1982;117(5):701.

38. Capella JF, Capella RF. The weight reduction operation of choice: vertical banded gastroplasty or gastric bypass? Am J Surg 1996;171(1):74–9.

39. Wilkinson LH. Reduction of gastric reservoir capacity. Am J Clin Nutr 1980;33: 515–7.

40. Wilkinson LH. Gastric (reservoir) reduction for morbid obesity. Arch Surg 1981; 116(5):602.

41. Näslund E, Granström L, Stockeld D, et al. Marlex mesh gastric banding: a 7-12 year follow-up. Obes Surg 1994;4(3):269–73.

42. Kuzmak LI. A review of seven years' experience with silicone gastric banding. Obes Surg 1991;1(4):403–8.

43. Szinicz G, Müller L, Erhart W, et al. "Reversible gastric banding" in surgical treatment of morbid obesity—results of animal experiments. Res Exp Med 1989; 189(1):55–60.

44. Belachew M, Legrand M, Vincent V, et al. Laparoscopic placement of adjustable silicone gastric band in the treatment of morbid obesity: how to do it. Obes Surg 1995;5(1):66–70.

45. Mcbride CL, Kothari V. Evolution of laparoscopic adjustable gastric banding. Surg Clin North Am 2011;91(6):1239–47.

46. Regan JP, Inabnet WB, Gagner M, et al. Early experience with two-stage laparoscopic Roux-en-y gastric bypass as an alternative in the super-super obese patient. Obes Surg 2003;13(6):861–4.

47. Gagner M, Gumbs AA, Milone L, et al. Laparoscopic sleeve gastrectomy for the super-super-obese (body mass index >60 kg/m2). Surg Today 2008;38(5): 399–403.

48. Spaniolas K, Kasten KR, Brinkley J, et al. The changing bariatric surgery landscape in the USA. Obes Surg 2015;25(8):1544–6.

49. Young MT, Gebhart A, Phelan MJ, et al. Use and outcomes of laparoscopic sleeve gastrectomy vs laparoscopic gastric bypass: analysis of the American College of Surgeons NSQIP. J Am Coll Surg 2015;220(5):880–5.

50. Alfredo G, Roberta M, Massimiliano C, et al. Long-term multiple intragastric balloon treatment—a new strategy to treat morbid obese patients refusing surgery: prospective 6-year follow-up study. Surg Obes Relat Dis 2014;10(2): 307–11.

51. Dumonceau J-M, François E, Hittelet A, et al. Single vs repeated treatment with the intragastric balloon: a 5-year weight loss study. Obes Surg 2010;20(6):692–7.

52. Ponce J, Woodman G, Swain J, et al. The REDUCE pivotal trial: a prospective, randomized controlled pivotal trial of a dual intragastric balloon for the treatment of obesity. Surg Obes Relat Dis 2015;11(4):874–81.

53. Sjöström L, Narbro K, Sjöström CD, et al. Effects of bariatric surgery on mortality in Swedish obese subjects. N Engl J Med 2007;357(8):741–52.

54. Longitudinal Assessment of Bariatric Surgery (LABS). Longitudinal Assessment of Bariatric Surgery (LABS). Available at: http://www.niddk.nih.gov/health-information/health-topics/weight-control/bariatric-surgery/pages/labs.aspx. Accessed November 18, 2015.

55. Longitudinal Assessment of Bariatric Surgery (LABS) Consortium, Flum DR, Belle SH, King WC, et al. Perioperative safety in the longitudinal assessment of bariatric surgery. N Engl J Med 2009;361(5):445–54.

56. Pratt GM, Mclees B, Pories WJ. The ASBS bariatric surgery centers of excellence program: a blueprint for quality improvement. Surg Obes Relat Dis 2006;2(5): 497–503.

57. Kuo LE, Simmons KD, Kelz RR. Bariatric centers of excellence: effect of centralization on access to care. J Am Coll Surg 2015;221(5):914–22.
58. Dimick JB, Nicholas LH, Ryan AM, et al. Bariatric surgery complications before vs after implementation of a national policy restricting coverage to centers of excellence. JAMA 2013;309(8):792.
59. Ogden CL, Carroll MD, Kit BK, et al. Prevalence of childhood and adult obesity in the United States, 2011-2012. JAMA 2014;311(8):806.
60. Statistics About Diabetes. American Diabetes Association. Available at: http://www.diabetes.org/diabetes-basics/statistics/. Accessed November 20, 2015.
61. Connect: the official news magazine of ASMBS. Connect: the official news magazine of ASMBS. Available at: http://connect.asmbs.org/may-2014-bariatric-surgery-growth.html. Accessed November 20, 2015.
62. Singh RP, Gans R, Kashyap SR, et al. Effect of bariatric surgery versus intensive medical management on diabetic ophthalmic outcomes. Diabetes Care 2015; 38(3):e32–3.
63. Mingrone G, Panunzi S, Gaetano AD, et al. Bariatric surgery versus conventional medical therapy for type 2 diabetes. N Engl J Med 2012;366(17):1577–85.
64. Ikramuddin S, Billington CJ, Lee W-J, et al. Roux-en-Y gastric bypass for diabetes (the Diabetes Surgery Study): 2-year outcomes of a 5-year, randomised, controlled trial. Lancet Diabetes Endocrinol 2015;3(6):413–22.
65. Carlsson LM, Peltonen M, Ahlin S, et al. Bariatric surgery and prevention of type 2 diabetes in Swedish obese subjects. N Engl J Med 2012;367(8):695–704.
66. Arterburn DE, Olsen MK, Smith VA, et al. Association between bariatric surgery and long-term survival. JAMA 2015;313(1):62–70.
67. Adams TD, Gress RE, Smith SC, et al. Long-term mortality after gastric bypass surgery. N Engl J Med 2007;357(8):753–61.
68. Benveniste GL. Alexis Carrel: the good, the bad, the ugly. ANZ J Surg 2013;83(9): 609–11.
69. Litynski GS. Laparoscopy—the early attempts: spotlighting Georg Kelling and Hans Christian Jacobaeus. JSLS 1997;1(1):83–5.
70. Bhattacharya K. Kurt Semm: a laparoscopic crusader. J Minim Access Surg 2007;3(1):35.
71. Bong MR, Koval KJ, Egol KA. The history of intramedullary nailing. Bull NYU Hosp Jt Dis 2006;64(3):94–7.

The Socioeconomic Impact of Morbid Obesity and Factors Affecting Access to Obesity Surgery

 CrossMark

Tammy Fouse, DO[a], Philip Schauer, MD[b],*

KEYWORDS

- Prevalence • Obesity • Economic impact • Bariatric and metabolic surgery
- Access to care

KEY POINTS

- From 1999 through 2014, obesity prevalence increased among adults and youth. However, among youth, prevalence did not change from 2003–2004 through 2013–2014.
- In 2010 dollars, the nationwide expenditure for obesity-related health care increased to more than $315 billion. These costs increase exponentially with an increase in body mass index greater than 35 kg/m^2.
- In general, the labor market consequences of obesity are greater for women than for men, and greater for white women than for other women.
- Bariatric surgery has been shown to be cost-effective and even cost-saving in certain patient subgroups, that is, type 2 diabetics. The resultant improvement in obesity-related comorbidities has led to reduced prescription drug costs after surgery.
- Patient access to surgical treatment for obesity remains a major economic dilemma in the United States. Of the eligible patients that qualify for bariatric surgery, less than 1% will actually undergo the procedure.

PREVALENCE OF OBESITY

Obesity remains a significant public health issue. It is a chronic disease associated with increased risks of cardiovascular disease, stroke, diabetes, certain cancers, and decreased quality of life. Individuals with severe obesity (body mass index, BMI, >35 kg/m^2) or obesity (>30 kg/m^2) have a 50% to 100% increased risk of premature death compared with individuals of a healthy weight.[1]

[a] Digestive Disease Institute, Department of General Surgery, Cleveland Clinic, 9500 Euclid Avenue, Cleveland, OH, USA; [b] Bariatric and Metabolic Institute, Cleveland Clinic Lerner College of Medicine, Cleveland Clinic, Cleveland, OH, USA
* Corresponding author.
E-mail address: schauep@ccf.org

Surg Clin N Am 96 (2016) 669–679
http://dx.doi.org/10.1016/j.suc.2016.03.002
0039-6109/16/$ – see front matter © 2016 Elsevier Inc. All rights reserved.
surgical.theclinics.com

Data recently published from the National Center for Health Statistics revealed during 2011 to 2014 the prevalence of obesity in the United States was more than 36% in adults and 17% in youth. From 1999–2000 through 2013–2014, a significant increase in obesity was observed in both adults and youth; however, over the past 4 years, the rate of increase in adult obesity has slowed whereas there has been no significant change in prevalence among youth (**Fig. 1**).[2]

According to this report, age, gender, and race are significant factors in the overall prevalence of obesity. Prevalence among middle-aged adults aged 40 to 59 (40.2%) and older adults aged 60 and over (37.0%) was higher than among younger adults aged 20 to 39 (32.3%) (**Fig. 2**).[2]

Overall, the prevalence of obesity among women (38.3%) was higher than among men (34.3%). For adults aged 20 to 39 and 40 to 59, the prevalence of obesity was higher among women than among men, but the difference between older women and men aged 60 and over was not significant.[2]

The prevalence of obesity was lowest among non-Hispanic Asian adults (11.7%), followed by non-Hispanic white (34.5%), Hispanic (42.5%), and non-Hispanic black (48.1%) adults. All differences were significant. The only gender differences found among the ethnic groups were among the non-Hispanic black and Hispanic adults. The prevalence of obesity among non-Hispanic black women was 56.9% compared with 37.5% in non-Hispanic black men. The prevalence of obesity was 45.7% among Hispanic women compared with 39.0% in Hispanic men (**Fig. 3**).[2]

The prevalence of obesity among US adults remains higher than the Healthy People 2020 goal of 30.5%[3]; however, the actual obesity rate among adults in 2010 was lower (35.7%) than the 2003 prediction by the Centers for Disease Control and Prevention (40%).

Although the overall prevalence of childhood obesity is higher than the Healthy People 2020 goal of 14.5%, the prevalence among children aged 2 to 5 years is less than

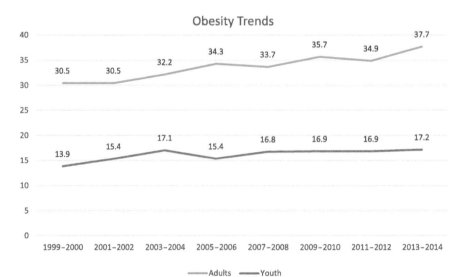

Fig. 1. Trends in obesity prevalence among adults aged 20 and older and youth aged 2 to 19 years: US, 1999–2000 through 2013–2014. (*Data from* Ogden CL, Carroll MD, Fryar CD, et al. Prevalence of obesity among adults and youth: United States, 2011–2014. NCHS Data Brief 2015;(219):1–8.)

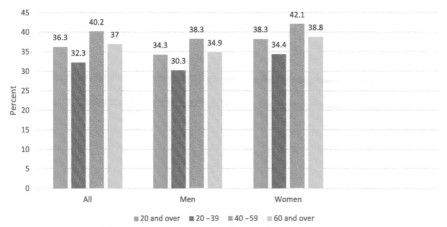

Fig. 2. Prevalence of obesity among adults aged 20 and older, by sex and age: United States, 2011 to 2014. (*Data from* Ogden CL, Carroll MD, Fryar CD, et al. Prevalence of obesity among adults and youth: United States, 2011–2014. NCHS Data Brief 2015;(219):1–8.)

the goal of 9.4%.[3] According to the 2012 American Heart Association Statistical Fact Sheet, overweight adolescents have a 70% probability of becoming overweight adults; this increases to 80% if at least one parent is overweight or obese (**Fig. 4**).[4]

Although the overall trajectory of obesity in the United States may have begun to flatten over the past 4 years, the overall change over the past 50 years clearly demonstrates a significant public health issue. More alarming than the overall prevalence is the impact by individual BMI categories. Measured BMI data from the 1960 to 1962 and 2009 to 2010 National Health and Nutrition Examination Surveys (NHANES)

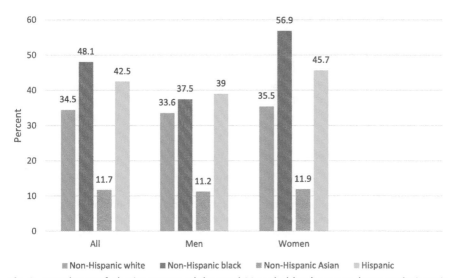

Fig. 3. Prevalence of obesity among adults aged 20 and older, by sex and race and Hispanic origin: United States, 2011 to 2014. (*Data from* Ogden CL, Carroll MD, Fryar CD, et al. Prevalence of obesity among adults and youth: United States, 2011–2014. NCHS Data Brief 2015;(219):1–8.)

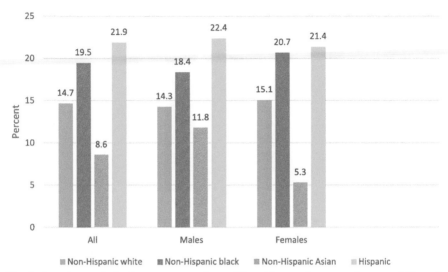

Fig. 4. Prevalence of obesity among youth aged 2 to 19 years, by sex and race and Hispanic origin: United States, 2011 to 2014. (*Data from* Ogden CL, Carroll MD, Fryar CD, et al. Prevalence of obesity among adults and youth: United States, 2011–2014. NCHS Data Brief 2015;(219):1–8.)

revealed the rapid expansion of obesity rates and extreme obesity (BMI>40) over this time period. In 1962, 31.5% of the population was overweight; 13.4% were obese, and less than 1% were in the extreme obesity range. In 2009 to 2010, rates of overweight were roughly the same but at the expense of those in the normal weight range, rates of obesity increased to 36.1%, and the rates of extreme obesity increased more than 6-fold to 6.6%. Among women, the rate of extreme obesity was 8.5%. Forecasts of obesity prevalence rates suggest that by 2030, the obesity rate will creep up to 42%, but the rate of extreme obesity will nearly double to 11.1%.[5]

ECONOMIC IMPACT OF OBESITY

The adverse health effects of obesity, and especially severe obesity, are well documented. Obesity adversely affects nearly every system of the human body, but has the most deleterious effects on rates of diabetes, cardiovascular diseases, and several cancers.[5]

Health Care Costs of Obesity

In 2009, Finkelstein and colleagues[6] released data estimating the costs of obesity for the United States across payers (Medicare, Medicaid, and private insurers) in separate categories for inpatient, non-inpatient, and prescription drug spending. Their analysis demonstrated an undeniable connection between rising rates of obesity and rising medical spending. This study relied on data from the 1998 and 2006 Medical Expenditure Panel Surveys (MEPS). Their results revealed that across all payers, per capita medical spending for the obese is $1429 higher per year, or roughly 42% higher, than for someone of normal weight. In aggregate, the annual medical burden of obesity has increased from 6.5% to 9.1% of annual medical spending and could be as high as $147 billion per year, in 2008 dollars. The results also provided new evidence of the important role of prescription drug spending in driving the costs of obesity. As a result of the Part D prescription drug benefit, the obesity-attributable prescription drug costs to Medicare were $7 billion for the noninstitutionalized patient.[6]

Cawley and Meyerhoefer,[7] in 2012, expanded on the work of Finkelstein and presented data that showed the previous estimates of the economic burden of obesity had been substantially underestimated. Their results were arrived at using the instrumental variables model using the 2000 to 2005 MEPS data. Their study provided the first estimates of the impact of obesity on medical costs that adjust for measurement error in weight. Their estimate of the national medical care costs of obesity-related illness in adults is $209.7 billion, or 20.6% of US national health expenditures, which is considerably higher than the previous estimate of 9.1%.

In 2015, Cawley and colleagues[8] updated and expanded their work from 2012 and included more recent MEPS data for 2000 to 2010. In 2010 dollars, the nationwide expenditure for obesity-related health care increased to more than $315 billion. In this study, they also evaluated the health care costs associated with different BMI values. They found the relationship of medical care costs over BMI is J-shaped, that is, expenditures decrease with BMI through the underweight and healthy weight categories, are relatively constant with BMI in the overweight category, and then increase exponentially with BMI through the obese category, especially at BMI levels greater than 35 kg/m² (**Fig. 5**).[8]

The nonlinearity of this relationship is important. It implies that, in the obese range, savings from a given reduction in weight will increase with the starting BMI. **Table 1** represents the reduction in annual medical care costs associated with a given percentage reduction in BMI (5%, 10%, 15%, or 20%) from a given starting BMI and cost-savings per person, per year.

As seen in **Table 1**, cost-savings are greater among the class 3 obese (BMI≥40 kg/m²) than among the class 2 obese (35 kg/m²≤BMI≥40 kg/m²), and in turn, the savings

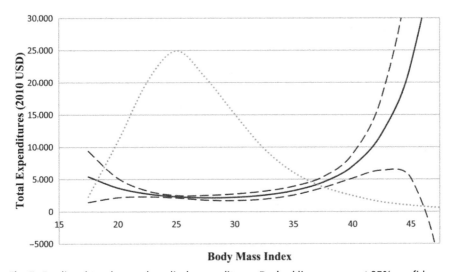

Fig. 5. Predicted total annual medical expenditures. Dashed lines represent 95% confidence intervals. Medical expenditures are denoted by the solid lines and are measured on the left axis. The dotted line indicates the distribution of individuals in the population. (*Data from* Cawley J, Meyerhoefer C, Biener A, et al. Savings in medical expenditures associated with reductions in body mass index among US adults with obesity, by diabetes status. Pharmacoeconomics 2015;33(7):707–22.)

Table 1
Predicted change in total annual medical expenditures ($US) from the instrumental variables model: costs are per person per year

Starting BMI (kg/m²)	Reduction in BMI			
	5%	10%	15%	20%
30	69.35	56.18	−41.36	−234.91
32	202.24	297.58	290.53	203.35
35	528.04	853.15	1030.07	1086.61
37	921.94	1495.47	1839.44	2018.76
40	2137.15	3401.82	4160.56	4606.71
42	3859.08	6017.45	7264.29	7993.11
45	10,030.69	15,071.78	17,742.27	20,229.05

among the class 2 obese are much greater than those among the class 1 obese (30 kg/m² $\leq$ BMI $\leq$ 35 kg/m²). The savings associated with a given reduction in weight can be nearly 13 times greater for those with a BMI of 44 kg/m² than for those with a BMI of 35 kg/m². A second observation from the table is that the annual medical care costs of the class 1 obese are not that much higher than those of the healthy weight or overweight. A third finding is that doubling the weight loss does not double the savings. Because medical expenditures increase exponentially with BMI in the obese region, the initial 5% weight loss results in more savings than subsequent additional increments of 5% weight loss.[8] These findings are significant because the fastest growing portion of the obese population is in the class 3 category. Public health policy decision-makers should take into consideration the impact of directing limited health care resources toward the class 3 obese population.

Work-Related Costs of Obesity

In 2010, Finkelstein and colleagues[9] published an analysis regarding the cost of obesity in the workplace. They evaluated data for full-time employees from the 2006 MEPS and the 2008 US National Health and Wellness Survey. In aggregate, the cost of obesity among US full-time employees was estimated to be $73.1 billion. Their results revealed that presenteeism (decreased productivity while on the job) was the single largest driver of cost of poor health among full-time employees regardless of BMI. For men, they estimated the cost of obesity in the workplace to be $33.8 billion. Work loss due to presenteeism accounted for 44% of the total. For women, the estimated work loss was $39.3 billion, with presenteeism accounting for 38% of the total.

A Gallup poll conducted in 2011 revealed a significantly higher cost due to absenteeism in unhealthy US full-time workers.[10] Their findings were based on Gallup-Healthways Well-Being Index data collected between January 2 and October 2, 2011. Gallup surveyed 109,875 full-time employees during that time period. Their survey revealed total costs due to absenteeism totaled $153 billion per year. Overweight and obese workers contributed an astonishing $113 billion, or 75% of the total loss. Chronic medical conditions associated with obesity (heart attack, high blood pressure, high cholesterol, cancer, diabetes, asthma, depression, or recurring physical pain in the neck, back, or knees) were found to be the major contributors to lost productivity. They found if the worker had no chronic medical conditions, loss due to absenteeism was 0.34 days per month; with 1 to 2 chronic conditions, loss of 1.1 days per month; 3 or more chronic conditions, a loss of 3.5 days per month was found. By projection, if overweight and obese workers were normal weight, the prevalence of 3+ chronic conditions would be cut in half, reducing losses from absenteeism by $40 billion or about 25%.

Although obesity adversely affects workplace productivity and absenteeism, it also appears to reduce employee earnings. Using data from the National Longitudinal Survey of Youth (NLSY) 1979 Cohort, Cawley[11] reported his findings in 2004 regarding the impact of obesity on overall earnings. His research revealed that weight lowers wages for women: an increase in weight of 2 standard deviations (roughly 64 pounds) is associated with 9% lower wages. The survey revealed the labor market consequences of obesity are greater for women than for men, and greater for white women than for other women. Based on NLSY data, it is impossible to say whether the labor market consequences of obesity are the result of relatively worse health impairing productivity, or to employer discrimination, but other studies suggest that discrimination plays an important role.

ECONOMIC IMPACT OF BARIATRIC AND METABOLIC SURGERY

Morbid obesity is associated with a myriad of serious comorbid conditions, including hypertension, type 2 diabetes mellitus, dyslipidemia, osteoarthritis, and gallbladder disease.[12,13] There have been numerous studies demonstrating the effectiveness in obtaining weight loss[14,15] and marked resolution of comorbidities with bariatric and metabolic surgery.[16] However, determination of the economic impact of these procedures has been challenging due to the complexity of assessing relative short- and long-term costs and cost-savings of bariatric surgery compared with nonsurgical treatment of severe obesity. Although the average initial cost of bariatric surgery in the United States is in the $11,500 to $26,000 range, the cost appears to be at least somewhat offset by reductions in subsequent overall health care costs related to obesity comorbidities.[17]

In 2009, Cremieux and colleagues[18] quantified the effect of bariatric surgery on direct medical costs. They evaluated the time required for third-party payers to recover the initial investment associated with bariatric surgery (ie, the return on investment). Their analysis revealed, after taking into account age, sex, and comorbidities, the initial investment is returned within 4 years for patients who undergo open surgery and within 2 years for patients who undergo laparoscopic surgery. They concluded that even ignoring potential quality-of-life and length-of-life benefits, as well as disability and work loss, third-party payers can rely on bariatric surgery paying for itself through decreased comorbidities within 2 to 4 years. These returns on investment result from reductions in prescription drug costs, physician visit costs, and hospital costs (including emergency department visits and inpatient and outpatient visits).

Diabetes appears to severely compound the costs related to obesity.[19] In 2011, Klein and colleagues[20] evaluated the economic impact of the clinical benefits of bariatric surgery on medical costs and return on investment of the surgery in patients with obesity (BMI>35 kg/m^2) and diabetes. At the time of their study, estimated yearly costs of managing a diabetic patient ($13,243) was more than 5 times that of a patient without diabetes ($2560). In this study, total surgery costs were fully recovered on average after 30 months in 1999 to 2007 for all types of surgeries. Clinical benefits appeared to be the underlying driver of the return on investment results. For diagnostic claims of diabetes, by the first 3-month period after surgery, 40.7% of surgery patients had a diabetes-related claim compared with 72.1% of control patients (P<.001). The drug utilization also had statistically significant results. By the first 3-month period after index, 45.6% of surgery patients had filled a prescription for diabetes medication in the previous 3 months, compared with 90.8% of control patients. At month 6, the percentages were 33.5% and 89.7%, respectively ($P<.001$). Among patients who had insulin claims before index date, insulin claims dropped to 42.8% for surgery patients and remained at 92.4% for control patients at month 3 after index ($P<.001$). Among surgery patients who had claims for noninsulin diabetes medications before surgery, 37.3% had claims for noninsulin medications at month 3, compared with 86.3% of control patients ($P<.001$); 84.5% of surgery patients who had claims for noninsulin medication at index had no claims for any diabetes medications by month 36. By the first 3-month period after index, the average total cost of diabetes medications and supplies for surgery patients was \$33 compared with \$123 for control patients ($P<.001$); this drug cost-savings trend was sustained for the duration of the study period.

In 2013, Neovius and colleagues[21] reported a long-term evaluation of health care use patterns using the ongoing Swedish Obese Subjects prospective, matched cohort. Previously, these investigators reported a 28% reduction in all-cause mortality after surgery compared with nonsurgical treatment of severe obesity. They assessed health care use over 20 years by obese patients treated conventionally or with bariatric surgery. Health care utilization was measured by hospital days, nonprimary care outpatient physician visits, and drug costs. In the 20 years following their bariatric procedure, surgery patients used a total of 54 mean cumulative hospital days compared with 40 used by those in the control group ($P = .03$). During the years 2 through 6, surgery patients had an accumulated annual mean of 1.7 hospital days versus 1.2 days among control patients ($P \le .001$). From year 7 to 20, both groups had a mean annual 1.8 hospital days ($P = .95$). Surgery patients had a mean annual 1.3 nonprimary care outpatient visits during the years 2 through 6 versus 1.1 among the controls ($P = .003$), but from year 7, the 2 groups did not differ. From year 7 to 20, the surgery group incurred a mean annual relative decreased cost (US \$930) compared with control patients (\$1123) ($P \le .001$). They concluded that, compared with controls, surgically treated patients used more inpatient and nonprimary outpatient care during the first 6-year period after undergoing bariatric surgery but not thereafter. Drug costs from years 7 through 20 were lower for surgery patients than for control patients. In a review of more than 12 cost assessment studies of bariatric surgery, investigators reported that all 12 studies demonstrated cost-effectiveness for bariatric surgery and one-third demonstrated cost-savings.[22]

FACTORS EFFECTING ACCESS TO BARIATRIC AND METABOLIC SURGERY

The evidence clearly demonstrates that bariatric and metabolic surgery is an effective treatment for obese patients, and in particular, obese patients with diabetes. However, approximately 11% of people with a BMI greater than 35 kg/m^2, almost 18 million in the United States alone, may be clinically eligible for surgery, but only 1% of those eligible have undergone surgery.[23] The reasons for this great disparity are multiple and represent complex socioeconomic issues surrounding the very problem that has led to the epidemic levels of obesity in this country.

In 2010, Martin and colleagues[24] reviewed the socioeconomic disparities between the portion of the population that was eligible for bariatric surgery and the patients that actually underwent the procedure. The national bariatric eligible population was identified from the 2005 to 2006 NHANES and compared with the adult noneligible population. The eligible cohort was then compared with the patients who had undergone bariatric surgery in the 2006 Nationwide Inpatient Sample. More than 22 million people were identified as bariatric eligible. Compared with the noneligible group, the bariatric eligible group had significantly lower family incomes, lower education levels, less access to health care, and a greater proportion of nonwhite race (all $P<.001$). Bariatric eligibility was associated with significant adverse economic and health-related markers, including days of work lost (5 vs 8, $P<.001$). More than one-third (35%) of bariatric-eligible patients were either uninsured or underinsured, and 15% had incomes less than poverty level. Almost 88,000 inpatient bariatric surgical procedures were performed in 2006. Three-fourths were performed in white patients with greater median incomes (80%) and private insurance (82%). Significant disparities associated with a decreased likelihood of undergoing bariatric surgery were noted by race, income, insurance type, and gender.

Bhogal and colleagues[25] published a systematic review and meta-analysis in 2015 that evaluated the inequity in the utilization of bariatric surgery. Nine studies providing data on more than 64 million patients were included in the meta-analysis. Of the patients eligible for bariatric surgery, only 260,677 (0.4%) patients received the surgery. Across studies, bariatric surgery-eligible patients who received surgery ranged from less than 1% (23–28) to 5% (29–31). Patients who received bariatric surgery were significantly more likely to be white than non-white (odds ratio [OR] 1.54; 95% confidence interval [CI], 1.08, 2.19), have private insurance than non-private insurance (OR 2.51; 95% CI 1.04, 6.05), and be female than male gender (OR 2.80; 95% CI 2.46, 3.22). Among those who were identified as being non-white, the majority were black (69%), followed by Hispanic (23.2%), other (7.4%), and Asian (0.4%). Additional analysis revealed that the odds of having bariatric surgery were more likely among those living in urban areas versus nonurban areas (OR 1.45; 95% CI 1.42, 1.48), and who were between the ages of 18 and 50 years versus 50 years of age and older (OR 2.39 95% CI 1.28, 4.48).

A study by Chawla and colleagues[26] aimed to further identify the barriers to bariatric and metabolic surgery, and second, to develop recommendations for stakeholders to improve patient access to surgery. In their review, they identified 6 categories that reflected significant barriers to patient access to bariatric surgery: (1) obesity bias: obese patients have been uniquely targeted as lacking willpower and ignoring healthy choices, resulting in a disproportionate focus on changes in patient behavior as a prerequisite to treatment; (2) patient-related barriers: cost, perceived risks associated with surgery, perception of one's own weight, and a lack of understanding of the impact of excess weight on life expectancy and morbidity; (3) current BMI-based selection criteria: the widespread use of a uniform BMI-centric criterion for patient selection across the world results in barriers to access. They recommend a shift away from a strict BMI-centric model to a comorbidity-centric model that would place the focus on complications rather than the weight itself; (4) access to Centers of Excellence or qualified surgeons; (5) infrequent clinical guideline updates and data gaps: approximately one-half of the guidelines (8/19) are largely based on the first US National Institutes of Health guideline, dating back to 1998. Guideline recommendations have not significantly changed in 16 years despite significant safety and efficacy data; (6) restrictive third-party payer coverage. Their study calls for updated public policies, patient education, updated reimbursement policies, and additional long-term data demonstrating the effectiveness of bariatric surgery.

SUMMARY

Based on scientific evidence, it is becoming increasingly clear and accepted that the only existing therapy for severe obesity that has been shown to result in clinically significant and durable weight loss is bariatric surgery. Furthermore, it has been shown that weight loss after bariatric surgery results in significant improvements in obesity comorbidity, quality of life, and reduced mortality. Short- and long-term complications of surgery, although not insignificant, appear to be reasonable and justifiable compared with the long-term risks of severe obesity. Economic analysis has demonstrated that bariatric surgery is cost-effective and perhaps cost-saving in certain subgroups such as those with type 2 diabetes. In addition, there is evidence that bariatric surgery may reduce indirect costs of obesity by improving workplace productivity and reducing absenteeism. Despite the aforementioned health and economic benefits of bariatric surgery, a relatively small percentage of patients who may benefit from surgery are receiving access to this very effective treatment. Much greater attention by health care providers, insurance carriers, and public health officials is required in order to address this tremendous disparity in access to the most effective treatment of severe obesity, perhaps the most threatening public health concern of our time.

REFERENCES

1. Weiner RA. Indications and principles of metabolic surgery. Chirurg 2010;81(4): 379–94 [in German].
2. Ogden CL, Carroll MD, Fryar CD, et al. Prevalence of obesity among adults and youth: United States, 2011-2014. NCHS Data Brief 2015;(219):1–8.
3. U.S. Department of Health and Human Services, Office of Disease Prevention and Health Promotion. Healthy People 2020 topics and objectives: nutrition and weight status. Washington, DC. Available at: http://www.healthypeople.gov/2020/topics-objectives/topic/nutrition-and-weight-status?topicid=29. Accessed February 1, 2016.
4. American Heart Association. Understanding childhood obesity. Available at: http://www.heart.org/HEARTORG/HealthyLiving/HealthyKids/ChildhoodObesity/What-is-childhood-obesity_UCM_304347_Article.jsp#.VqzVYo-cHid. Accessed February 1, 2016.
5. Finkelstein EA. How big of a problem is obesity? Surg Obes Relat Dis 2014;10(4): 569–70.
6. Finkelstein EA, Trogdon JG, Cohen JW, et al. Annual medical spending attributable to obesity: payer- and service-specific estimates. Health Aff (Millwood) 2009;28(5):w822–31.
7. Cawley J, Meyerhoefer C. The medical care costs of obesity: an instrumental variables approach. J Health Econ 2012;31(1):219–30.
8. Cawley J, Meyerhoefer C, Biener A, et al. Savings in medical expenditures associated with reductions in body mass index among US adults with obesity, by diabetes status. Pharmacoeconomics 2015;33(7):707–22.
9. Finkelstein EA, DiBonaventura Md, Burgess SM, et al. The costs of obesity in the workplace. J Occup Environ Med 2010;52(10):971–6.
10. Gallup. Available at: http://www.gallup.com/poll/150026/unhealthy-workers-absenteeism-costs-153-billion.aspx. Accessed February 1, 2016.
11. Cawley J. The impact of obesity on wages. J Hum Resour 2004;39(2):451–74. Body Weight and Women's Labor Market Outcomes, NBER Working Paper No. 7841.
12. National Heart, Lung, and Blood Institute Web site. The practical guide: identification, evaluation, and treatment of overweight and obesity in adults. 2000. Available at: http://www.nhlbi.nih.gov/guidelines/obesity/prctgd_c.pdf. Accessed June 12, 2007.
13. Hensrud DD, Klein S. Extreme obesity: a new medical crisis in the United States. Mayo Clin Proc 2006;81(Suppl 10):S5–10.

14. Zhao Y, Encinosa W. Bariatric surgery utilization and outcomes in 1998 and 2004. Rockville (MD): Agency for Healthcare Research and Quality; 2007. Statistical brief 23.
15. Kendrick ML, Daken GF. Surgical approaches to obesity. Mayo Clin Proc 2006; 81(Suppl 10):S18–24.
16. Buchwald H, Avidor Y, Braunwald E, et al. Bariatric surgery: a systematic review and meta-analysis. JAMA 2004;292(14):1724–37 [Erratum appears in JAMA 2005;293(14):1728].
17. Salem L, Jensen Flum CC, Flum DR. Are bariatric surgical outcomes worth their cost? A systematic review. J Am Coll Surg 2005;200(2):270–8.
18. Cremieux PY, Buchwald H, Shikora SA, et al. A study on the economic impact of bariatric surgery. Am J Manag Care 2008;14(9):589–96.
19. Campbell RK, Martin TM. The chronic burden of diabetes. Am J Manag Care 2009;15:S248–54.
20. Klein S, Ghosh A, Cremieux PY, et al. Economic impact of the clinical benefits of bariatric surgery in diabetes patients with BMI $\geq$35 kg/m^2. Obesity (Silver Spring) 2011;19(3):581–7.
21. Neovius M, Narbro K, Keating C, et al. Health care use during 20 years following bariatric surgery. JAMA 2012;308(11):1132–41.
22. Chang SH, Stoll C, Colditz GA. Cost effectiveness of bariatric surgery: should it be universally available? Maturitas 2011;69(3):230–8.
23. Dixon JB. Adjustable gastric banding and conventional therapy for type 2 diabetes. JAMA 2008;299(3):316–23.
24. Martin M, Beekley A, Kjorstad R, et al. Socioeconomic disparities in eligibility and access to bariatric surgery: a national population-based analysis. Surg Obes Relat Dis 2010;6(1):8–15.
25. Bhogal SK, Reddigan JI, Rotstein OD, et al. Inequity to the utilization of bariatric surgery: a systematic review and meta-analysis. Obes Surg 2015;25(5):888–99.
26. Chawla AS, Hsiao CW, Romney MC, et al. Gap between evidence and patient access: policy implications for bariatric and metabolic surgery in the treatment of obesity and its complications. Pharmacoeconomics 2015;33(7):629–41.

Obesity, Type 2 Diabetes, and the Metabolic Syndrome

Pathophysiologic Relationships and Guidelines for Surgical Intervention

Laurent Genser, MD[1], James Rossario Casella Mariolo, MD[1],
Lidia Castagneto-Gissey, MD[1], Spyros Panagiotopoulos, MD, PhD,
Francesco Rubino, MD*

KEYWORDS

- Obesity • Metabolic syndrome • Diabetes • Bariatric metabolic surgery
- Insulin resistance • Gut • Microbiota

KEY POINTS

- Visceral obesity is associated with systemic low-grade inflammation leading to insulin resistance, β-cell dysfunction, and cardiometabolic diseases.
- The gastrointestinal tract is a key organ in metabolic regulation; hence, it is a biologically rational target for interventions aimed at treating metabolic syndrome, obesity, and type 2 diabetes (ie, metabolic surgery).
- Recent randomized clinical trials show that bariatric/metabolic surgery causes greater improvement of type 2 diabetes and reduction of cardiovascular risk compared with lifestyle modification and medical therapies.
- Based on such clinical and mechanistic evidence, several international professional organizations and government agencies have recently suggested expanding the indications for bariatric/metabolic surgery to include patients with inadequately controlled type 2 diabetes and a body mass index as low as 30 kg/m^2 and 27.5 kg/m^2 for Asians.

Conflicts of Interests: None.
Funding: L. Genser is a research fellow and was supported by the Institute of Cardiometabolism and Nutrition (ICAN), Société Française de Chirurgie Digestive (SFCD), Fondation Obélisque and APPERT Institute (UPPIA).
Bariatric and Metabolic Surgery, Division of Diabetes and Nutritional Sciences, King's College London and King's College Hospital, London SE5 9RS, UK
[1] These authors equally contributed to the present work.
* Corresponding author.
E-mail address: Francesco.rubino@kcl.ac.uk

Surg Clin N Am 96 (2016) 681–701
http://dx.doi.org/10.1016/j.suc.2016.03.013
0039-6109/16/$ – see front matter © 2016 Elsevier Inc. All rights reserved.
surgical.theclinics.com

INTRODUCTION

Obesity represents one of the primary causes of preventable deaths. In 2014, an estimated 1.9 billion adults were considered overweight and more than 600 million were obese, translating to 13% of the worldwide adult population.[1,2] Also, the prevalence of morbid obesity (defined by a body mass index [BMI] >40 kg/m^2) has almost doubled since 1980.[1] Such increase in the prevalence of obesity and morbid obesity has been related to a variety of factors including sedentary lifestyle, disproportionate caloric intake, stress, socioeconomic status, in addition to ethnicity and genetic susceptibility. Obese men and women are at significantly higher risk of developing type 2 diabetes mellitus (T2DM).[3,4] In fact, the prevalence of T2DM has increased in parallel with the augmented prevalence of obesity. Currently, T2DM affects about 285 million people worldwide, a number predicted to almost double by 2030.[5]

The term "metabolic syndrome" (MS) is generally used to indicate the cluster of central obesity, insulin resistance (IR), hypertension, and hyperlipidemia. Metabolic syndrome results in a greater risk of developing T2DM and cardiovascular disease, 2 of the principal causes of death worldwide.[6]

Bariatric surgery causes significant and sustained weight loss and can considerably reduce IR, with dramatic clinical improvement or remission of insulin-resistant states (ie, dyslipidemia, hypertension, hyperuricemia, sleep apnea). Experimental evidence from animals shows that the effects of bariatric surgery on insulin sensitivity and glucose homeostasis are not just the consequence of mechanical reduction of food intake or energy absorption but derive from a variety of physiologic mechanisms, including changes in gut hormones, biliary acids metabolism, nutrient sensing, and microbiota.[7]

This knowledge corroborates evidence of a critical role of the gut in glucose and energy homeostasis and supports consideration of the gastrointestinal (GI) tract as a rational biological target for interventions aimed at treating obesity, diabetes, and metabolic disorders.[8] Recent randomized clinical trials show that bariatric surgery results in better control of T2DM and greater reduction of cardiovascular risk factors compared with a variety of lifestyle interventions and medical therapies.[9–12] Based on such mounting mechanistic and clinical evidence, conventional bariatric procedures are now increasingly being proposed not only as mere surgical management of obesity but also as a valuable approach to intentionally treat T2DM—a new concept and practice referred to as "metabolic surgery."[13–15]

Obesity and the Adipose Tissue

Obesity has become a pandemic and has received increasing attention over the past decades for the implications it carries in the development of numerous chronic diseases. In the last 30 years, the average BMI has increased at a rate of 0.4 kg/m^2 per decade worldwide.[16] Among high-income countries, the United States has the highest prevalence of obesity, with one third of the population having a BMI of 30 or greater.[17] Even though the prevalence of obesity in the United States tended to stabilize after 2005, the prevalence of severe (BMI >35 kg/m^2) and morbid (BMI >40 kg/m^2) obesity has continued to increase. Between 1986 and 2000, the prevalence of subjects with a BMI of 40 or greater quadrupled and that of subjects with a BMI of 50 or greater quintupled.[17,18]

Obesity is a condition characterized by an excess of body adiposity and for practical reasons is commonly measured by BMI, an expression of body weight as a nonlinear function of height. A BMI $\geq$30 kg/m^2 indicates the presence of obesity; when BMI exceeds 40 kg/m^2, the subject is regarded as morbidly obese.[19]

However, using BMI as a unit of measure assumes that adipose tissue has an even distribution throughout the body, because it does not take into account the diverse topographic deposition of body fat among individuals. Thus, BMI is not a measure of dysfunctional adipose tissue nor an accurate metrics of metabolic disease. In fact, an excessive and preferential accumulation of fat in visceral depots may not be necessarily associated with a high BMI; nonetheless, it strongly correlates with those metabolic disturbances that increase the risk of developing cardiovascular disease.[20] A significant number of individuals present hyperglycemia, hyperinsulinemia, IR, hyperlipidemia, and hypertension despite a lean body type and a normal BMI, a phenotype often referred to as "metabolically obese but normal weight subjects."[21,22] Conversely, many persons categorized as obese by BMI lack all the components of MS and display average risk of developing cardiovascular disease compared with the general population; this group of subjects is referred to as "metabolically healthy obese."[23]

It has been shown that subcutaneous adipose tissue (SAT) distribution, common in women, is related to metabolic protection, conversely to central or intra-abdominal obesity, typical of men, which frequently accompanies MS.[24,25] In addition, ectopic fat accumulation in organs such as liver, skeletal muscles, heart, kidneys, pancreas is associated with metabolic comorbidities.[26] In consideration of the importance of fat distribution in metabolic disease, waist circumference (WC) is widely considered a more reliable predictor of cardiometabolic risk than BMI. A WC $\geq$ 88 cm in women and WC $\geq$ 102 cm in men is considered an independent risk factor for developing cardiovascular disease and atherogenic dyslipidemia, and a rough measure of the degree of IR.[19]

The exact reasons behind the differential deposition of adipose tissue in the various regions of the body are unclear; both modifiable factors (eg, physical activity, nutritional status, growth hormone, glucocorticoids, sex steroids) and nonmodifiable factors (such as gender, age, ethnicity, and genetic susceptibility) seem to play a role.[19]

The adipose tissue exerts metabolic and endocrine functions and is characterized by great pliability and expandability. Whereas adipocytes in the subcutaneous tissue can become both hyperplasic and hypertrophic, visceral adipose tissue (VAT) appears to have a limited capacity of recruitment and differentiation of new adipose cells and is more prone to develop hypertrophic cells with impaired adipocyte function.[27] Such dysfunctional adipocytes cause altered secretion of adipocytokines (ie, adipokines) and an elevation of free fatty acids (FFAs) release into the circulation that ultimately leads to the onset of obesity-related IR, the common denominator of MS and other metabolic disorders.[19,28,29]

Metabolic Syndrome: Definitions and Pathophysiologic Aspects

In the late 1970s, the term "metabolic syndrome" was proposed to identify a cluster of interrelated factors, comprising visceral obesity, IR, hypertension, and dyslipidemia, that were associated with an augmented risk of developing T2DM and cardiovascular disease.[30] In the 1980s, Reaven[31] proposed that IR could be the primary defect of the syndrome, arguing that insulin-resistant subjects could develop MS even though they were not obese. The World Health Organization (WHO)[1] and the American Heart Association subsequently recognized MS[32] as a distinct clinical entity with its own code (277.7) in the WHO's ICD-9 classification. However, in the following years, other scientists and clinicians have challenged the idea of MS as a separate clinical entity. In 2012, a joint statement by the American Diabetes Association (ADA) and the European Association for the Study of Diabetes was particularly critical of the idea of MS as a distinct clinical entity.[33] In particular, this statement argued that existing definitions of MS are based on ambiguous or unclear criteria and that the cutoff points used to define abnormal levels of the individual components ignore the continuum in risk associated with glucose, blood pressure, and lipids levels. This statement also questioned the evidence that the syndrome as a whole adds to cardiovascular disease prediction beyond the contribution of the individual component risk factors.

Despite this, MS continues to be considered a distinct entity by many researchers that investigate the link between IR and metabolic disease, whereas clinical cardiologists rely on MS for their assessment of cardiometabolic morbidity and mortality in individual patients. One of the most commonly used definitions of MS was proposed in 2001 by the National Cholesterol Education Program (NCEP) Adult Treatment Panel III (ATP III)[34] and includes criteria such as WC, triglycerides, high-density lipoprotein (HDL)-cholesterol, blood pressure, and fasting glycemia. The presence of abnormal levels of 3 of these 5 variables, listed in **Table 1**, is used for a diagnosis of MS.

The definition of MS by the International Diabetes Federation (IDF) slightly differs from the one reported because it recommends considering a different cutoff for WC in relation to the ethnicity of the individual; this is based on knowledge that persons of Asian descent can have abdominal obesity and an elevated risk for cardiovascular disease at lower BMI levels compared with individuals of other ethnicities.[35] Using the NCEP-ATP III definition, the prevalence of MS among US adults was estimated to range from 22%[36] to 34% and up to 39% when using the IDF criteria.[37]

Prospective population studies showed that the relative risk for the development of atherosclerotic cardiovascular disease in patients with MS is twice as high as that of the general population; the risk of developing T2DM is 5-fold greater.[38–44]

A diet rich in lipids and carbohydrates contributes to the emergence of 2 of the essential factors for the diagnosis of MS: visceral obesity and IR. The increased VAT contains hypertrophic, dysfunctional adipocytes at increased lypolytic activity; this can cause high release of FFAs in the splanchnic circulation, thus directly reaching the liver.[45] It is also thought that when peripheral adipocytes have surpassed their capacity and are no longer capable of storing triglycerides, these will be deposited in other tissues (mainly liver and skeletal muscle), favoring the establishment of peripheral and hepatic IR.

Table 1
Criteria for diagnosis of metabolic syndrome according to National Cholesterol Education Program–Third Adult Treatment Panel, International Diabetes Federation, World Health Organization

Criteria	NCEP: ATP III Three of the Following:	IDF Central Obesity (as WC Gender/Ethnicity-Specific) + 2 of the Following:	WHO Hyperinsulinemia + 2 of the Following:
waist circumference (cm/inches)	>102/40 in men >88/35 in women	>94/37 in men >80/31.5 in women	>94/37 in men and/or BMI >30 kg/m^2
Triglycerides	≥150 mg/dL	≥150 mg/dL	≥150 mg/dL
Cholesterol-HDL	<40 mg/dL men <50 mg/dL women	<40 mg/dL men <50 mg/dL women	<35 mg/dL men <39 mg/dL women
Blood pressure	≥130/85 mm Hg	≥130/85 mm Hg	≥140/90 mm Hg
Fasting plasma glucose	≥110 mg/dL	FPG ≥5.6 mmol/L or T2DM	—
Microalbuminuria	—	—	>30 mg/g

The augmented flow of FFAs to the liver causes an increase in hepatic neoglucogenesis contributing to the development of hyperglycemia.[46,47] In addition, in the presence of IR, high circulating levels of FFAs induce hepatic triglyceride synthesis leading to hypertriglyceridemia and overproduction of very low-density lipoproteins (LDL), rich in Apo B and triglycerides.[48] In the setting of hypertriglyceridemia, LDL and HDL undergo alterations of their composition. LDL triglyceride content increases at the expense of phospholipids, and esterified and nonesterified cholesterol. As a result, LDL particles become smaller in size and denser, possibly becoming more atherogenic. Similarly, the cholesterol portion of the HDL lipoprotein core is reduced with an inconstant increase in triglycerides, resulting once again in small, dense particles that undergo a higher rate of clearance from the circulation.[49–51] In fact, reduced serum levels of HDL, elevated triglycerides, and small, dense LDL represent the typical lipidic profile present in MS-related dyslipidemia.

Hypertension is one of the components of MS with the latest onset. Adipocytes are capable of producing several biologically active peptides, including angiotensinogen, angiotensin converting enzyme, and cathepsins. An expanded adipose tissue could result in increased production of angiotensinogen, which in turn may lead to the onset of obesity-associated hypertension. Moreover, IR might also contribute to the development of hypertension because of reduced stimulation of nitric oxide, causing a decreased vasodilation.[52,53]

LINKING OBESITY TYPE 2 DIABETES MELLITUS AND METABOLIC SYNDROME: PATHOPHYSIOLOGIC EVIDENCE

Obesity, T2DM, and cardiometabolic disorders are associated with IR.[31] Nevertheless, most obese subjects with IR do not develop hyperglycemia. Physiologically, the pancreatic islet β cells present adaptative features allowing an increased insulin release to overcome IR and maintain normal glucose tolerance. However in patients with T2DM, IR is not completely compensated by B cells.[54,55] Herein, the principal pathophysiologic mechanisms associated with obesity, T2DM, and other metabolic disorders are presented.

Insulin Resistance

IR is considered the most important pathophysiologic aspect linking obesity and cardiometabolic diseases.[31,56] IR is an impairment of insulin action on insulin-sensitive tissues characterized by a decreased glucose access in muscles and an increased neoglucogenesis in the liver, resulting in fasting as well as postprandial hyperglycemia. IR has systemic impact causing arterial endothelial dysfunction, atherosclerosis, increased lipolysis, sarcopenia, decreased bone mass, and β-cell mass.[27,57]

Pancreatic β-Cell Dysfunction and Defective Insulin Secretion

Studies have shown that the basal insulin secretion rate and the insulin output in response to an oral glucose tolerance test grow in a linear fashion as BMI increases.[58] A hyperbolic correlation instead has been found between β-cell function and insulin sensitivity.[59] Hence, on a background of IR, the β cell must enhance its insulin release in order to compensate and maintain a state of euglycemia.[60]

β-Cell failure is a requisite for the development of T2DM, whereas skeletal muscle IR is evident decades before β-cell failure and overt hyperglycemia occur.[61,62] High-risk individuals with IR who are prone to develop diabetes show a progressively reduced β-cell function over time, whereas "nonprogressors" can maintain increased insulin secretion that compensates for the worsening insulin sensitivity.[62]

This capacity of β cells to adjust their secretive function to the grade of insulin sensitivity is known as disposition index (DI). DI is calculated as the product of β-cell sensitivity multiplied by the insulin sensitivity. The disposition curve typically follows a hyperbolic function[59]; this implies that the product of insulin sensitivity and secretion should yield a constant for a given degree of glucose tolerance and thereby provide a measure of β-cell function.

Progression from normal glucose tolerance to impaired fasting glycemia, impaired glucose tolerance, and finally, T2DM, is likely the result of various contributing factors, including high-caloric diet, lack of physical activity, and genetic predisposition. In a first compensatory phase, the insulin-resistant state causes an increase in total insulin secretion rate, determining hyperinsulinemia.[63] In this stage, greater insulin secretion is mainly due to β-cell hyperplasia and to a lesser extent hypertrophy, globally contributing to an increased islet mass, as found in human autopsies.[63–65] Subsequently, as a consequence of increasing glucose levels (ie, glucotoxicity hypothesis), a loss of acute glucose-stimulated insulin secretion develops, resulting in the inability to promptly respond to glycemic increments. The prolonged exposure to hyperglycemia and increased circulating FFAs favor a constant, low-grade inflammation, leading to stress of endoplasmic reticulum, altered function of mitochondria, increased release of reactive oxygen species, and ultimately, oxidative stress in the β cell. Oxidative stress in the β cell in turn is responsible for changes observed in β-cell phenotype, differentiation, and gene expression, which might be responsible for such loss of acute secretory action.[66–69] Moreover, a higher insulin request, caused by a state of IR, conduces to increase cosecretion of insulin and islet amyloid polypeptide. The presence of amyloid in high concentrations is toxic and contributes to inducing β-cell apoptosis.[70,71] Chronic hyperglycemia and worsening of IR cause a critical decline in β-cell mass, ultimately leading to overt diabetes.[71]

Inside the β cells, insulin granules ready for the secretion are docked to the cell membrane; when glucose binds to the glucose transporter isoform GLUT2, they fuse with the membrane and secrete packages of insulin. Diabetic subjects lose the capacity to promptly secrete such already synthesized insulin granules and therefore characteristically lack the first phase of insulin secretion in response to a glucose load; they also usually show an exaggerated second phase of insulin secretion. Although loss of first-phase insulin secretion was thought to be an irreversible defect, bariatric metabolic surgery (BMS) has been shown to promptly restore the first phase of insulin secretion within 1 month of the operation, suggesting that such defect is instead a reversible phenomenon rather than a structural defect of the β cell.[72,73]

The Adipose Tissue in Metabolic Diseases

Adipose tissue affects metabolism by releasing FFAs and adipocytokines. The oversecretion of some of these cytokines may act as a potential mediator of inflammation leading to IR.

Factors with deleterious effects on metabolism

Free fatty acids Increased FFAs levels are observed in human obesity and T2DM and are strongly correlated with the level of IR.[54,74] FFAs have anti-insulin action and are produced during the metabolism of lipids. When reaching insulin-sensitive tissues, increased FFAs levels lead to increased liver glucose production and muscular lipid storage, leading to IR state in T2DM patients.[74,75] In obesity, which is considered a low-grade inflammatory state, increased circulating levels of FFAs appear to be positively correlated with plasma levels of pro-inflammatory cytokines, which are known to be associated with IR and T2DM.[74]

Proinflammatory adipocytokines

Obesity and T2DM are associated with the overproduction of proinflammatory cytokines such as Tumor necrosis factor-a (TNF-a) Interleukin-6 (IL-6).[76] These cytokines are produced by the adipocytes among many other cell types and inhibit insuling signaling which in turn promote IR. TNF-alfa may also have direct deleterious effect on Beta-cells by inhibiting insulin secretion and promoting B-cell apoptosis as observed in-vitro.[76,77] An associaton has been demonstrated between IL-6 signaling pathway in the adipose tissue and IR, with a positive correlation between IL-6 serum levels and IR levels.[77,78] Other cytokines such as IL-1 beta, Resistin, Retinol binding Protein-4, Visfatin, Plasminogen Activator-1 (PAI-1), Monocyte Chemoattractant Protein-1, fibrinogen and angiotensin are increasingly produced by the adipose tissue in obesity and T2DM. These cytokines contribute to inflammation, lipid accumulation and participate to the develoment of endothelial dysfunctions and therefore myocardial infarction, stroke and cardiomyopathy.[76]

Protective adipocyte-derived factors

Leptin is an adipocytokine that reduces appetite and IR along with improvement of metabolic disturbances associated with T2DM. Increase in tissue sensitivity of insulin by leptin may be due to its action on oxidation of FFAs, leading to decreased FFAs in the circulation.[78] Unlike other adipocytokines, serum levels of adiponectin are decreased in obesity and T2DM. This cytokine has insulin-sensitizing and antiatherogenic actions. In human obesity and T2DM, this adipocytokine has been shown to stimulate FFAs oxidation, and therefore decrease plasma FFAs oxidation, reduce lipid accumulation and increase insulin sensitivity. Adiponectin reduces endothelial dysfunction by increasing nitric-oxide synthesis and decreasing the expression of adhesion molecules and also prevents atherosclerosis by inhibiting LDL oxidation.[79,80] Other adipocytokines, such as Apelin, appear to have antiobesity and antidiabetic actions, because of its possible positive role in energy metabolism and insulin sensitivity.[78]

Body fat distribution

Another critical factor involved in IR and metabolic diseases is body fat distribution. All definitions of MS include a measure of WC (**Table 1**). Obesity is often associated with IR; however, insulin sensitivity varies markedly in lean individuals and in obese subjects because of differences in body fat distribution.[19] Lean individuals with a more peripheral type of fat distribution (ie, SAT) are more insulin sensitive than obese subjects who have predominantly central fat distribution (ie, VAT).[54] VAT is more resistant to the antilipolytic action of insulin than SAT, which may explain the association between VAT, IR, and T2DM.[81,82]

Tissular and Systemic Inflammation

Obesity, T2DM, and MS are associated with low-grade systemic[83,84] and tissular inflammation in the adipose tissue, the liver, the pancreas, and the intestine.[85–87] Infiltration of immune cells, including macrophages, mast cells, and lymphocytes, was found in these tissues with a modification in cell population into a proinflammatory profile. These cells produce proinflammatory cytokines that interfere with insulin signaling in insulin-sensitive tissues, cause β-cell dysfunction, and consequently, insulin deficiency. Obese and T2DM patients show increased white blood cell counts, plasma levels of coagulation factors (fibrinogen and PAI-1), C-reactive protein (CRP), serum amyloid A, and proinflammatory cytokines (TNF-α, IL-1β, and IL-6).[78] The overexpression of these cytokines, and especially CRP, contribute to systemic inflammation and lipid accumulation, which in turn have deleterious effects on blood vessels, leading to endothelial dysfunction, myocardial infarction, cardiomyopathy, and death in the general population as well as in patients presenting with MS.[79] These markers are strongly associated with central adiposity,[88] IR, and MS.[87]

Obstructive Sleep Apnea Syndrome

Obstructive sleep apnea (OSA) is linked to obesity and affects 15% of men and 6% of women.[89] OSA is characterized by airway obstruction during sleep, responsible for chronic hypoxia; this leads to the activation of the hypothalamic-pituitary-adrenal axis, causing oxidative stress, systemic and tissular inflammation (adipose tissue and liver), and increased secretion of proinflammatory adipocytokines (Resistin, TNF-α, IL-6, plasminogen activator-1). These disturbances result in decreased insulin sensitivity and pancreatic β-cell dysfunction. OSA is known as a critical independent risk factor of cardiovascular disease, hypertension, MS, and T2DM.[90,91]

Sympathetic Nervous System Overdrive

Recent evidence from experimental and human studies has linked obesity, T2DM, and other metabolic comorbidities to a chronic activation of sympathetic nervous system (SNS), possibly caused by different types of stimuli (ie, food intake, hyperinsulinemia, glucose consumption, increased adiposity, and hyperleptinemia; hypothalamic-pituitary-adrenal axis activation).[92] Chronic activation of SNS results in increased adrenergic outflow with high levels of circulating catecholamines and glucocorticoids, leading to IR. SNS activation increases glucose release from the liver, reduces insulin, increases glucagon release by the pancreas, and increases lipolysis in the adipose tissue.[92] These effects are associated with vasoconstriction in peripheral arteries, which also results in impaired glucose uptake in skeletal muscle.[92] The effects of chronic SNS activation can therefore predispose to IR, hypertension, renal disease, and cardiac dysfunctions (ie, diastolic dysfunction, left ventricular hypertrophy).[93]

THE GUT AS A BIOLOGICALLY RATIONAL TARGET FOR THE TREATMENT OF CARDIOMETABOLIC DISEASES
Mechanisms Linking the Gut to Cardiometabolic Diseases

A growing body of evidence has accumulated, especially in the last decade, supporting a role of the gut in the physiology of metabolic regulation and in the pathophysiology of cardiometabolic disorders. This evidence comes from physiologic studies as well as from investigations regarding the mechanisms of weight loss and glycemic improvement after bariatric/metabolic surgery. Here the role of various aspects of intestinal physiology in metabolic regulation and metabolic disease is briefly reviewed.

Gut microbiota

The human gut microbiota (GM) is a complex entity composed of more than 1000 species of comensal microorganisms.[94] GM is present across the GI tract with greater concentrations in the ileum and colon. In physiologic conditions, the GM contributes to intestinal system maturation, host defense against pathogens, degradation of non-digestible polysaccharides and plays an important role in body fat distribution and control of energy homeostasis.[95] The GM is influenced by diet, lifestyle, physical exercise, antibiotics, and genetic background.[96] GM modulates energy harvesting from dietary fibers, fat storage, lipopolysaccharides (LPS) content, and the production of short-chain fatty acids which in turn regulate host food intake, insulin signaling and generate low-grade inflammation.[88,97–99] Interestingly, germ-free mice appear to be protected from high-fat diet (HFD)-induced obesity and metabolic alterations.[100] In addition, mice transplanted with GM isolated from obese donors develop increased body fat content and IR.[101,102] Metformin administration in mice is associated with an increase of *Akkermansia muciniphila*, a mucin-degrading bacteria known to positively impact obesity and diabetes,[103] resulting in improved weight loss, glycemic control, and reduced systemic inflammation.[104,105] In humans, obesity and T2DM have been associated with altered GM composition, reduced diversity, and gene richness.[106,107] Recently, metabolomics studies of human plasma samples allowed the identification of GM products, such as trimethylamine-*N*-oxide, involved in atherogenesis and therefore linked to cardiovascular risk.[108]

Alterations of intestinal permeability and metabolic endotoxemia

Intestinal permeability, a feature of the intestinal barrier, regulates the passage of molecules from the lumen into the interstitium. This function is finely regulated by GM and other local factors.[109] In rodent models of diet-induced obesity (ie, HFD), modifications of GM are associated with altered intestinal permeability characterized by a reduced expression of tight junction proteins (ie, zonula occludens-1, occludin, claudins) in the intestinal epithelial cells and an increase in the passage of nutrients and/or bacterial antigens/components (ie, LPS) responsible for systemic inflammation (ie, endotoxemia) and IR.[110] Consistent with this model, GM composition modulation induced by antibiotics or prebiotics/probiotics in rodents improves gut permeability and reduces metabolic endotoxemia and glucose intolerance.[103] However, despite encouraging results[111] intestinal permeability alterations and its role in the crosstalk between GM and inflammation at systemic and tissular levels are still poorly characterized in human obesity and metabolic diseases.[111]

Gut Adaptation to Bariatric/Metabolic Surgery

BMS is currently the most effective treatment for severe obesity and T2DM, providing sustained weight loss as well as reduction and prevention of obesity-related cardio-metabolic comorbidities.[9,15] Given its dramatic clinical effectiveness, BMS provides an opportunity to better understand the role of the gut in physiology and disease. In addition to weight loss, BMS can cause changes in various mechanisms of GI physiology, including changes in satiety-promoting gut hormones (ie, glucose-dependent insulinotropic peptide, glucagon-like peptide 1 [GLP-1], peptide YY, and Oxyntomodulin) and increased gastric emptying. Certain bariatric/metabolic procedures such as Roux-en-Y gastric bypass (RYGB) and sleeve gastrectomy (SG) cause a shift in bile acids (BAs) metabolism composition, bile flow, and increased BAs signaling through the BAs nuclear receptor Farnesoid X (FXR). GI modifications imposed by certain procedures, particularly those involving a re-re-routing of the small intestine (ie, RYGB, duodenal-jejunal bypass, DJB), can cause changes in microbiota composition and nutrient sensing; all of these effects appear to be involved in the metabolic benefits of BMS.[112–114]

Gastrointestinal hormones

RYGB and SG are characterized by an excessive postprandial response of the enteroendocrine intestinal L cells responsible for a rapid increase in postprandial GI hormones.[115] The increase in GLP-1 causes a rapid postprandial "incretin effect," increasing insulin secretion. This mechanism is thought to be at least in part responsible for the improvement of glucose tolerance observed after these procedures.[116] However, the underlying mechanisms supporting this phenomenon remain unclear and debated. Specifically, it is unclear whether the increased secretion and/or release of hormones from intestinal L cells after GI surgery is due to changes in the characteristics (ie, number, functions) of the enteroendocrine cell population,[117] due to stimulation of cells located in the distal small bowel by relatively undigested nutrients (due to a shortcut or expedited gastric emptying and intestinal transit), or if it is secondary to the lack of physiologic gastric modulation on L-cell activity.[118] The role of GLP-1 in the antidiabetic effects of RYGB and SG also has been recently called into question by experiments showing that the improvement of glucose metabolism after surgery is substantially preserved in humans after treatment with GLP-1 receptor (GLP-1-R) agonist[119] as well as in GLP-1R knockout mice models.[120] Ghrelin, a hunger-promoting hormone, is mostly produced in the stomach. Although no specific pattern was observed regarding Ghrelin serum level changes following gastric banding, RYGB, and biliopancreatic diversion, serum levels appeared consistently reduced after SG.[116]

Bile acids
Beyond their role in the absorption of fat-soluble vitamins and dietary lipids, BAs are key regulators of glucose and lipid metabolism as well as energy expenditure thanks to the interaction with GM.[7] The BAs are produced from cholesterol in the liver (primary BA). Primary BAs are transformed into secondary BAs by GM in the intestine; these are absorbed in the terminal ileum, returned to the liver, and are then secreted again into the bile (enterohepatic cycle). Through FXR, BAs stimulate postprandial ileal production of fibroblast growth factor 19, which inhibits hepatic expression of cholesterol 7 alpha hydroxylase 1 (CYP7A1), thus regulating the conversion of cholesterol into BAs.[121] BAs exert positive effects on metabolism by interaction with FXR and the membrane BA receptor TGR5, which inhibits neoglucogenesis and promotes insulin signaling thus controlling glucose of glucose metabolism in the liver[122] and stimulating the intestinal secretion of GLP-1.[123] Increased BA serum levels are observed after RYGB and SG, but not following gastric banding, suggesting that elevated serum BAs levels in procedures that modify GI anatomy could improve insulin sensitivity, incretin secretion, and postprandial glycemia. However, changes in BAs may only partly explain metabolic improvements after RYGB.[7,122,124]

Gut microbiota
BMS induces modifications of microbiome ecology,[125] which could mediate the metabolic effects of surgery and contribute to modulation of fat mass deposition.[114] Recent studies in mice revealed that transfer of the GM from RYGB-treated mice to germ-free mice was associated with significant weight loss, when compared with similar recipients receiving the GM from sham operated mice.[126] These findings support the notion that changes in the GM following RYGB could contribute to weight loss.

Intestinal remodeling
Jejunoileal bypass as well as RYGB are known to induce adaptive intestinal hyperplasia and hypertrophy of intestinal villi in humans.[127–129] In rodents undergoing RYGB, the intestinal remodeling of the alimentary (Roux) limb was associated with a modification of the intestinal glucose metabolism characterized by an upregulation of the intestinal glucose transporter GLUT-1 and increased glucose disposal toward metabolic pathways involved in tissue growth.[130] Moreover, an increase in enteroendocrine cell morphology and number (L cells) has been recently characterized in rodent models of RYGB.[131,132] These observations could contribute to the improvement in glucose

homeostasis observed after RYGB; however, the relevance of this mechanism for the clinical effects of RYGB in humans remains unclear.

Intestinal nutrient sensing

Recent studies have shown that nutrients activate sensing mechanisms in the duodenum, triggering a gut-brain-liver negative feedback mechanism that inhibits hepatic glucose production and food intake to maintain homeostasis.[133] Such nutrient sensing mechanism appears to be dysfunctional in diabetes and obesity, failing to lower food intake and glucose production. Interestingly, the jejunum appears to be able to recover nutrient sensing after DJB, with resulting inhibition of glucose production,[134] suggesting that enhancement of nutrient sensing might contribute to the glucose-lowering effects of GI bypass procedures.

Changes in food preference: the gut-brain axis

Bariatric procedures reduce food intake and change food choices and preferences. In a randomized trial comparing RYGB to vertical gastroplasty, Olbers and colleagues[135] reported a significantly decreased consumption of sweeteners after RYGB, but also of fatty foods with increased fibers and vegetable consumption. Some patients experience after-ingestive disabling symptoms with sweets (ie, dumping syndrome) and fatty food and in turn adapt their eating behaviors, suggesting a beneficial switch in food preferences and choices after RYGB.[136] However even if encouraging functional brain imaging studies demonstrated an involvement of different cerebral pathways in the modification of food preferences observed after RYGB.[136,137] However, the key players responsible for these modifications are unknown.

GUIDELINES FOR SURGICAL TREATMENT OF OBESITY AND DIABETES

The role of the GI tract in the digestion and absorption of nutrients supported the idea that modifications of gastric or intestinal anatomy could be used to reduce energy intake/absorption and, therefore, produce weight loss. In the 1950s, such a concept provided a biological rationale for the use of GI surgery as a weight loss therapy for patients with morbid obesity ("bariatric surgery"). Despite ample documentation of additional metabolic benefits, obesity remained the only indication for bariatric surgery for more than 5 decades. Coherently, clinical guidelines for bariatric surgery have been merely based on weight-centric criteria.

Over the last decade, however, the use of bariatric surgery as an intentional treatment of T2DM[138] has become increasingly popular in academic circles and in the media. This idea is based on consistent clinical observations of the dramatic improvement of hyperglycemia in patients with T2DM and on the experimental evidence that rearrangements of GI anatomy similar to those in some bariatric procedures directly and weight-independently affect glucose homeostasis.[139]

Numerous recent randomized controlled trials (level 1 evidence) have shown superior glycemic control after bariatric/metabolic surgery than with conventional medical and lifestyle approaches for the treatment of obese patients with T2DM.[10,12,140,141]

Further research on mechanisms of action of these procedures and the increasing recognition of the complex and crucial role of the gut in metabolism, as described above, provide a biological rationale for the use of GI-based interventions to treat T2DM.[142] Such conceptual evolution is reflected in most recent guidelines by professional organizations and government agencies that recognize the role of surgery as a treatment of T2DM and advocate the use of disease-based criteria beyond just BMI. These guidelines are contributing to transforming a weight loss intervention (bariatric surgery) into a surgical practice shaped around the goal to improve metabolism and reduce cardiometabolic risk. Such concept and practice is referred to as "metabolic surgery."[13]

A summary of available guidelines for surgical treatment of obesity and T2DM is presented in **Table 2**.

A National Institutes of Health (NIH) Consensus conference in 1991 produced the first guidelines published in bariatric surgery. These BMI-based recommendations state that patients with BMI of 40 kg/m^2 or greater or BMI 35 kg/m^2 or greater with concomitant high-risk morbidities (eg, T2DM, OSA, obesity-related cardiomyopathy) may be considered candidates for bariatric surgery.[8] In 2007, delegates from the first Diabetes Surgery Summit (DSS-I), an international consensus conference, recommended expanding the use and study of GI surgery to treat diabetes, including among only mildly obese persons. Specifically, the DSS-I recommended that "diabetes surgery" should be considered in diabetic, obese patients with BMI 35 kg/m^2 or greater and also in carefully selected candidates with BMI 30 to 35 kg/m^2 and poorly controlled T2DM by lifestyle and medical interventions. Importantly, the DSS-I encouraged

Table 2
According to all committees, bariatric surgery should be considered only after failure to lose weight through lifestyle modifications and weight loss programs

Bariatric Surgery Guidelines	Eligible	Conditional Eligibility	Ethnicity
NIH (1991)	• BMI >40 kg/m^2	• BMI ≥35 kg/m^2 + • Concomitant high-risk morbidities (eg, T2DM, severe OSA)	—
DSS-I (2007)	• BMI >35 kg/m^2	• BMI 30–35 kg/m^2	—
IDF (2011)	• BMI >40 kg/m^2 or • BMI >35 kg/m^2 and T2DM (HbA1c <7% of 53 mmol/mol) unresponsive to medical therapy	• BMI 30–35 kg/m^2 + • Inadequately controlled T2DM by full conventional therapy (HbA1c <7.5% or 58 mmol/mol) or • Other weight-related comorbidities (eg, dyslipidemia, hypertension) possibly responsive to surgical treatment	• BMI lowered by 2.5 kg/m^2 in Asian subjects
ADA (2014)	• BMI >40 kg/m^2	• BMI >35 kg/m^2 if inadequate control of T2DM or other co-morbidities difficult to control with lifestyle and pharmacologic therapy • Insufficient data are available to recommend surgery for BMI <35 kg/m^2	—
NICE (2014)	• BMI >35 kg/m^2 and Tier 3 services[a] (or equivalent)	• BMI 30–35 kg/m^2 + • Recent onset of T2DM and Tier 3 services (or equivalent)	• BMI lowered by according to ethnicity

[a] Tier 3 service: a community/primary care–based multidisciplinary team to provide an intensive level of input to patients.

further studies on the role of surgery in diabetes care as an important research priority.[143] In the ensuing years, several randomized controlled trials have been launched in this area, and most major worldwide bariatric surgery societies have changed their names to include the word "metabolic."

In 2009, the ADA for the first time introduced bariatric surgery in its Standards of Care for the treatment of T2DM, limiting its use, however, to patients with BMI > 35 kg/m^2, because of the lack of sufficient evidence in lower BMI patients.[144,145] In 2011, a position statement by the IDF suggested expanding the indications for bariatric/metabolic surgery to include patients with inadequately controlled T2DM and a BMI as low as 30 kg/m^2, or down to 27.5 kg/m^2 for Asians.[146] More recently, in November 2014, the National Institute for Health and Care Excellence in the United Kingdom (NICE), amended its 2006 guidelines on obesity management, advising assessment for bariatric/metabolic surgery in patients with BMI as low as 30 kg/m^2 and recent onset of T2DM.[147]

On the 28th to 30th of September 2015, the 2nd Diabetes Surgery Summit (DSS-II) was organized in partnership with leading international diabetes organizations and held in London, United Kingdom, in conjunction with the 3rd World Congress on Interventional Therapies for Type 2 Diabetes. The aim of the DSS-II was to review available evidence and develop global recommendations that introduce surgical therapies in a rational treatment algorithm for T2DM. The DSS-II expert committee included a large group of 47 international scholars, representing various medical specialties such as endocrinology/dialectology, internal medicine, cardiology, gastroenterology, primary care, nutrition, and surgery, including official representatives of partner diabetes organizations. A report with the recommendations and guidelines developed through the DSS-II is expected to be published in the spring of 2016.

SUMMARY

Cardiometabolic disorders are characterized by a complex pathophysiology and increased risk of mortality. Experimental evidence shows that some rearrangements of GI anatomy can directly affect glucose homeostasis, insulin sensitivity, and inflammation, supporting the idea that the GI tract is a biologically rational target for interventions aimed at correcting pathophysiologic aspects of obesity and T2DM. Recent randomized controlled trials show that GI surgery results in superior glycemic control compared with conventional medical and lifestyle approaches in patients with T2DM. Such mechanistic and clinical evidence is transforming traditional bariatric surgery, focused on weight reduction, into a new surgical discipline aimed at the improvement of metabolic regulation and reduction of cardiometabolic risk ("metabolic surgery"). Future studies designed to further elucidate the mechanisms of action of metabolic surgery can inform decisions regarding the choice of procedures for individual patients, may help optimize surgical design, and could also identify targets for novel device-based and/or pharmaceutical approaches to obesity and T2DM.

REFERENCES

1. World Health Organization (WHO), Fact Sheet No. 311. 2013. Media Center; Obesity and Overweight. Available at: http://www.who.int/mediacentre/factsheets/fs311/en/. Accessed April 2013.
2. Ng M, Fleming T, Robinson M, et al. Global, regional, and national prevalence of overweight and obesity in children and adults during 1980-2013: a systematic analysis for the Global Burden of Disease Study 2013. Lancet 2014; 384(9945):766–81.

3. Colditz GA, Willett WC, Rotnitzky A, et al. Weight gain as a risk factor for clinical diabetes mellitus in women. Ann Intern Med 1995;122(7):481–6.

4. Chan JM, Rimm EB, Colditz GA, et al. Obesity, fat distribution, and weight gain as risk factors for clinical diabetes in men. Diabetes Care 1994;17(9): 961–9.

5. Unwin N, Gan D, Whiting D. The IDF Diabetes Atlas: providing evidence, raising awareness and promoting action. Diabetes Res Clin Pract 2010; 87(1):2–3.

6. O'Neill S, O'Driscoll L. Metabolic syndrome: a closer look at the growing epidemic and its associated pathologies. Obes Rev 2015;16(1):1–12.

7. Dixon JB, Lambert EA, Lambert GW. Neuroendocrine adaptations to bariatric surgery. Mol Cell Endocrinol 2015;418(Pt 2):143–52.

8. NIH conference. Gastrointestinal surgery for severe obesity. Consensus Development Conference Panel. Ann Intern Med 1991;115(12):956–61.

9. Dixon JB, O'Brien PE, Playfair J, et al. Adjustable gastric banding and conventional therapy for type 2 diabetes: a randomized controlled trial. JAMA 2008; 299(3):316–23.

10. Schauer PR, Bhatt DL, Kirwan JP, et al. Bariatric surgery versus intensive medical therapy for diabetes–3-year outcomes. N Engl J Med 2014;370(21): 2002–13.

11. Ikramuddin S, Korner J, Lee W-J, et al. Roux-en-Y gastric bypass vs intensive medical management for the control of type 2 diabetes, hypertension, and hyperlipidemia: the Diabetes Surgery Study randomized clinical trial. JAMA 2013;309(21):2240–9.

12. Mingrone G, Panunzi S, De Gaetano A, et al. Bariatric-metabolic surgery versus conventional medical treatment in obese patients with type 2 diabetes: 5 year follow-up of an open-label, single-centre, randomised controlled trial. Lancet 2015;386(9997):964–73.

13. Rubino F, Shukla A, Pomp A, et al. Bariatric, metabolic, and diabetes surgery: what's in a name? Ann Surg 2014;259(1):117–22.

14. Norris SL, Zhang X, Avenell A, et al. Efficacy of pharmacotherapy for weight loss in adults with type 2 diabetes mellitus: a meta-analysis. Arch Intern Med 2004; 164(13):1395–404.

15. Colquitt JL, Pickett K, Loveman E, et al. Surgery for weight loss in adults. Cochrane Database Syst Rev 2014;(8):CD003641.

16. Finucane MM, Stevens GA, Cowan MJ, et al. National, regional, and global trends in body-mass index since 1980: systematic analysis of health examination surveys and epidemiological studies with 960 country-years and 9·1 million participants. Lancet 2011;377(9765):557–67.

17. Sturm R. Increases in clinically severe obesity in the United States, 1986-2000. Arch Intern Med 2003;163(18):2146–8.

18. Sturm R, Hattori A. Morbid obesity rates continue to rise rapidly in the United States. Int J Obes (Lond) 2013;37(6):889–91.

19. Tchernof A, Després J-P. Pathophysiology of human visceral obesity: an update. Physiol Rev 2013;93(1):359–404.

20. Lapidus L, Bengtsson C, Larsson B, et al. Distribution of adipose tissue and risk of cardiovascular disease and death: a 12 year follow up of participants in the population study of women in Gothenburg, Sweden. Br Med J (Clin Res Ed) 1984;289(6454):1257–61.

21. Ruderman NB, Schneider SH, Berchtold P. The "metabolically-obese," normal-weight individual. Am J Clin Nutr 1981;34(8):1617–21.

22. Ruderman N, Chisholm D, Pi-Sunyer X, et al. The metabolically obese, normal-weight individual revisited. Diabetes 1998;47(5):699–713.
23. Samocha-Bonet D, Dixit VD, Kahn CR, et al. Metabolically healthy and unhealthy obese–the 2013 Stock Conference report. Obes Rev 2014;15(9): 697–708.
24. Snijder MB, Visser M, Dekker JM, et al. Low subcutaneous thigh fat is a risk factor for unfavourable glucose and lipid levels, independently of high abdominal fat. The Health ABC Study. Diabetologia 2005;48(2):301–8.
25. Wajchenberg BL. Subcutaneous and visceral adipose tissue: their relation to the metabolic syndrome. Endocr Rev 2000;21(6):697–738.
26. Castro AVB, Kolka CM, Kim SP, et al. Obesity, insulin resistance and comorbidities? Mechanisms of association. Arq Bras Endocrinol Metabol 2014;58(6): 600–9.
27. Jo J, Gavrilova O, Pack S, et al. Hypertrophy and/or hyperplasia: dynamics of adipose tissue growth. PLoS Comput Biol 2009;5(3):e1000324.
28. Björntorp P. "Portal" adipose tissue as a generator of risk factors for cardiovascular disease and diabetes. Arteriosclerosis 1990;10(4):493–6.
29. Virtue S, Vidal-Puig A. Adipose tissue expandability, lipotoxicity and the metabolic syndrome–an allostatic perspective. Biochim Biophys Acta 2010; 1801(3):338–49.
30. Haller H. Epidermiology and associated risk factors of hyperlipoproteinemia. Z Gesamte Inn Med 1977;32(8):124–8 [in German].
31. Reaven GM. Banting lecture 1988. Role of insulin resistance in human disease. Diabetes 1988;37(12):1595–607.
32. Grundy SM, Brewer HB, Cleeman JI, et al. Definition of metabolic syndrome: report of the National Heart, Lung, and Blood Institute/American Heart Association conference on scientific issues related to definition. Circulation 2004;109(3): 433–8.
33. Kahn R, Buse J, Ferrannini E, et al. The metabolic syndrome: time for a critical appraisal: joint statement from the American Diabetes Association and the European Association for the Study of Diabetes. Diabetes Care 2005;28(9): 2289–304.
34. Grundy SM, Cleeman JI, Daniels SR, et al. Diagnosis and management of the metabolic syndrome: an American Heart Association/National Heart, Lung, and Blood Institute scientific statement: executive summary. Crit Pathw Cardiol 2005;4(4):198–203.
35. The IDF consensus worldwide definition of the metabolic syndrome. International Diabetes Federation. Available at: http://www.idf.org/webdata/docs/MetS_def_update2006.pdf.
36. Ford ES, Giles WH, Dietz WH. Prevalence of the metabolic syndrome among US adults: findings from the third National Health and Nutrition Examination Survey. JAMA 2002;287(3):356–9.
37. Ford ES. Prevalence of the metabolic syndrome defined by the International Diabetes Federation among adults in the U.S. Diabetes Care 2005;28(11):2745–9.
38. Lakka H-M, Laaksonen DE, Lakka TA, et al. The metabolic syndrome and total and cardiovascular disease mortality in middle-aged men. JAMA 2002; 288(21):2709–16.
39. Isomaa B, Almgren P, Tuomi T, et al. Cardiovascular morbidity and mortality associated with the metabolic syndrome. Diabetes Care 2001;24(4):683–9.

40. Hu G, Qiao Q, Tuomilehto J, et al. Prevalence of the metabolic syndrome and its relation to all-cause and cardiovascular mortality in nondiabetic European men and women. Arch Intern Med 2004;164(10):1066–76.
41. Alexander CM, Landsman PB, Teutsch SM, et al. NCEP-defined metabolic syndrome, diabetes, and prevalence of coronary heart disease among NHANES III participants age 50 years and older. Diabetes 2003;52(5):1210–4.
42. Ford ES. The metabolic syndrome and mortality from cardiovascular disease and all-causes: findings from the National Health and Nutrition Examination Survey II Mortality Study. Atherosclerosis 2004;173(2):309–14.
43. Hunt KJ, Resendez RG, Williams K, et al. National Cholesterol Education Program versus World Health Organization metabolic syndrome in relation to all-cause and cardiovascular mortality in the San Antonio Heart Study. Circulation 2004;110(10):1251–7.
44. McNeill AM, Rosamond WD, Girman CJ, et al. The metabolic syndrome and 11-year risk of incident cardiovascular disease in the atherosclerosis risk in communities study. Diabetes Care 2005;28(2):385–90.
45. Eckel RH. Lipoprotein lipase. A multifunctional enzyme relevant to common metabolic diseases. N Engl J Med 1989;320(16):1060–8.
46. Jensen MD, Caruso M, Heiling V, et al. Insulin regulation of lipolysis in nondiabetic and IDDM subjects. Diabetes 1989;38(12):1595–601.
47. Kim Y-B, Shulman GI, Kahn BB. Fatty acid infusion selectively impairs insulin action on Akt1 and protein kinase C lambda/zeta but not on glycogen synthase kinase-3. J Biol Chem 2002;277(36):32915–22.
48. Manzato E, Zambon S, Zambon A, et al. Levels and physicochemical properties of lipoprotein subclasses in moderate hypertriglyceridemia. Clin Chim Acta 1993;219(1–2):57–65.
49. Halle M, Berg A, Baumstark MW, et al. Influence of mild to moderately elevated triglycerides on low density lipoprotein subfraction concentration and composition in healthy men with low high density lipoprotein cholesterol levels. Atherosclerosis 1999;143(1):185–92.
50. Kwiterovich PO. Clinical relevance of the biochemical, metabolic, and genetic factors that influence low-density lipoprotein heterogeneity. Am J Cardiol 2002;90(8A):30i–47i.
51. Eckel RH, Alberti KGMM, Grundy SM, et al. The metabolic syndrome. Lancet 2010;375(9710):181–3.
52. Egan BM, Greene EL, Goodfriend TL. Insulin resistance and cardiovascular disease. Am J Hypertens 2001;14(6 Pt 2):116S–25S.
53. Higashi Y, Sasaki S, Nakagawa K, et al. Effect of obesity on endothelium-dependent, nitric oxide-mediated vasodilation in normotensive individuals and patients with essential hypertension. Am J Hypertens 2001;14(10):1038–45.
54. Kahn SE, Hull RL, Utzschneider KM. Mechanisms linking obesity to insulin resistance and type 2 diabetes. Nature 2006;444(7121):840–6.
55. Kahn SE. Clinical review 135: the importance of beta-cell failure in the development and progression of type 2 diabetes. J Clin Endocrinol Metab 2001;86(9):4047–58.
56. Taniguchi CM, Emanuelli B, Kahn CR. Critical nodes in signalling pathways: insights into insulin action. Nat Rev Mol Cell Biol 2006;7(2):85–96.
57. Castro AV, Kolka CM, Kim SP, et al. Obesity, insulin resistance and comorbidities? Mechanisms of association. Arq Bras Endocrinol Metabol 2014;58(6):600–9.
58. Ferrannini E, Mari A. β-Cell function in type 2 diabetes. Metabolism 2014;63(10):1217–27.

59. Kahn SE, Prigeon RL, McCulloch DK, et al. Quantification of the relationship between insulin sensitivity and beta-cell function in human subjects. Evidence for a hyperbolic function. Diabetes 1993;42(11):1663–72.

60. Porte D. Normal physiology and phenotypic characterization of beta-cell function in subjects at risk for non-insulin-dependent diabetes mellitus. Diabet Med 1996;13(9 Suppl 6):S25–32.

61. Lillioja S, Mott DM, Howard BV, et al. Impaired glucose tolerance as a disorder of insulin action. Longitudinal and cross-sectional studies in Pima Indians. N Engl J Med 1988;318(19):1217–25.

62. Warram JH, Martin BC, Krolewski AS, et al. Slow glucose removal rate and hyperinsulinemia precede the development of type II diabetes in the offspring of diabetic parents. Ann Intern Med 1990;113(12):909–15.

63. Butler AE, Janson J, Bonner-Weir S, et al. Beta-cell deficit and increased beta-cell apoptosis in humans with type 2 diabetes. Diabetes 2003;52(1):102–10.

64. Bonner-Weir S. Life and death of the pancreatic beta cells. Trends Endocrinol Metab 2000;11(9):375–8.

65. Maclean N, Ogilvie RF. Quantitative estimation of the pancreatic islet tissue in diabetic subjects. Diabetes 1955;4(5):367–76.

66. Weir GC, Laybutt DR, Kaneto H, et al. Beta-cell adaptation and decompensation during the progression of diabetes. Diabetes 2001;50(Suppl 1):S154–9.

67. Prentki M, Corkey BE. Are the beta-cell signaling molecules malonyl-CoA and cystolic long-chain acyl-CoA implicated in multiple tissue defects of obesity and NIDDM? Diabetes 1996;45(3):273–83.

68. Jonas JC, Sharma A, Hasenkamp W, et al. Chronic hyperglycemia triggers loss of pancreatic beta cell differentiation in an animal model of diabetes. J Biol Chem 1999;274(20):14112–21.

69. Laybutt DR, Kaneto H, Hasenkamp W, et al. Increased expression of antioxidant and antiapoptotic genes in islets that may contribute to beta-cell survival during chronic hyperglycemia. Diabetes 2002;51(2):413–23.

70. Höppener JWM, Jacobs HM, Wierup N, et al. Human islet amyloid polypeptide transgenic mice: in vivo and ex vivo models for the role of hIAPP in type 2 diabetes mellitus. Exp Diabetes Res 2008;2008:697035.

71. Höppener JWM, Lips CJM. Role of islet amyloid in type 2 diabetes mellitus. Int J Biochem Cell Biol 2006;38(5–6):726–36.

72. Salinari S, Bertuzzi A, Asnaghi S, et al. First-phase insulin secretion restoration and differential response to glucose load depending on the route of administration in type 2 diabetic subjects after bariatric surgery. Diabetes Care 2009;32(3):375–80.

73. Salinari S, Bertuzzi A, Guidone C, et al. Insulin sensitivity and secretion changes after gastric bypass in normotolerant and diabetic obese subjects. Ann Surg 2013;257(3):462–8.

74. Boden G. Obesity, insulin resistance and free fatty acids. Curr Opin Endocrinol Diabetes Obes 2011;18(2):139–43.

75. Eckel RH, Grundy SM, Zimmet PZ. The metabolic syndrome. Lancet 2005;365(9468):1415–28.

76. Chakraborti CK. Role of adiponectin and some other factors linking type 2 diabetes mellitus and obesity. World J Diabetes 2015;6(15):1296–308.

77. Bastard J-P, Maachi M, Lagathu C, et al. Recent advances in the relationship between obesity, inflammation, and insulin resistance. Eur Cytokine Netw 2006;17(1):4–12.

78. Hajer GR, van Haeften TW, Visseren FLJ. Adipose tissue dysfunction in obesity, diabetes, and vascular diseases. Eur Heart J 2008;29(24):2959–71.

79. Leon BM, Maddox TM. Diabetes and cardiovascular disease: epidemiology, biological mechanisms, treatment recommendations and future research. World J Diabetes 2015;6(13):1246–58.

80. Shoelson SE, Lee J, Goldfine AB. Inflammation and insulin resistance. J Clin Invest 2006;116(7):1793–801.

81. Roden M, Price TB, Perseghin G, et al. Mechanism of free fatty acid-induced insulin resistance in humans. J Clin Invest 1996;97(12):2859–65.

82. Fain JN, Madan AK, Hiler ML, et al. Comparison of the release of adipokines by adipose tissue, adipose tissue matrix, and adipocytes from visceral and subcutaneous abdominal adipose tissues of obese humans. Endocrinology 2004; 145(5):2273–82.

83. Poitou C, Dalmas E, Renovato M, et al. CD14dimCD16+ and CD14+CD16+ monocytes in obesity and during weight loss: relationships with fat mass and subclinical atherosclerosis. Arterioscler Thromb Vasc Biol 2011;31(10):2322–30.

84. Magalhaes I, Pingris K, Poitou C, et al. Mucosal-associated invariant T cell alterations in obese and type 2 diabetic patients. J Clin Invest 2015;125(4):1752–62.

85. Monteiro-Sepulveda M, Touch S, Mendes-Sá C, et al. Jejunal T cell inflammation in human obesity correlates with decreased enterocyte insulin signaling. Cell Metab 2015;22(1):113–24.

86. Dalmas E, Venteclef N, Caer C, et al. T cell-derived IL-22 amplifies IL-1β-driven inflammation in human adipose tissue: relevance to obesity and type 2 diabetes. Diabetes 2014;63(6):1966–77.

87. Esser N, Legrand-Poels S, Piette J, et al. Inflammation as a link between obesity, metabolic syndrome and type 2 diabetes. Diabetes Res Clin Pract 2014;105(2): 141–50.

88. Cox AJ, West NP, Cripps AW. Obesity, inflammation, and the gut microbiota. Lancet Diabetes Endocrinol 2015;3(3):207–15.

89. Peppard PE, Young T, Barnet JH, et al. Increased prevalence of sleep-disordered breathing in adults. Am J Epidemiol 2013;177(9):1006–14.

90. Foster GD, Sanders MH, Millman R, et al. Obstructive sleep apnea among obese patients with type 2 diabetes. Diabetes Care 2009;32(6):1017–9.

91. Rajan P, Greenberg H. Obstructive sleep apnea as a risk factor for type 2 diabetes mellitus. Nat Sci Sleep 2015;7:113–25.

92. Schlaich M, Straznicky N, Lambert E, et al. Metabolic syndrome: a sympathetic disease? Lancet Diabetes Endocrinol 2015;3(2):148–57.

93. Mancia G, Bousquet P, Elghozi JL, et al. The sympathetic nervous system and the metabolic syndrome. J Hypertens 2007;25(5):909–20.

94. Palm NW, de Zoete MR, Flavell RA. Immune-microbiota interactions in health and disease. Clin Immunol 2015;159(2):122–7.

95. Cerf-Bensussan N, Gaboriau-Routhiau V. The immune system and the gut microbiota: friends or foes? Nat Rev Immunol 2010;10(10):735–44.

96. Chen J, Li Y, Tian Y, et al. Interaction between microbes and host intestinal health: modulation by dietary nutrients and gut-brain-endocrine-immune axis. Curr Protein Pept Sci 2015;16(7):592–603.

97. Miele L, Giorgio V, Alberelli MA, et al. Impact of gut microbiota on obesity, diabetes, and cardiovascular disease risk. Curr Cardiol Rep 2015;17(12):120.

98. Tremaroli V, Bäckhed F. Functional interactions between the gut microbiota and host metabolism. Nature 2012;489(7415):242–9.

99. Caesar R, Tremaroli V, Kovatcheva-Datchary P, et al. Crosstalk between gut microbiota and dietary lipids aggravates WAT inflammation through TLR signaling. Cell Metab 2015;22(4):658–68.
100. Bäckhed F, Manchester JK, Semenkovich CF, et al. Mechanisms underlying the resistance to diet-induced obesity in germ-free mice. Proc Natl Acad Sci U S A 2007;104(3):979–84.
101. Turnbaugh PJ, Ley RE, Mahowald MA, et al. An obesity-associated gut microbiome with increased capacity for energy harvest. Nature 2006;444(7122):1027–31.
102. Turnbaugh PJ, Bäckhed F, Fulton L, et al. Diet-induced obesity is linked to marked but reversible alterations in the mouse distal gut microbiome. Cell Host Microbe 2008;3(4):213–23.
103. Everard A, Lazarevic V, Derrien M, et al. Responses of gut microbiota and glucose and lipid metabolism to prebiotics in genetic obese and diet-induced leptin-resistant mice. Diabetes 2011;60(11):2775–86.
104. Shin N-R, Lee J-C, Lee H-Y, et al. An increase in the Akkermansia spp. population induced by metformin treatment improves glucose homeostasis in diet-induced obese mice. Gut 2014;63(5):727–35.
105. Everard A, Belzer C, Geurts L, et al. Cross-talk between Akkermansia muciniphila and intestinal epithelium controls diet-induced obesity. Proc Natl Acad Sci U S A 2013;110(22):9066–71.
106. Le Chatelier E, Nielsen T, Qin J, et al. Richness of human gut microbiome correlates with metabolic markers. Nature 2013;500(7464):541–6.
107. Qin J, Li Y, Cai Z, et al. A metagenome-wide association study of gut microbiota in type 2 diabetes. Nature 2012;490(7418):55–60.
108. Wang Z, Klipfell E, Bennett BJ, et al. Gut flora metabolism of phosphatidylcholine promotes cardiovascular disease. Nature 2011;472(7341):57–63.
109. Bischoff SC, Barbara G, Buurman W, et al. Intestinal permeability–a new target for disease prevention and therapy. BMC Gastroenterol 2014;14:189.
110. Cani PD, Bibiloni R, Knauf C, et al. Changes in gut microbiota control metabolic endotoxemia-induced inflammation in high-fat diet-induced obesity and diabetes in mice. Diabetes 2008;57(6):1470–81.
111. Vors C, Pineau G, Drai J, et al. Postprandial endotoxemia linked with chylomicrons and lipopolysaccharides handling in obese versus lean men: a lipid dose-effect trial. J Clin Endocrinol Metab 2015;100(9):3427–35.
112. Miras AD, le Roux CW. Mechanisms underlying weight loss after bariatric surgery. Nat Rev Gastroenterol Hepatol 2013;10(10):575–84.
113. Ryan KK, Tremaroli V, Clemmensen C, et al. FXR is a molecular target for the effects of vertical sleeve gastrectomy. Nature 2014;509(7499):183–8.
114. Tremaroli V, Karlsson F, Werling M, et al. Roux-en-Y gastric bypass and vertical banded gastroplasty induce long-term changes on the human gut microbiome contributing to fat mass regulation. Cell Metab 2015;22(2):228–38.
115. Laferrère B, Teixeira J, McGinty J, et al. Effect of weight loss by gastric bypass surgery versus hypocaloric diet on glucose and incretin levels in patients with type 2 diabetes. J Clin Endocrinol Metab 2008;93(7):2479–85.
116. Sweeney TE, Morton JM. Metabolic surgery: action via hormonal milieu changes, changes in bile acids or gut microbiota? A summary of the literature. Best Pract Res Clin Gastroenterol 2014;28(4):727–40.
117. Elliott JA, le Roux CW, Ph D FR. How long should we make the biliopancreatic limb during Roux-en-Y gastric bypass? Surg Obes Relat Dis 2015;11(6):1246–7.

118. Patel RT, Shukla AP, Ahn SM, et al. Surgical control of obesity and diabetes: the role of intestinal vs. gastric mechanisms in the regulation of body weight and glucose homeostasis. Obesity (Silver Spring) 2014;22(1):159–69.

119. Gómez-Huelgas R, Azriel S, Puig-Domingo M, et al. Glucagon-like peptide-1 receptor agonists as insulin add-on therapy in patients with inadequate glycemic control in type 2 diabetes mellitus: lixisenatide as a new therapeutic option. Int J Clin Pharmacol Ther 2015;53(3):230–40.

120. Habegger KM, Heppner KM, Amburgy SE, et al. GLP-1R responsiveness predicts individual gastric bypass efficacy on glucose tolerance in rats. Diabetes 2014;63(2):505–13.

121. Cătoi AF, Pârvu A, Mureşan A, et al. Metabolic mechanisms in obesity and type 2 diabetes: insights from bariatric/metabolic surgery. Obes Facts 2015;8(6):350–63.

122. Pournaras DJ, Glicksman C, Vincent RP, et al. The role of bile after Roux-en-Y gastric bypass in promoting weight loss and improving glycaemic control. Endocrinology 2012;153(8):3613–9.

123. Kohli R, Bradley D, Setchell KD, et al. Weight loss induced by Roux-en-Y gastric bypass but not laparoscopic adjustable gastric banding increases circulating bile acids. J Clin Endocrinol Metab 2013;98(4):E708–12.

124. Steinert RE, Peterli R, Keller S, et al. Bile acids and gut peptide secretion after bariatric surgery: a 1-year prospective randomized pilot trial. Obesity (Silver Spring) 2013;21(12):E660–8.

125. Aron-Wisnewsky J, Doré J, Clement K. The importance of the gut microbiota after bariatric surgery. Nat Rev Gastroenterol Hepatol 2012;9(10):590–8.

126. Liou AP, Paziuk M, Luevano J-M, et al. Conserved shifts in the gut microbiota due to gastric bypass reduce host weight and adiposity. Sci Transl Med 2013; 5(178):178ra41.

127. Iversen BM, Schjonsby H, Skagen DW, et al. Intestinal adaptation after jejuno-ileal bypass operation for massive obesity. Eur J Clin Invest 1976;6(5):355–60.

128. Dudrick SJ, Daly JM, Castro G, et al. Gastrointestinal adaptation following small bowel bypass for obesity. Ann Surg 1977;185(6):642–8.

129. Casselbrant A, Elias E, Fändriks L, et al. Expression of tight-junction proteins in human proximal small intestinal mucosa before and after Roux-en-Y gastric bypass surgery. Surg Obes Relat Dis 2015;11(1):45–53.

130. Saeidi N, Meoli L, Nestoridi E, et al. Reprogramming of intestinal glucose metabolism and glycemic control in rats after gastric bypass. Science 2013; 341(6144):406–10.

131. Hansen CF, Bueter M, Theis N, et al. Hypertrophy dependent doubling of L-cells in Roux-en-Y gastric bypass operated rats. PLoS One 2013;8(6):e65696.

132. Mumphrey MB, Patterson LM, Zheng H, et al. Roux-en-Y gastric bypass surgery increases number but not density of CCK-, GLP-1-, 5-HT-, and neurotensin-expressing enteroendocrine cells in rats. Neurogastroenterol Motil 2013;25(1):e70–9.

133. Breen DM, Rasmussen BA, Côté CD, et al. Nutrient-sensing mechanisms in the gut as therapeutic targets for diabetes. Diabetes 2013;62(9):3005–13.

134. Breen DM, Rasmussen BA, Kokorovic A, et al. Jejunal nutrient sensing is required for duodenal-jejunal bypass surgery to rapidly lower glucose concentrations in uncontrolled diabetes. Nat Med 2012;18(6):950–5.

135. Olbers T, Björkman S, Lindroos A, et al. Body composition, dietary intake, and energy expenditure after laparoscopic Roux-en-Y gastric bypass and laparoscopic vertical banded gastroplasty: a randomized clinical trial. Ann Surg 2006;244(5):715–22.

136. Behary P, Miras AD. Food preferences and underlying mechanisms after bariatric surgery. Proc Nutr Soc 2015;74(4):419–25.

137. Ochner CN, Kwok Y, Conceição E, et al. Selective reduction in neural responses to high calorie foods following gastric bypass surgery. Ann Surg 2011;253(3): 502–7.

138. Rubino F, Gagner M. Potential of surgery for curing type 2 diabetes mellitus. Ann Surg 2002;236(5):554–9.

139. Rubino F, Forgione A, Cummings DE, et al. The mechanism of diabetes control after gastrointestinal bypass surgery reveals a role of the proximal small intestine in the pathophysiology of type 2 diabetes. Ann Surg 2006;244(5):741–9.

140. Look AHEAD Research Group, Wing RR. Long-term effects of a lifestyle intervention on weight and cardiovascular risk factors in individuals with type 2 diabetes mellitus: four-year results of the Look AHEAD trial. Arch Intern Med 2010; 170(17):1566–75.

141. Vest AR, Heneghan HM, Agarwal S, et al. Bariatric surgery and cardiovascular outcomes: a systematic review. Heart 2012;98(24):1763–77.

142. Rubino F, Amiel SA. Is the gut the "sweet spot" for the treatment of diabetes? Diabetes 2014;63(7):2225–8.

143. Rubino F, Kaplan LM, Schauer PR, et al. The Diabetes Surgery Summit Consensus Conference: recommendations for the evaluation and use of gastrointestinal surgery to treat type 2 diabetes mellitus. Ann Surg 2010;251(3): 399–405.

144. Inzucchi SE, Bergenstal RM, Buse JB, et al. Management of hyperglycemia in type 2 diabetes: a patient-centered approach: position statement of the American Diabetes Association (ADA) and the European Association for the Study of Diabetes (EASD). Diabetes Care 2012;35(6):1364–79.

145. American Diabetes Association. 7. Approaches to glycemic treatment. Diabetes Care 2015;38(Suppl 1):S41–8.

146. Dixon JB, Zimmet P, Alberti KG, et al. Bariatric surgery: an IDF statement for obese type 2 diabetes. Diabet Med 2011;28(6):628–42.

147. Obesity prevention | Guidance and guidelines | NICE. Available at: http://www. nice.org.uk/guidance/cg43. Accessed November 27, 2015.

The Effects of Metabolic Surgery on Fatty Liver Disease and Nonalcoholic Steatohepatitis

Jesse Clanton, MD[a],*, Michael Subichin, MD[b]

KEYWORDS

- Fatty liver disease • NAFLD • NASH • Bariatric surgery

KEY POINTS

- Nonalcoholic fatty liver disease (NAFLD) is a severe and under-recognized hepatic manifestation of insulin resistance and the metabolic syndrome.
- NAFLD is typically asymptomatic, even in the setting of nonalcoholic steatohepatitis (NASH) and high-grade fibrosis.
- A significant number of retrospective and prospective observational cohort studies have demonstrated bariatric surgery to be effective for improving and even completely resolving NAFLD.
- Bariatric surgery acts on NAFLD not only by inducing rapid and substantial weight loss but also through a host of other indirect effects that improve liver steatosis and steatohepatitis.

INTRODUCTION

Nonalcoholic fatty liver disease (NAFLD) is a drastically underappreciated consequence of morbid obesity. Fatty liver disease represents a spectrum of disease from simple fat deposition in hepatic steatosis to inflammation and fibrosis in nonalcoholic steatohepatitis (NASH) with potential progression to cirrhosis.[1] This process is thought to develop through complex interactions of obesity, insulin resistance, and inflammation. Over the last 20 years, NAFLD has become the most common liver disease in the western world, surpassing both alcoholic and viral liver disease.[2]

In samples of nonobese patients, the prevalence of NAFLD is very low, generally less than 3%.[3] However, fatty liver disease in the obese and morbidly obese

Disclosure Statement: The authors have no conflicts of interest or financial relationships to disclose.
[a] Department of Surgery, West Virginia University Charleston Division, 3100 MacCorkle Avenue, Medical Staff Office Building, Suite 700, Charleston, WV 25304, USA; [b] Department of Surgery, Summa Health System, Akron City Hospital, 55 Arch Street, Suite 2F, Akron, OH 44304, USA
* Corresponding author.
E-mail address: jclanton82@gmail.com

http://dx.doi.org/10.1016/j.suc.2016.03.008
0039-6109/16/$ – see front matter © 2016 Elsevier Inc. All rights reserved.
surgical.theclinics.com

populations is significant. Large studies suggest that NAFLD affects greater than 80% of morbidly obese patients.[4] Even more significant is that nearly 15% of obese patients demonstrate severe liver disease, including NASH or fibrosis, on histologic review.[4] Today, 70% of American adults are overweight and 35% are classified as obese, putting most of the US population at risk for developing fatty liver disease or worse.[5] Increased recognition and understanding has led to the realization that fatty liver disease is also present in the pediatric population.[6] As the obesity epidemic continues, NAFLD will likely affect more than half of the United States population in the years to come. This surge in liver disease would predispose the population to unprecedented levels of cirrhosis, cancer risk, and the morbidity and mortality associated with these syndromes.

NAFLD is a sinister disease process. Although many patients are asymptomatic, NAFLD has the potential to progress to NASH, cirrhosis, and even end-stage liver disease. Additionally, most patients with NAFLD have normal liver enzymes even in the setting of NASH or cirrhosis.[4,7] These factors make it challenging to determine which patients are at risk for developing progressive fatty liver disease. It is important to accurately classify these patients because those with NAFLD have an increased mortality compared with those with normal liver disease, even when controlling for other patient comorbidities.[8,9] It is now recognized that many individuals previously diagnosed with cryptogenic cirrhosis actually suffered from progressive NASH.[10] It is not surprising that NASH is rapidly growing as an indication for liver transplantation and may even overtake viral hepatitis as the primary indication for liver transplant before 2030.[11]

Comorbidities such as diabetes and coronary artery disease are well known to be associated with obesity. These conditions also increase in severity and prevalence as BMI increases.[12] However, only recently has pathophysiology of NAFLD begun to be understood. Although NAFLD is associated with obesity, unlike other comorbidities associated with the metabolic syndrome, the severity of obesity does not seem to affect the severity or prevalence of NAFLD.[4] Fatty liver disease has also been independently associated with insulin resistance and dyslipidemia. Although there can be severe consequences from the development of NAFLD, most patients will not develop progressive liver disease. Nevertheless, a sizable minority of patients will progress to severe liver disease, which can significantly shorten life. Scoring systems have been developed to estimate the risk of disease presence and progression.[13] Unfortunately, these scoring systems lack sensitivity and specificity to accurately and effectively dichotomize patients. As a result, both the duration of quiescence and the factors for disease progression remain largely unknown.

NAFLD and even NASH have potential for improvement and even reversibility with weight loss.[14] Importantly, repeat liver biopsies have shown recovery of even high-grade steatosis and steatohepatitis after significant weight loss.[15] The unique ability of the liver to regenerate in the setting of severe disease has significant implications for the workup and treatment of NAFLD. This is especially important concerning the use of bariatric surgery in these patients.

Bariatric surgery and liver disease have a long history together. Elevated liver enzymes were commonly observed after certain types of early bariatric surgery, especially the jejunoileal bypass procedure. Early reports and anecdotal evidence suggested that this procedure may even lead to steatohepatitis and subsequent hepatic failure.[16–18] These reports raised concerns on the safety of bariatric surgery. It also simultaneously drew increased attention to the risks of fatty liver disease, and the relationship between NAFLD and bariatric surgery. For a comprehensive understanding of the effects of bariatric surgery, this article reviews the biologic development and progression of NAFLD and discusses treatment options that are currently available.

PATHOPHYSIOLOGY

Understanding of the biologic mechanisms that lead to NAFLD and NASH have considerably improved over the last few decades but much is still unknown. Because obesity affects the entire body, it also affects metabolic homeostasis across organ systems at the microscopic level. Although the initial insult may not cause significant results, the compounding effect throughout the body can become catastrophic. Once these disruptions in metabolism occur, the pathophysiology of fatty liver disease begins. The development of NAFLD and the progression to steatohepatitis have several proposed mechanisms that warrant discussion, including insulin resistance, the inflammatory state of metabolic syndrome, and genetic predisposition. This process is outlined in **Fig. 1**.

Insulin Resistance

Insulin resistance is extremely common in the morbidly obese because body mass index (BMI) directly correlates with the risk of developing insulin resistance.[12] The mechanism of insulin resistance begins as a decreased signaling of transmembrane insulin receptors.[19] This manifests as a loss of sensitivity to serum insulin by the peripheral tissues. The clinical result is a compensatory increase in serum insulin levels to overcome this loss in sensitivity. Over time, as the body loses the ability to compensate with increased insulin levels, type 2 diabetes results.[20]

In peripheral adipose tissue, insulin drives lipogenesis and prevents lipolysis. As these tissues become insulin resistant, the antilipolytic effect of insulin fades, resulting in lipolysis and release of fatty acids.[21] The increase of free fatty acids, even in the setting of dietary fat intake, leads to hepatic fatty acid deposition and other ectopic fat deposition caused by lipotoxicity.[22]

NAFLD is increasingly considered the hepatic manifestation of insulin resistance and metabolic syndrome.[23] As hepatic fat deposition occurs, this process gradually replaces normal liver tissue. Without fibrosis, function is preserved in the remaining

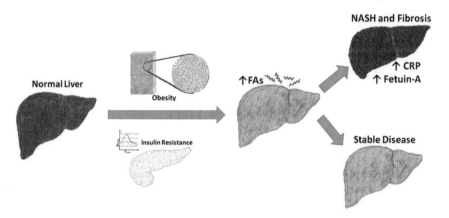

Fig. 1. Pathophysiology of NAFLD. The normal liver, after prolonged exposure to inflammatory cytokines from excessive adipose tissue and subsequent insulin resistance, begins to demonstrate fatty deposition, hepatocellular ballooning, and lobular inflammation. The increased fatty acids (FAs) in the liver further contribute to the inflammatory metabolic state. Although many patients remain asymptomatic with stable disease, others have a more profound inflammatory response, which promotes fibrosis in the liver and progression to NASH. CRP, C reactive protein. (*Courtesy of* Michael Subichin, MD, Summa Health System, Akron, OH.)

liver tissue and there is no effect on overall hepatic function early in the disease process. In a subset of patients with NAFLD, an inflammatory process begins with fat deposition that can lead to NASH and fibrosis development.

Inflammatory State of Metabolic Syndrome

Although simple steatosis with fat deposition can be well understood through the physiology of insulin resistance, the biology of progressive NAFLD is far better understood through the scope of inflammation in metabolic syndrome. The liver is a key organ in the acute inflammatory response. Fatty deposition in the liver and relative lipid toxicity cause systemic oxidative stress.[24] Not only is the excess adipose tissue a source of inflammatory cytokines but the oxidative stress leads to the hepatic release of inflammatory proteins, including C reactive protein, fetuin-A, interleukin (IL)-6, and tumor necrosis factor (TNF)-alpha.[25] These proteins cause a long-term inflammatory state that has systemic effects, including increased rates of coronary artery disease and strokes in patients with metabolic syndrome.[26] Overproduction of TNF-alpha itself has also been shown to be associated with development of NAFLD.[27] The adipose tissue from patients with NAFLD and NASH has been shown to produce increased levels of these inflammatory cytokines and demonstrate increased expression of genes that regulate inflammation compared with adipose tissues from controls.[28]

This inflammatory state is likely responsible for progression of NAFLD to NASH and even cirrhosis. Inflammation and progression is seen as lobular inflammation, hepatocyte ballooning, hepatocyte death, and eventual fibrosis. Most patients with NAFLD seem to only develop simple, nonprogressive steatosis. However, once hepatic inflammation is noted on liver biopsy, there is a high chance for the development of NASH.[29] The specific trigger that predisposes some patients to NASH while others remain with only mild NAFLD remains largely unknown.

Adiponectin is another factor that has gained increased recognition for its role in obesity and the metabolic syndrome. Adiponectin is a protein secreted by adipocytes with significant protective anti-inflammatory and antifibrotic effects.[30] Despite arising from fat cells, adiponectin levels are paradoxically much lower in obese subjects than the rest of the population. Low adiponectin to leptin ratios have been shown to be directly associated with steatosis and NASH, independent from insulin resistance.[31]

Genetic Predisposition

Mechanisms for insulin resistance include both metabolic and genetic factors. Identified mutations for insulin resistance include WFS1, TCF7L2, KCNJ11, PPARG, and SCL30A8.[32] With their susceptibility to insulin resistance, these mutations certainly have some effect on the development of NAFLD. However, several studies have demonstrated specific genetic mutations for the development of NAFLD.[32–37]

The major genetic mutation affecting the development of NAFLD is PNPLA3.[33] PNPLA3 encodes for adiponutrin, a protein expressed on hepatocytes and lipid droplets.[34] PNPLA3 seems partially responsible for the breakdown of triglycerides, although specific substrate research is ongoing. A missense mutation of PNPLA3 limits the breakdown of triglycerides, leading to fat deposition and, subsequently, NAFLD.[35] This process seems independent of obesity and insulin resistance.

Additional genes predisposing patients to NAFLD include familial hypobetalipoproteinemia, NCAN, and DGAT among others.[36,37] These genes all seem to affect lipid metabolism but the underlying mechanisms of these mutations are unknown. Some genetic mutations have also shown to predict progression of NAFLD to steatohepatitis. Mutation of PNPLA3, discussed earlier, has also been shown to predict liver disease progression from NAFLD to NASH.[38] As lipid biology is more understood and genetic research improves, these mutations and their significance will become more widely known.

CLINICAL PRESENTATION AND DIAGNOSIS

Patients with NAFLD most often present without symptoms or serum chemical abnormalities. Due to its insidious nature, this disease process is present in patients for years without diagnosis. As previously addressed, patients with obesity and diabetes most often will have NAFLD in the background as an unrecognized comorbidity. Some of these patients may have advanced disease but greater than 80% present with the diagnosis of NAFLD without other systemic hepatic effects.[39] For these patients, this disease quiescence will most likely be lifelong. Almost all patients with NAFLD will have stable steatosis and not progress to a more aggressive liver disease.[8] Patients with aggressive liver disease, even if asymptomatic and with normal laboratory values, should be referred for medical or surgical treatment because they have a high risk of progression.

The most recognized group of NAFLD patients are those who present as asymptomatic but also have elevated serum liver function tests on laboratory evaluation. It was once believed that this represented most patients with NAFLD. However, with increased recognition and biopsy rates, it is now known that most patients with NAFLD will actually have no abnormal findings and only a minority of patients present with significant abnormal liver function studies.[40] Many scoring systems are being developed to stratify these patients' risk for developing NASH but none have become widely used in practice.[13] This group of patients can present in a variety of states. Some undergo extensive workup for liver function test abnormalities, ultimately resulting in liver biopsy, whereas most just undergo serial laboratory examination.

Patients who have asymptomatic abnormal liver enzymes should undergo testing to exclude other causes of elevated liver enzymes, including alcohol, hepatitis, and intrinsic liver diseases. Unfortunately, although imaging is helpful, NAFLD is not possible to confirm without a tissue biopsy. Patients with elevated liver function tests do seem to have an increased risk of progression to NASH.[41] This likely stems from the presence of increased inflammation and hepatic turnover demonstrated with the elevated liver function tests. Liver biopsy in these patients frequently shows isolated NAFLD but can show more progressive disease. Patients with increased liver function tests are those who can be identified and followed. These patients have a great opportunity for attempt at medical management, including lifestyle and pharmacologic modalities to help prevent progression. This can be monitored with repeat liver enzymes.

A minority of NAFLD patients have minor hepatic symptoms but present with advanced liver disease. These patients can have grossly abnormal liver function tests, low platelets, anemia, or may be completely asymptomatic. In a series of 1000 subjects with more than 800 NAFLD subjects, 20 subjects who had severe NASH or cirrhosis on liver biopsy were relatively asymptomatic before liver biopsy at the time of bariatric surgery.[4] These subjects potentially have the most benefit from bariatric surgery because they have risk for continued progression of disease without drastic intervention.

Finally, a growing group of patients present with advanced disease. These are patients who present with signs and symptoms of cirrhosis, including ascites, encephalopathy, and worsening liver function. This group must have other causes of liver failure excluded and a continued broad metabolic workup. Most often, these patients will require hepatic optimization before any treatment can be considered and should likely be referred for at least initial evaluation by a liver transplant team. With optimization, some of these patients will stabilize. Unfortunately, except for the most optimized of patients, those with advanced liver disease have advanced cirrhosis on biopsy and are generally not candidates for bariatric surgery.

Accurate diagnosis is important for the work-up and management of NAFLD. The current gold standard for diagnosis is via histologic evaluation of liver tissue, from either a percutaneous core biopsy or surgical biopsy. Evaluation in this manner carries the added benefit of being able to accurately grade the degree of liver disease. Routine use of liver function testing and ultrasound evaluation is ineffective in detecting NAFLD due to poor accuracy.[42] Several noninvasive diagnostic tests have been developed, including transient elastography, acoustic radiation force impulse measurement, evaluation of serum biomarkers, and various scoring systems to predict or exclude NAFLD. No single test has emerged as superior to the others at this time, and further research and evaluation is ongoing.

Because NAFLD is so prevalent among the obese, and undiagnosed and untreated NAFLD can lead to progressive disease, including cirrhosis and liver failure, accurate diagnosis is of paramount importance. Most bariatric surgeons agree that liver biopsy at the time of bariatric surgery is mandatory because routine biopsy identifies significantly more patients with significant liver abnormalities than selective biopsy.[43] Once diagnosis has been established, and the degree of liver disease has been assessed, a treatment strategy can be determined.

MEDICAL MANAGEMENT OF FATTY LIVER DISEASE

The first-line therapy for patients with asymptomatic NAFLD is lifestyle modification and medical management. Lifestyle modifications, including diet and exercise, are recommended as primary first-line treatments and weight loss has been shown to be the gold standard for treating NAFLD.[44] Most studies have demonstrated improvements in NAFLD after implementation of diet, exercise, or lifestyle programs only when weight loss was achieved. A diet or exercise program that does not result in weight loss is unlikely to result in improvement of liver disease. Nearly all patients who lose greater than 10% of excess weight demonstrate improved histology.[45–47] Additionally, biochemical and histologic improvement of the liver is proportional to the degree of weight loss. When successful, lifestyle modification can be a definitive treatment of NAFLD. However, additional treatments are often necessary for patients with NASH because there is a considerably higher risk of progression to clinically significant fibrosis and cirrhosis.[48] Additional medical treatments include avoidance of hepatotoxic substances and the addition of pharmacologic agents.

Many pharmacologic treatments for NAFLD and NASH have been studied and it is important to be aware of the existing medical treatments. There are convincing data to suggest that vitamin E, pioglitazone, and pentoxifylline may all improve liver histology.[49] Additionally, angiotensin receptor blockers, antioxidants such as N-acetylcysteine or oral betaine glucoronate, fibrates, L-carnitine, metformin, omega-3 fatty acids, orlistat, simvastatin, and ursodeoxycholic acid have all been studied and show some promise in reducing liver injury that is a result of obesity. Almost all of these studies have been nonrandomized observational studies, often of small sample sizes. Currently, even the highest quality studies demonstrated only moderate effect and showed a high response rate in the comparison placebo groups. Randomized controlled trials of a larger scale still need to be undertaken to determine the ultimate long-term effects of medical therapy on NAFLD, as well as the agent of choice.

SURGICAL MANAGEMENT OF FATTY LIVER DISEASE

The literature clearly demonstrates that weight loss is the primary means of achieving improvements in both abnormal liver enzymes and liver histology that results from fatty liver disease. Bariatric surgery remains the most consistent and effective method of achieving weight loss in the morbidly obese. Bariatric surgery is typically superior to exercise and weight loss programs for creating and maintaining weight loss; therefore, bariatric surgery is also a most effective treatment for improving NAFLD and NASH. Additionally, typical diet and exercise regimes in the literature have been short-term, whereas extended data have shown that lifestyle modifications are typically not effective for maintaining long-term weight loss. This makes bariatric surgery a serious consideration as effective and long-lasting treatment of fatty liver disease.

There are many potential benefits of using bariatric surgery to treat fatty liver disease. The effects of bariatric surgery on the metabolic state can have both direct and indirect consequences to the liver. Besides the obvious weight loss effects, bariatric surgery can also directly improve some of the factors thought to cause NAFLD, namely insulin resistance and the proinflammatory state created by obesity. Improvement in insulin resistance is a well-known and immediate effect of bariatric surgery as demonstrated by high rates of diabetes remission and improvements of insulin sensitivity demonstrated almost directly after surgery. A large meta-analysis comprising 136 studies of bariatric surgery demonstrated a remission rate of type 2 diabetes of 84% after Roux-en-Y gastric bypass.[50]

Bariatric surgery has also been shown to improve the inflammatory state present in the metabolic syndrome. Serum levels of TNF-α and IL-6, as well as C reactive protein, are reduced following bariatric surgery.[51,52] Interestingly, recent studies have even shown that bariatric surgery may acutely change the expression of inflammatory and lipogenic genes in adipose tissue.[53] Significantly increased levels of adiponectin have also been observed at 3, 6, and 12 months after bariatric surgery.[52] Because adiponectin is a known anti-inflammatory protein involved in regulating glucose, increased levels may help improve the inflammatory state created by excess adipose tissue. An increased adiponectin environment has also been shown to promote a more anti-inflammatory state in the liver, directly as well as systemically.[54]

To date, there are no randomized controlled trials evaluating the efficacy of bariatric surgery on NAFLD. A 2010 Cochrane review of the effect of bariatric surgery on NASH in obese subjects was unable to come to a conclusion about the benefits or harms of this treatment because of the lack of adequate trials and the concern for bias among the existing studies.[55] However, the many retrospective and prospective observational cohort studies in the literature have demonstrated improvement in liver enzymes, as well as liver histology, after bariatric surgery. A summary of the results of these studies are presented in **Table 1**.[56–68] This table reviews the significant studies examining the effects of bariatric surgery on liver disease over the last 2 decades. Inclusion is limited to only high-quality studies with a sample size of greater than 50 subjects.

The largest study to date was a prospective evaluation of liver histology after surgery in 381 subjects.[64] Subjects underwent a variety of bariatric surgeries, including biliopancreatic diversion with duodenal switch, adjustable gastric banding, or Roux-en-Y gastric bypass procedures. There was an observed decrease in liver steatosis from 37.4% to 16% after surgery, as well as a reduction in the average NAFLD score from 1.97 to 1. Additionally, the percentage of subjects with probable or definite NASH decreased significantly over 5 years, from 27.4% to 14.2%. Another large retrospective review included 236 subjects who underwent laparoscopic sleeve

Table 1
Summary of studies examining the effect of bariatric surgery on nonalcoholic fatty liver disease

Study	Type of Study	Number of Subjects	Type of Surgery	Primary Outcome	Follow-up (mo)
Silverman et al,[56] 1995	Retrospective cohort	91	RYGB	Steatosis improved or resolved in 91%	18.4
Luyckx et al,[57] 1998	Retrospective cohort	69	GP	Steatosis reduced from 83% to 38%, with severe steatosis reduced from 42% to 15%	27 ± 15
Kral et al,[58] 2004	Prospective cohort	104	BPD	Severe fibrosis decreased in 27% but mild fibrosis appeared in 40% of subjects after surgery	41 ± 25
Keshishian et al,[59] 2005	Retrospective cohort	78	BPD-DS	60% improvement in steatosis and up to 3 grades in severity of NASH	6–36
Mattar et al,[60] 2005	Prospective cohort	70	RYGB	Improvement of 83% in grade and 39% in stage of liver disease	15 ± 9
Mottin et al,[61] 2005	Retrospective cohort	90	RYGB	82% had improvement or resolution of steatosis	12
Stratopoulos et al,[62] 2005	Prospective cohort	51	VBG	Steatosis and fibrosis improved in 84.3% and 47.0% of subjects, respectively	18 ± 9.6
Dixon et al,[63] 2006	Prospective cohort	60	AGB	Reduced high-grade steatosis from 77% to 20% and fibrosis from 52% to 22%	29.5 ± 16
Mathurin et al,[64] 2009	Prospective cohort	381	BIB, RYGB, AGB	Decreased steatosis from 37.4% to 16% and NAFLD score from 1.97 to 1	50 ± 7.8
Weiner,[65] 2010	Retrospective cohort	116	RYGB, AGB, and BPD-DS	Complete regression of NAFLD in 83% of subjects	18.6 ± 8.3
Karcz et al,[66] 2011	Retrospective cohort	236	LSG	Transaminase levels reduced >50% in those with NASH	12
Moretto et al,[67] 2012	Retrospective cohort	78	RYGB	Decreased prevalence of fibrosis from 45% to 31%	Unavailable
Cazzo et al,[68] 2015	Prospective cohort	63	RYGB	Resolution rate of advanced fibrosis of 55% by fibrosis score	12

Abbreviations: AGB, adjustable gastric banding; BIB, biliointestinal bypass; BPD, biliary-pancreatic diversion; DS, duodenal switch; GP, gastroplasty; LSG, laparoscopic sleeve gastrectomy; RYGB, Roux-en-Y gastric bypass; VBG, vertical band gastroplasty.
Data from Refs.[56–68]

gastrectomy.[66] Liver biopsy was performed at the time of surgery and subsequent serum assessment of liver enzymes was followed for up to 3 years after surgery. A strong correlation was observed between high transaminase levels and histologically diagnosed NASH. Among subjects with NASH (87 of 236), transaminase levels were reduced more than 50% within 6 months. All of the remaining published articles that prospectively evaluated liver histology before and after bariatric surgery have shown a significant improvement in the presence and grading of liver histology in regard to steatosis, ballooning, steatohepatitis, fibrosis, and cirrhosis.

A recent systematic review and meta-analysis was conducted by Mummadi and colleagues[69] in 2008. Fifteen studies (766 paired liver biopsies) met inclusion criteria and revealed alarming rates of steatosis and steatohepatitis of 83.2% and 39.0%, respectively, in the morbidly obese. Even when the analysis was restricted to studies with prospective designs that followed strict classification for steatosis and steatohepatitis grading, these results did not significantly change. An overwhelming number of subjects in the pooled analysis demonstrated improvement in liver histology. This included improvement or resolution in steatosis of 91.6%, in steatohepatitis of 81.3%, in fibrosis of 65.5%, and the rate of complete resolution of NASH was 69.5%. The overwhelming conclusion from the current literature is that steatosis, steatohepatitis, and fibrosis all improve or even completely resolve after bariatric surgery.

It is difficult to determine which effect of bariatric surgery most effects NAFLD. It is unknown if these histologic changes are solely from the rapid and often substantial weight loss that occurs as a result of bariatric surgery, or if surgery more directly influences improvement in fatty liver disease. Although weight loss is a key part of medical management of NAFLD, the improvements in insulin resistance and inflammatory proteins as described likely also help improve liver disease. This suggests that there are both direct and indirect effects of bariatric surgery that lead to the observed reduction in steatosis, NASH, and fibrosis.

Although the presence of advanced cirrhosis is a contraindication to bariatric surgery, the risk of surgery in the presence of NASH is not as clear. Many investigators have suggested that NASH does not increase the rate of complications of bariatric surgery,[70] whereas others have noted an increased risk of death in patients with NASH who undergo bariatric surgery compared with those with no liver disease.[71,72] This underscores the importance of liver biopsy during bariatric surgery, sometimes with intraoperative frozen section evaluation. A thorough preoperative evaluation for risk factors and the presence of cirrhosis should always be undertaken before any surgery, especially bariatric surgery. Based on the known evidence, the authors believe that NAFLD should be considered a comorbidity that lowers the BMI threshold for bariatric surgery (BMI >35). However, further studies are needed to determine whether the presence of advanced NAFLD, including NASH, should be an absolute indication for bariatric surgery.

SUMMARY

Morbid obesity is the greatest risk factor for developing NAFLD and subsequent NASH. Weight loss before the development of significant liver disease is the treatment of choice for avoiding transformation into fibrosis and cirrhosis. Not only is bariatric surgery the most proven method for achieving significant and long-term weight loss but there is also a host of additional indirect effects of bariatric surgery that may improve and even cure NAFLD. There is a need for well-designed randomized controlled studies to further clarify the efficacy of bariatric surgery for treating steatosis and NASH in the morbidly obese patient population.

REFERENCES

1. Bugianesi E, Leone N, Vanni E, et al. Expanding the natural history of nonalcoholic steatohepatitis: from cryptogenic cirrhosis to hepatocellular carcinoma. Gastroenterology 2002;123(1):134–40.
2. Clark JM. The epidemiology of nonalcoholic fatty liver disease in adults. J Clin Gastroenterol 2006;40(Suppl 1):S5–10.
3. Wanless IR, Lentz JS. Fatty liver hepatitis (steatohepatitis) and obesity: an autopsy study with analysis of risk factors. Hepatology 1990;12(5):1106–10.
4. Subichin M, Clanton J, Makuszewski M, et al. Liver disease in the morbidly obese: a review of 1000 consecutive patients undergoing weight loss surgery. Surg Obes Relat Dis 2015;11(1):137–41.
5. Flegal KM, Carroll MD, Kit BK, et al. Prevalence of obesity and trends in the distribution of body mass index among US adults, 1999-2010. JAMA 2012;307(5):491–7.
6. Schwimmer JB, Deutsch R, Kahen T, et al. Prevalence of fatty liver in children and adolescents. Pediatrics 2006;118(4):1388–93.
7. Uchil D, Pipalia D, Chawla M, et al. Non-alcoholic fatty liver disease (NAFLD)–the hepatic component of metabolic syndrome. J Assoc Physicians India 2009;57: 201–4.
8. Dam-Larsen S, Franzmann M, Andersen IB, et al. Long term prognosis of fatty liver: risk of chronic liver disease and death. Gut 2004;53(5):750–5.
9. Dunn W, Xu R, Wingard DL, et al. Suspected nonalcoholic fatty liver disease and mortality risk in a population-based cohort study. Am J Gastroenterol 2008; 103(9):2263–71.
10. Caldwell SH, Crespo DM. The spectrum expanded: cryptogenic cirrhosis and the natural history of non-alcoholic fatty liver disease. J Hepatol 2004;40(4): 578–84.
11. Agopian VG, Kaldas FM, Hong JC, et al. Liver transplantation for nonalcoholic steatohepatitis: the new epidemic. Ann Surg 2012;256(4):624–33.
12. Bays HE, Chapman RH, Grandy S, SHIELD Investigators' Group. The relationship of body mass index to diabetes mellitus, hypertension and dyslipidaemia: comparison of data from two national surveys. Int J Clin Pract 2007;61(5):737–47.
13. Angulo P, Hui JM, Marchesini G, et al. The NAFLD fibrosis score: a noninvasive system that identifies liver fibrosis in patients with NAFLD. Hepatology 2007; 45(4):846–54.
14. Promrat K, Kleiner DE, Niemeier HM, et al. Randomized controlled trial testing the effects of weight loss on nonalcoholic steatohepatitis. Hepatology 2010;51(1):121–9.
15. Furuya CK Jr, de Oliveira CP, de Mello ES, et al. Effects of bariatric surgery on nonalcoholic fatty liver disease: preliminary findings after 2 years. J Gastroenterol Hepatol 2007;22(4):510–4.
16. Grimm IS, Schindler W, Haluszka O. Steatohepatitis and fatal hepatic failure after biliopancreatic diversion. Am J Gastroenterol 1992;87:775–9.
17. Castillo J, Fabrega E, Escalante CF, et al. Liver transplantation in a case of steatohepatitis and subacute hepatic failure after biliopancreatic diversion for morbid obesity. Obes Surg 2001;11:640–2.
18. Holzbach RT. Hepatic effects of jejunoileal bypass for morbid obesity. Am J Clin Nutr 1977;30(1):43–52.
19. Weyer C, Tataranni PA, Bogardus C, et al. Insulin resistance and insulin secretory dysfunction are independent predictors of worsening of glucose tolerance during each stage of type 2 diabetes development. Diabetes Care 2001;24(1):89–94.

20. Weyer C, Bogardus C, Mott DM, et al. The natural history of insulin secretory dysfunction and insulin resistance in the pathogenesis of type 2 diabetes mellitus. J Clin Invest 1999;104(6):787–94.
21. Arner P. Insulin resistance in type 2 diabetes: role of fatty acids. Diabetes Metab Res Rev 2002;18(Suppl 2):S5–9.
22. Machado MV, Ferreira DM, Castro RE, et al. Liver and muscle in morbid obesity: the interplay of fatty liver and insulin resistance. PLoS One 2012;7(2):e31738.
23. Gastaldelli A. Fatty liver disease: the hepatic manifestation of metabolic syndrome. Hypertens Res 2010;33(6):546–7.
24. Bugianesi E, Gastaldelli A, Vanni E, et al. Insulin resistance in non-diabetic patients with non-alcoholic fatty liver disease: sites and mechanisms. Diabetologia 2005;48(4):634–42.
25. Park SH, Kim BI, Yun JW, et al. Insulin resistance and C-reactive protein as independent risk factors for non-alcoholic fatty liver disease in non-obese Asian men. J Gastroenterol Hepatol 2004;19(6):694–8.
26. Weikert C, Stefan N, Schulze MB, et al. Plasma fetuin-a levels and the risk of myocardial infarction and ischemic stroke. Circulation 2008;118(24):2555–62.
27. Ahmed MH, Byrne CD. Non-alcoholic fatty liver disease. In: Byrne CD, Wild SH, editors. The Metabolic Syndrome. 2nd edition. Oxford (United Kingdom): Wiley-Blackwell; 2011. p. 245–77.
28. du Plessis J, van Pelt J, Korf H, et al. Association of adipose tissue inflammation with histologic severity of nonalcoholic fatty liver disease. Gastroenterology 2015; 149(3):635–48.
29. Argo CK, Northup PG, Al-Osaimi AM, et al. Systematic review of risk factors for fibrosis progression in non-alcoholic steatohepatitis. J Hepatol 2009;51(2): 371–9.
30. Gatselis NK, Ntaios G, Makaritsis K, et al. Adiponectin: a key playmaker adipocytokine in non-alcoholic fatty liver disease. Clin Exp Med 2014;14(2):121–31.
31. Lemoine M, Ratziu V, Kim M, et al. Serum adipokine levels predictive of liver injury in non-alcoholic fatty liver disease. Liver Int 2009;29:1431–8.
32. Stancáková A, Kuulasmaa T, Paananen J, et al. Association of 18 confirmed susceptibility loci for type 2 diabetes with indices of insulin release, proinsulin conversion, and insulin sensitivity in 5,327 nondiabetic Finnish men. Diabetes 2009;58(9):2129–36.
33. Kantartzis K, Peter A, Machicao F, et al. Dissociation between fatty liver and insulin resistance in humans carrying a variant of the patatin-like phospholipase 3 gene. Diabetes 2009;58(11):2616–23.
34. Kotronen A, Johansson LE, Johansson LM, et al. A common variant in PNPLA3, which encodes adiponutrin, is associated with liver fat content in humans. Diabetologia 2009;52(6):1056–60.
35. Bugianesi E, Pagotto U, Manini R, et al. Plasma adiponectin in nonalcoholic fatty liver is related to hepatic insulin resistance and hepatic fat content, not to liver disease severity. J Clin Endocrinol Metab 2005;90(6):3498–504.
36. Amaro A, Fabbrini E, Kars M, et al. Dissociation between intrahepatic triglyceride content and insulin resistance in familial hypobetalipoproteinemia. Gastroenterology 2010;139(1):149–53.
37. Kantartzis K, Machicao F, Machann J, et al. The DGAT2 gene is a candidate for the dissociation between fatty liver and insulin resistance in humans. Clin Sci (Lond) 2009;116(6):531–7.
38. Sookoian S, Pirola CJ. Meta-analysis of the influence of I148M variant of patatin-like phospholipase domain containing 3 gene (PNPLA3) on the susceptibility and

histological severity of nonalcoholic fatty liver disease. Hepatology 2011;53(6): 1883–94.

39. Milić S, Stimac D. Nonalcoholic fatty liver disease/steatohepatitis: epidemiology, pathogenesis, clinical presentation and treatment. Dig Dis 2012;30(2):158–62.

40. Kunde SS, Lazenby AJ, Clements RH, et al. Spectrum of NAFLD and diagnostic implications of the proposed new normal range for serum ALT in obese women. Hepatology 2005;42(3):650–6.

41. Harrison SA, Torgerson S, Hayashi PH. The natural history of nonalcoholic fatty liver disease: a clinical histopathological study. Am J Gastroenterol 2003;98(9):2042–7.

42. Cazzo E, de Felice Gallo F, Pareja JC, et al. Nonalcoholic fatty liver disease in morbidly obese subjects: correlation among histopathologic findings, biochemical features, and ultrasound evaluation. Obes Surg 2014;24(4):666–8.

43. Shalhub S, Parsee A, Gallagher SF, et al. The importance of routine liver biopsy in diagnosing nonalcoholic steatohepatitis in bariatric patients. Obes Surg 2004; 14(1):54–9.

44. Ratziu V, Bellentani S, Cortez-Pinto H, et al. A position statement on NAFLD/NASH based on the EASL 2009 special conference. J Hepatol 2010;53(2):372–84.

45. Harrison SA, Fecht W, Brunt EM, et al. Orlistat for overweight subjects with nonalcoholic steatohepatitis: A randomized, prospective trial. Hepatology 2009;49(1):80–6.

46. Vilar-Gomez E, Martinez-Perez Y, Calzadilla-Bertot L, et al. Weight loss through lifestyle modification significantly reduces features of nonalcoholic steatohepatitis. Gastroenterology 2015;149(2):367–78.e5.

47. Wong VW, Chan RS, Wong GL, et al. Community-based lifestyle modification programme for non-alcoholic fatty liver disease: a randomized controlled trial. J Hepatol 2013;59(3):536–42.

48. Matteoni CA, Younossi ZM, Gramlich T, et al. Nonalcoholic fatty liver disease: a spectrum of clinical and pathological severity. Gastroenterology 1999;116(6):1413–9.

49. Rinella ME. Nonalcoholic fatty liver disease: a systematic review. JAMA 2015; 313(22):2263–73.

50. Buchwald H, Avidor Y, Braunwald E, et al. Bariatric surgery: a systematic review and meta-analysis. JAMA 2004;292(14):1724–37.

51. Viana EC, Araujo-Dasilio KL, Miguel GP, et al. Gastric bypass and sleeve gastrectomy: the same impact on IL-6 and TNF-α. Prospective clinical trial. Obes Surg 2013;23(8):1252–61.

52. Illán-Gómez F, Gonzálvez-Ortega M, Orea-Soler I, et al. Obesity and inflammation: change in adiponectin, C-reactive protein, tumour necrosis factor-alpha and interleukin-6 after bariatric surgery. Obes Surg 2012;22(6):950–5.

53. Ortega FJ, Vilallonga R, Xifra G, et al. Bariatric surgery acutely changes the expression of inflammatory and lipogenic genes in obese adipose tissue. Surg Obes Relat Dis 2016;12(2):357–62.

54. Moschen AR, Molnar C, Wolf AM, et al. Effects of weight loss induced by bariatric surgery on hepatic adipocytokine expression. J Hepatol 2009;51(4):765–77.

55. Chavez-Tapia NC, Tellez-Avila FI, Barrientos-Gutierrez T, et al. Bariatric surgery for non-alcoholic steatohepatitis in obese patients. Cochrane Database Syst Rev 2010;(1):CD007340.

56. Silverman EM, Sapala JA, Appelman HD. Regression of hepatic steatosis in morbidly obese persons after gastric bypass. Am J Clin Pathol 1995;104(1): 23–31.

57. Luyckx FH, Desaive C, Thiry A, et al. Liver abnormalities in severely obese subjects: effect of drastic weight loss after gastroplasty. Int J Obes Relat Metab Disord 1998;22(3):222–6.

58. Kral JG, Thung SN, Biron S, et al. Effects of surgical treatment of the metabolic syndrome on liver fibrosis and cirrhosis. Surgery 2004;135(1):48–58.

59. Keshishian A, Zahriya K, Willes EB. Duodenal switch has no detrimental effects on hepatic function and improves hepatic steatohepatitis after 6 months. Obes Surg 2005;15(10):1418–23.

60. Mattar SG, Velcu LM, Rabinovitz M, et al. Surgically-induced weight loss significantly improves nonalcoholic fatty liver disease and the metabolic syndrome. Ann Surg 2005;242(4):610–7.

61. Mottin CC, Moretto M, Padoin AV, et al. Histological behavior of hepatic steatosis in morbidly obese patients after weight loss induced by bariatric surgery. Obes Surg 2005;15(6):788–93.

62. Stratopoulos C, Papakonstantinou A, Terzis I, et al. Changes in liver histology accompanying massive weight loss after gastroplasty for morbid obesity. Obes Surg 2005;15(8):1154–60.

63. Dixon JB, Bhathal PS, O'Brien PE. Weight loss and non-alcoholic fatty liver disease: falls in gamma-glutamyl transferase concentrations are associated with histologic improvement. Obes Surg 2006;16(10):1278–86.

64. Mathurin P, Hollebecque A, Arnalsteen L, et al. Prospective study of the long-term effects of bariatric surgery on liver injury in patients without advanced disease. Gastroenterology 2009;137(2):532–40.

65. Weiner RA. Surgical treatment of non-alcoholic steatohepatitis and non-alcoholic fatty liver disease. Dig Dis 2010;28(1):274–9.

66. Karcz WK, Krawczykowski D, Kuesters S, et al. Influence of Sleeve Gastrectomy on NASH and Type 2 Diabetes Mellitus. J Obes 2011;2011:765473.

67. Moretto M, Kupski C, da Silva VD, et al. Effect of bariatric surgery on liver fibrosis. Obes Surg 2012;22(7):1044–9.

68. Cazzo E, Jimenez LS, Pareja JC, et al. Effect of Roux-en-Y gastric bypass on nonalcoholic fatty liver disease evaluated through NAFLD fibrosis score: a prospective study. Obes Surg 2015;25(6):982–5.

69. Mummadi RR, Kasturi KS, Chennareddygari S, et al. Effect of bariatric surgery on nonalcoholic fatty liver disease: systematic review and meta-analysis. Clin Gastroenterol Hepatol 2008;6(12):1396–402.

70. Dallal RM, Mattar SG, Lord JL, et al. Results of laparoscopic gastric bypass in patients with cirrhosis. Obes Surg 2004;14(1):47–53.

71. Weingarten TN, Swain JM, Kendrick ML, et al. Nonalcoholic steatohepatitis (NASH) does not increase complications after laparoscopic bariatric surgery. Obes Surg 2011;21(11):1714–20.

72. Goossens N, Hoshida Y, Song WM, et al. Non-alcoholic steatohepatitis is associated with increased mortality in obese patients undergoing bariatric surgery. Clin Gastroenterol Hepatol 2015 [pii:S1542-3565(15)01406-8]; [Epub ahead of print].

Resolution of Comorbidities and Impact on Longevity Following Bariatric and Metabolic Surgery

Tammy Fouse, DO, Stacy Brethauer, MD*

KEYWORDS

- Obesity • Mortality • Bariatric surgery • Metabolic syndrome • Cancer mortality

KEY POINTS

- Overweight is a modifiable risk factor directly linked to 3 of the 5 leading causes of death. This effect is seen most notably at body mass indexes greater than 35 (class II and III).
- Multiple studies have been conducted demonstrating the reduction in mortality associated with bariatric surgery. Most studies have been conducted on young females; however, the results have been reproducible in older, male patients within the Veterans Affairs health system.
- Recent systematic reviews and meta-analyses have shown dramatic reduction in rates of cardiovascular events, myocardial infarction, and stroke in patients undergoing bariatric surgery. Lower levels of medication use associated with hypertension have also been found in bariatric surgical patients.
- The increase in incidence of type II diabetes is rising commensurate with the increase in obesity rates. Bariatric surgery has been shown in multiple studies to be superior to medical management for treatment and remission of diabetes.
- Several cancers have been identified that are associated with obesity. Data are accumulating demonstrating reduction.

IMPACT OF OBESITY ON MORTALITY

Obesity is a global epidemic with well-documented links to decreased life expectancy. Overweight and obesity are linked to more deaths worldwide than underweight. According to the most recent data from the World Health Organization, most of the world's population live in countries where overweight and obesity result in more deaths than being underweight.[1]

Digestive Disease Institute, Department of General Surgery, Cleveland Clinic, 9500 Euclid Avenue, Cleveland, OH 44195, USA
* Corresponding author.
E-mail address: brethas@ccf.org

Surg Clin N Am 96 (2016) 717–732
http://dx.doi.org/10.1016/j.suc.2016.03.007
0039-6109/16/$ – see front matter © 2016 Elsevier Inc. All rights reserved.

Among the 5 leading causes of death in the United States, being overweight is a major modifiable risk factor for 3 (cardiovascular, cancer, stroke).[2] In a comprehensive, quantitative assessment of the mortality burden of key modifiable risk factors, Harvard researchers found that, in those younger than 70 years, overweight and obesity causes more deaths than did high blood pressure. This modifiable risk factor was second only to tobacco smoking.[3]

The risk of increased mortality due to excess weight seems to vary based on the severity of the disease. In a 2013 meta-analysis, there was a significant increase in mortality among higher grades of obesity. Grades 2 and 3 obesity (body mass index [BMI] >35) were found to have an adjusted hazard ratio [HR] of 1.34 compared with 0.97 and 0.94 in grade 1 obesity (BMI between 30 and 35) and overweight (BMI between 25 and 30), respectively. Further analysis revealed that the overweight group was associated with a significantly lower overall mortality relative to the normal weight category (BMI 20–25) with an overall summary HR of 0.94.[4] The cause for this decrease in HR in the overweight and grade 1 obese population is not clear. Possible explanations for this protective effect of overweight and mild obesity have included earlier presentation of heavier patients,[5] greater likelihood of receiving optimal medical treatment,[6–8] cardioprotective metabolic effects of increased body fat,[9,10] and benefits of higher metabolic reserves.[11]

The increase in rates of obesity over the past several decades in the United States are well understood. What is not frequently discussed though is that during the period between 1960 and 2006, the total US population has also increased. Therefore, the total number of Americans affected has also increased. Looking at the numbers of people affected, the overweight population has doubled, the obese population has increased 5-fold, and the population with extreme or morbid obesity has increased by a factor of nearly 12 (**Figs. 1** and **2**).[12,13]

Given the detrimental effect of grade II and III obesity on mortality, coupled with the significant change in absolute numbers of Americans involved, it is clear that this is a public health crisis. Bariatric surgery remains the most cost-effective treatment of

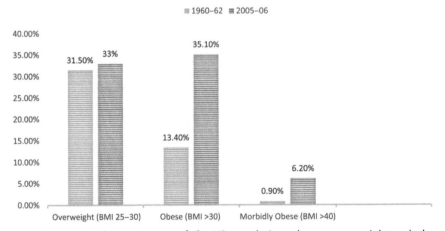

Fig. 1. Changes in the percentage of the US population who are overweight and obese over the last 4 decades. (*Data from* The Downey Obesity Report. Downey fact sheet 2 – quick facts. Available at: http://www.downeyobesityreport.com/2009/09/fact-sheet-2-quick-facts/.)

GREATER POPULATION, GREATER PROBLEM

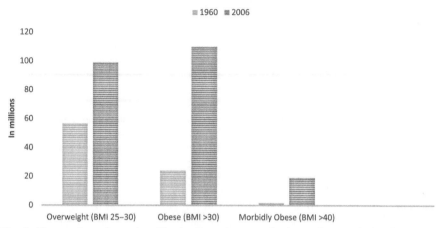

Fig. 2. The number of people with obesity and severe obesity as the population has grown over the last 4 decades. (*Data from* The Downey Obesity Report. Downey fact sheet 2 – quick facts. Available at: http://www.downeyobesityreport.com/2009/09/fact-sheet-2-quick-facts/.)

most patients with clinically severe obesity with a safety profile better than many commonly performed general surgery procedures.[14]

EFFECT OF BARIATRIC AND METABOLIC SURGERY ON ALL-CAUSE MORTALITY

There are almost 2 decades of published data regarding the impact that bariatric surgery has on reducing mortality. In 2015, Adams and colleagues[15] published a review of 28 articles, reporting on mortality rates at least 2 years after bariatric surgery. As expected, these studies have included a wide variety of methodological approaches.

In one of the earlier published studies, Flum and Dellinger[16] conducted a retrospective cohort study in 2004, using the Washington State Comprehensive Hospital Abstract Reporting System database and the Vital Statistics database. They demonstrated after 15 years of follow-up, 16.3% of nonoperated patients had died, compared with 11.8% of patients who had undergone a Roux-en-Y gastric bypass (RYGB). In this study, using Cox proportional hazards, when patient survival was compared starting at 1 year after hospitalization, the hazard for death was significantly less for operated patients than for those who did not have the procedure (HR, 0.67; 95% confidence interval [CI], 0.54–0.85) after adjusting for age, sex, and comorbidity index. In their study, 80.5% of the operated patients were female with a mean age (standard deviation [SD]) of 43.1 years (±10.1).[16]

During the same year, Christou and colleagues[17] conducted an observational 2-cohort study demonstrating a significant decrease in overall mortality in patients who had an RYGB compared with a well-matched cohort that did not undergo the surgery. During the 5-year follow-up period, the mortality rate in the bariatric surgery cohort was 0.68% compared with 6.17% for controls (relative risk [RR] 0.11; 95% CI 0.04–0.27). The mean age (SD) of the surgical group was 45.1 (±11.6) years. This finding was similar to the population in the Flum and Dellinger[16] study. The percentage of female patients was slightly lower, however, at 65.6%. In addition to the mortality results, Christou and colleagues[17] also found, on average, the total direct health care cost for the nonoperated control group was 45% higher compared with the bariatric surgery patients.

In 2007, 2 key studies were published that further demonstrated the association between decreased overall mortality in bariatric surgery patients. To date, the Swedish Obesity Subjects (SOS) study is the only prospective matched cohort study. This study involved 4047 obese subjects. The surgery group consisted of 2010 subjects who underwent gastric bypass (13%), vertical banded gastroplasty (68%), or adjustable gastric band (19%). During a 16-year follow-up period, subjects in the surgery group had a mortality HR of 0.76, as compared with the control group (95% CI, 0.59–0.99). After multivariate adjustments for baseline conditions, the risk reduction was almost 30%. During the follow-up period, 6.3% in the control group died, compared with 5.0% in the surgery group. The surgical population in this study was more than 70% female with a mean (SD) age of 46.1 ($\pm$5.8) years.[18]

The second key study published in 2007 by Adams and colleagues[19] evaluated the rates of death over a 7-year follow-up period between subjects who had undergone gastric bypass compared with severely obese control subjects from the general population in Utah. After covariate adjustment, the rate of death from any cause was 40% lower in the surgery group than in the control group (HR 0.60; 95% CI, 0.45–0.67); without covariate adjustment, the rate of death was 34% lower in the surgery group. The surgical arm was 86% female with an average age (SD) of 39.3 ($\pm$10.3) years. Interestingly, the researchers also reported deaths not caused by disease (including suicide, accidents not related to drugs, poisonings of undetermined intent, and other deaths) were 1.58 times as great in the surgery group as in the control group, though the overall number of these events was low ($P = .04$). The researchers suggested that further research is warranted to explore the optimal approach to evaluating candidates for surgery, including aggressive psychological evaluation before and after surgery.[19]

In comparison with the previous studies conducted in predominately younger, white, female populations, 2 studies have been published analyzing results in bariatric surgery patients within the Veterans Affairs (VA) medical centers. In 2011, Maciejewski and colleagues[20] evaluated the association of survival and bariatric surgery in a cohort of older, high-risk male patients. The mean age (SD) was 49.5 ($\pm$8.3) years in the surgical cohort, and 74% of the patients were male. In propensity score-adjusted analyses of 2 cohorts of 847 patients, bariatric surgery compared with usual care, was not associated with decreased mortality during a mean 6.7 years of follow-up (HR 0.83; 95% CI, 0.61–1.14). These findings were attributed to the possibility of higher perioperative mortality for RYGB in veteran cohorts. The 30-day mortality rates of 1.3% observed in this study was 4-fold higher than that reported in a multicenter Longitudinal Assessment of Bariatric Surgery study, which included a younger, predominantly female cohort.[21]

In a second study of VA bariatric centers published in 2015, Arterburn and colleagues[14] found contrasting results compared with the Maciejewski study after following patients for a longer time. They hypothesized that longer follow-up and a larger sample size of patients might yield findings similar to prior studies, given that it took 10 years to observe a significant relationship between bariatric surgery and survival in the SOS study.[18] In Arterburn and colleagues'[14] study, the mean age was 52 years with 74% male in the surgical group. Among the bariatric patients, 74% had RYGB, 15% had sleeve gastrectomy, 10% had adjustable gastric banding, and 1% had another procedure. The Kaplan-Meier estimated mortality rates were 2.4% at 1 year, 6.4% at 5 years, and 13.8% at 10 years for surgical patients; for matched controls, the estimated mortality rates were 1.7% at 1 year, 10.4% at 5 years, and 23.9% at 10 years. In multivariate-adjusted Cox regression, bariatric surgery was not associated with a difference in all-cause mortality in the first year of follow-up (HR 1.28, 95% CI, 0.98–1.68) but was associated with lower mortality after 1 to 5 years (HR 0.45, 95% CI, 0.36–0.56) and 5 or more years of follow-up (HR 0.47, 95% CI, 0.39–0.58).[14] By extending the follow-up period from 5 to 10 years, the findings were consistent with several observational studies that examined lower-risk, predominantly female cohorts.[16,18,19]

A 2015 study from New York by Telem and colleagues[22] reported on long-term mortality rates of patients undergoing surgery and, additionally, identified specific patient risk factors for long-term mortality. The New York State Planning and Research Cooperative System longitudinal administrative data were used to identify 7862 adult patients undergoing a primary bariatric surgery from 1999 to 2005. Of the surgical cohort, 7.5% underwent sleeve gastrectomy, 57.2% RYGB, 26.8% adjustable gastric band, and 8.5% had vertical banded gastroplasty. Patients who had bariatric procedures had significantly decreased long-term mortality compared with the general or obese populations. The estimated mortality rate from 1999 to 2010 for the general population as derived from the Centers for Disease Control and Prevention (CDC) Web site was 2.1% versus 1.5% for the bariatric surgery population ($P = .006$). Comparison of the actual predictions for the obese population during this time frame to the bariatric surgery population also demonstrates significant improvement in long-term mortality (2.3% vs 1.5%, $P = .0008$). This study is the first to demonstrate, regardless of procedure, the positive impact of surgery on long-term mortality as compared with both obese controls and the general population.[22]

Bariatric surgery is associated with improved long-term survival compared with matched cohorts. In the studies reviewed, the benefits can be seen as early as 2.5 years across several types of procedures and in both female and male cohorts. Importantly, there are no studies that demonstrate an increase in all-cause long-term mortality after bariatric surgery compared with obese controls (**Table 1**).

EFFECT OF BARIATRIC AND METABOLIC SURGERY ON WEIGHT-RELATED COMORBIDITIES AND DISEASE-SPECIFIC MORTALITY
Cardiovascular Disease

Myocardial infarction and stroke, either separately or in combination, were predefined secondary end points in the SOS trial.[23] In January 2012, Sjöström and colleagues[24] reported that bariatric surgery is associated with a reduced number of cardiovascular deaths and with a lower number of total first-time (fatal or nonfatal) cardiovascular events.

The same year, Vest and colleagues[25] published a systematic review that evaluated the impact of bariatric surgery on cardiovascular risk factors and on cardiac structure and function. Seventy-three cardiovascular risk factor studies involving 19,543 subjects were included (mean age 42 years, 76% female). Baseline prevalence of hypertension, diabetes, and hyperlipidemia were 44%, 24%, and 44%, respectively. The mean follow-up was 57.8 months. Postoperative resolution/improvement of hypertension occurred in 63% of patients, of diabetes in 73%, and hyperlipidemia in 65%. Echocardiographic data demonstrated statistically significant improvement in 713 patients that data were available.

A second systematic review and meta-analysis, published a year later by Gloy and colleagues[26] aimed to summarize the effects of bariatric surgery on cardiovascular risk factors and other end points in patients with a BMI of 30 or greater compared with patients who had nonsurgical treatment. The meta-analysis included 11 studies with 796 individuals. They were unable to show a significant difference between bariatric surgery and nonsurgical treatment for changes in blood pressure and levels

Table 1
Bariatric surgery studies evaluating long-term mortality

Author	Type	Start Year	Surgical n (M/F)	Control n	Follow-up, Years Surgery	Follow-up, Years Controls	Types of Surgery	Mortality Results	Comments
Christou et al,[17] 2004	Retrospective cohort	1986	1035 (356/679)	5746 (2068/3678)	2.5	2.5	RYGB	HR, 0.11 (95% CI, 0.04–0.27)	Control data extracted from hospital records (ICD codes); surgeries Canada
Flum & Dellinger,[16] 2004	Retrospective cohort	1987	233 (46/187)	11,132 (3975/7157)	10	10	RYGB	HR, 0.67 (95% CI, 0.54–0.85)	Control data extracted from hospital records (ICD codes); surgeries United States
Zhang[43]	Retrospective cohort	1986	18.972 (2526/16,446)	None	8.3	NA	Simple or complex	Death rate of 3.4%	Data extracted from 55 data sites (77 surgeons) using IBSR data collection system
Sjöström et al,[18] 2007	Prospective cohort	1990	2010 (590/1420)	2037 (590/1447)	10	10	VBG, band, RYGB	HR, 0.76 (95% CI, 0.59–0.99; P = .04)	Only prospective long-term mortality study; preclinical and postclinical data available; surgeries Sweden
Adams et al,[19] 2007	Retrospective cohort	1984	7925 (1268/6657)	7925 (1268/6657)	7.1	7.1	RYGB	HR, 0.60 (95% CI, 0.45–0.67; P<.001)	Control data extracted from driver's license applications; surgeries United States

	Design	Year	N (surgical/control)				Surgery type	Mortality	Comments
Marsk[44]	Retrospective cohort	1980	12,379 (2756/9614)	None	10.9	NA	VBG, RYGB, jejunoileal bypass, other	Mortality rate 60 per 10,000 person-years; estimated mortality rate ratio 1.8 (95% CI, 1.5–2.1)	Longer-term mortality greater in men than women; surgeries Sweden
Perry[45]	Retrospective cohort	2001	11,903 (2665/9238)	190,488 (42,669/ 147,819)	2	2	RYGB, band, VBG	Mortality rate 4.5% vs 8.6% for surgical vs nonsurgical (P<.001) for <65 y; 8.0% vs 12.2% (P<.001) for surgery vs nonsurgery >65 y	Surgical and control groups were severely obese Medicare patients; surgeries United States
Maciejewski[20]	Retrospective cohort	2000	850 (628/222)	41,244 (37,840/3404)	6.7	6.7	None indicated	HR, 0.64 (95% CI 0.51–0.80) unmatched; HR, 0.83 (95% CI, 0.61–1.14, not significant) propensity matched	All subject data (surgical and nonsurgical) from VA medical centers; unmatched and propensity matched; propensity matched no significant mortality reduction; surgeries United States

(continued on next page)

Table 1
(continued)

Author	Type	Start Year	Surgical n (M/F)	Control n	Follow-up, Years Surgery	Follow-up, Years Controls	Types of Surgery	Mortality Results	Comments
Telem et al,[22] 2015	Retrospective cohort	1999	7862 (sex not indicated)	General and estimated obese population	4–6	4–6	RYGB (57%), band (27%), VBG (9%), sleeve (8%)	Observed mortality rate of bariatric surgery 1.5% vs predicted general population (NY state) 2.1% (P = .005) Mortality rate of bariatric surgery 1.5% vs 2.3% estimated obese population (NY state) (P = .0008)	Bariatric surgeries in NY state; comparative data included actuarial projections for NY mortality rates (CDC) for obese population assumed one-third NY population obese; surgeries United States
Arterburn et al,[14] 2015	Retrospective cohort	2000	2500 (1850/650)	7462 (5542/1920)	6.9	6.6	RYGB, band, BD, sleeve, VBG	After 1–5 y surgery, HR, 0.45 (95% CI, 0.36–0.56) 5–14 y after surgery, HR, 0.47 (95% CI, 0.39–0.58)	Expanded follow-up of previous study (Maciejewski, 2011); 74% male surgical patients; data (surgical and nonsurgical) from VA medical centers; surgeries United States

Abbreviations: BD, biliopancreatic diversion; F, female; ICD, International Classification of Diseases; M, male; NA, not applicable.

Adapted from Adams TD, Mehta TS, Davidson LE, et al. All-cause and cause-specific mortality associated with bariatric surgery: a review. Curr Atheroscler Rep 2015;17:74; with permission.

of total or low-density lipoprotein cholesterol, although some studies in the analysis were able to demonstrate concomitant reductions in drug use for these conditions. They were, however, able to demonstrate higher rates of remission of type 2 diabetes and metabolic syndrome. One reported limitation of this meta-analysis was that they were not able to investigate the effect of bariatric surgery on cardiovascular morbidity and mortality.

In 2014, Kwok and colleagues[27] published a third systematic review and meta-analysis to evaluate the impact of bariatric surgery on long-term incident cardiovascular disease and mortality. Fourteen studies met their inclusion criteria with 195,408 participants. The bariatric surgery cohort consisted of 29,208 subjects compared with 166,200 nonsurgical controls, with an overall mean age of 48 years (70% female). At the time of publication, it was the first meta-analysis to demonstrate that bariatric surgery is associated with a reduced risk of myocardial infarction, stroke, and composite adverse cardiovascular events. The reduction in risk of these events was approximately 50% after surgery compared with nonoperated cohorts. In terms of absolute event rates, they found that there was a lower fraction of events in the surgery group for all outcomes (mortality 3.6% vs 11.4%, cardiovascular events 2.4% vs 4.0%, myocardial infarction 1.3% vs 2.5%, and stroke 0.8% vs 1.5%). These findings suggest that patients who are both candidates for bariatric surgery and are at high risk of cardiovascular events should undergo bariatric surgery.

Diabetes

According to the American Diabetes Association National Diabetes Statistics Report, released in 2014, 29.1 million Americans, 9.3% of the US population, have diabetes. More than 95% of these cases are type 2 diabetes. In 2012, 86 million Americans aged 20 years and older had prediabetes; this is up from 79 million in 2010. According to this report, diabetes remains the seventh leading cause of death in the United States and affects almost 37% of the population either as a definitive diagnosis or as prediabetes. Most patients with type 2 diabetes are obese or, if not obese by traditional BMI calculations, have increased body fat distributed in the abdominal region.[28]

Metabolic surgery has been recommended as an effective treatment option for obese patients with type 2 diabetes mellitus who do not achieve satisfactory control with only lifestyle changes.[29] According to the 2010 position statement from the Diabetes Surgery Summit, surgery should be accepted as an option in patients with diabetes and a BMI of 35 or greater and be considered as an option with a BMI of 30 to 35 when diabetes is poorly controlled, particularly in the presence of other major comorbidities.[30]

In 2012, Arterburn and colleagues[31] conducted a retrospective cohort study of adults with uncontrolled or medication-controlled type 2 diabetes who underwent gastric bypass. A total of 4434 adults underwent gastric bypass over a 13-year period and 68.2% (95% CI, 66% and 70%) experienced complete diabetes remission within 5 years after surgery. Among these, 35.1% (95% CI, 32% and 38%) redeveloped diabetes within 5 years. Significant predictors of complete remission and relapse were poor preoperative glycemic control, insulin use, and longer diabetes duration.

Mingrone and colleagues,[32] in 2012, reported results from one of 2 prospective, randomized trials comparing RYGB and biliopancreatic diversion (BPD) with medical therapy for the treatment of diabetes. In this trial, the primary end point was the rate of diabetes remission at 2 years (defined as a fasting glucose level <100 mg/dL and a glycated hemoglobin level of <6.5% in the absence of pharmacologic therapy). Sixty patients were randomized; at 2 years, diabetes remission had occurred in no patients in the medical-therapy group vs 75% in the gastric-bypass group and 95% in the biliopancreatic-diversion group (P<.001 for both comparisons). At the end of the study period, baseline glycated hemoglobin level (8.65 ±1.45%) had decreased in all groups, but patients in the two surgical groups had the greatest degree of improvement (average glycated hemoglobin levels, 7.69 ±0.57% in the medical-therapy group, 6.35 ±1.42% in the gastric bypass group, and 4.95 ±0.49% in the BPD group). Preoperative BMI and weight loss did not predict the improvement in hyperglycemia after these procedures.

The second prospective, randomized trial in 2012 by Schauer and colleagues[33] assessed outcomes of 150 obese patients with uncontrolled type 2 diabetes who were randomized to receive either intensive medical therapy alone or intensive medical therapy plus RYGB or sleeve gastrectomy. Their primary end point was a glycated hemoglobin level of 6.0% or less. Three-year outcomes were reported in 2014 demonstrating intensive medical therapy plus bariatric surgery resulted in glycemic control in significantly more patients than did medical therapy alone.

In an attempt to assess diabetic remission rates after bariatric surgery compared with usual care on a longer-term basis, Sjostrom and colleagues[34] provided an update in 2014 from the ongoing prospective SOS intervention study. In this observational study, the prevalence of diabetes remission after 2, 10, and 15 years was evaluated. The proportion in remission after 2 years was 72.3% in the surgery group and 16.4% in the control group. The difference at 2 years between the two groups remained significant after multivariate adjustments (odds ratio [OR], 40.5; 95% CI, 21.0–78.2; P<.001). The proportion of surgery patients in remission decreased to 38.1% and 30.4% after 10 and 15 years, respectively, but remained higher than in the controls (10 years: OR 5.3; 95% CI, 2.9–9.8, and 15 years: OR 6.3; 95% CI 2.1–18.9). In further analysis, the study showed that short diabetes duration at baseline was associated with higher diabetes remission rates in surgery patients after 2, 10, and 15 years of follow-up.[34]

The impact on glycemic control after bariatric surgery is well studied; however, the question whether this improves life expectancy is not well understood. A study published in 2015 by Schauer and colleagues[35] developed a Markov state transition model from data obtained from 3 large cohorts: (1) 159,000 severely obese diabetic patients (4185 had bariatric surgery) from 3 HMO Research Network sites; (2) 23,000 subjects from the Nationwide Inpatient Sample; and (3) 18,000 subjects from the National Health Interview Survey linked to the National Death Index. In their analysis, they found a 45-year-old woman with diabetes and a BMI of 45 gained an additional 6.7 years of life expectancy with bariatric surgery. Sensitivity analysis revealed that the gain in life expectancy decreased with increasing BMI, until a BMI of 62 is reached, at which point nonsurgical treatment was associated with greater life expectancy. Similar results were seen for both men and women in all age groups. However, only 2.7% of the surgical cases had a BMI of 60 or more. It is possible though that diabetic patients with a BMI more than 60 may reap benefits from surgery, such as improved quality of life and reduced burden of obesity-associated diseases, which were not modeled.[35]

Cancer

In 2015, the World Cancer Research Fund has estimated that up to one-third of the cancer cases that occur in economically developed countries like the United States are related to overweight or obesity, physical inactivity, and/or poor nutrition and, thus, could be prevented.[36] Being overweight or obese is clearly linked with an increased risk of many cancers, including cancers of the breast in postmenopausal women, colon and rectum, endometrium, esophagus, kidney, and pancreas. In addition, having too much visceral fat (that is, a larger waistline), regardless of body weight, is linked with an increased risk of colon and rectal cancer and is probably linked to a higher risk of cancers of the pancreas, endometrium, and breast cancer (in women past menopause).[37]

Bariatric surgery patients have lower cancer rates and lower cancer mortality when compared with obese patients who have not had this surgery.[38]

In addition to the decrease in all-cause mortality reported by Adams and colleagues[19] in the previous discussion, their study also reported on the rate of death from cancer. After all deaths from cancer that occurred within the first 5 years after baseline were excluded, the reduction in the rate of death from any cause in the surgery group was 36% (P<.001) and the reduction in the rate of death from cancer was 46% (P<.05). After matching the surgery and nonsurgery groups and excluding prevalent cancers at baseline, the reduction in the rate of death from any cause was 38% (HR 0.62, 95% CI, 0.51–0.74) and the reduction in the rate of death from cancer was 61% (HR 0.39, 95% CI, 0.24–0.64).[19]

In 2013, Sjöström[39] published a review of the key results from the SOS trial. Although cancer was not a predefined secondary end point of the trial, it was found to be the most common cause of death among the study participants. The number of first-time cancers after inclusion was lower in the surgery group than in the control group (HR 0.67, 95% CI 0.53–0.85). The effect was more significant in women, with no effect of surgery on cancer-related mortality seen in men.[39]

A review and meta-analysis by Tee and colleagues[40] evaluated the RR of cancer in obese patients undergoing bariatric surgery versus obese control subjects. Six observational studies, including 51,740 subjects, found the RR in obese patients after undergoing surgery was 0.55 (95% CI, 0.41–0.73). The effect of bariatric surgery on cancer risk was modified by sex (P = .021). The pooled RR in women was 0.68 (95% CI 0.60–0.77) and in men was 0.99 (95% CI 0.74–1.32), again demonstrating the effect of bariatric surgery on oncologic outcomes is protective in women but not in men.

A second systematic review and meta-analysis released in 2014 by Casagrande and colleagues[41] also demonstrated reduced cancer risk in obese patients treated with bariatric surgery. Four controlled studies were selected with 11,087 patients in the bariatric surgery group and 20,720 patients in the control group. In these studies, bariatric surgery was associated with a reduction in the risk of cancer (OR 0.42, 95% CI 0.24–0.73). After adjusting for heterogeneity, the association between bariatric surgery and low cancer risk was maintained. Data from the surgery group of controlled[4] and uncontrolled[9] studies displayed a cancer incidence density rate of 1.06 cases per 1000 person-years in a postoperative follow-up period of 2 to 23 years.[41]

Although there is a lack of randomized controlled trials, there is an association between bariatric surgery and risk reduction for cancer. This association seems to affect women in a greater way.

Obesity's link to cardiovascular disease, diabetes, and certain cancers is clear and well documented. Obesity is also associated with an increased risk of numerous other comorbidities. In general, the risk of a comorbidity increases as the degree of obesity increases. The risk of developing a comorbidity with increasing weight varies by sex, racial/ethnic group, and genetic factors.[42] The figures depict the body systems that are impacted with obesity (**Fig. 3**).

A

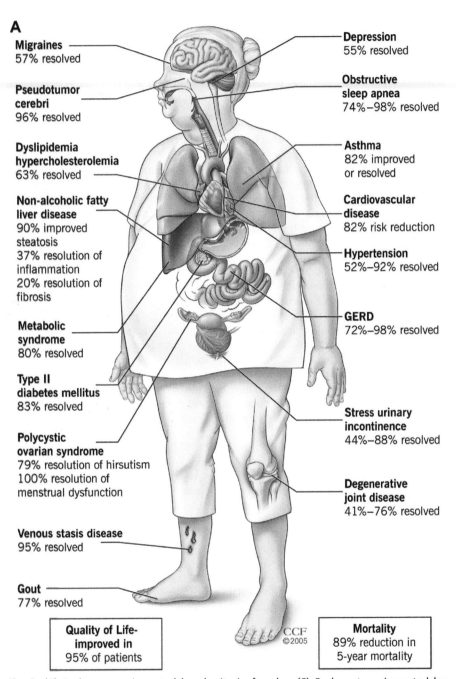

Migraines
57% resolved

Pseudotumor
cerebri
96% resolved

Dyslipidemia
hypercholesterolemia
63% resolved

Non-alcoholic fatty
liver disease
90% improved
steatosis
37% resolution of
inflammation
20% resolution of
fibrosis

Metabolic
syndrome
80% resolved

Type II
diabetes mellitus
83% resolved

Polycystic
ovarian syndrome
79% resolution of hirsutism
100% resolution of
menstrual dysfunction

Venous stasis disease
95% resolved

Gout
77% resolved

Depression
55% resolved

Obstructive
sleep apnea
74%–98% resolved

Asthma
82% improved
or resolved

Cardiovascular
disease
82% risk reduction

Hypertension
52%–92% resolved

GERD
72%–98% resolved

Stress urinary
incontinence
44%–88% resolved

Degenerative
joint disease
41%–76% resolved

Quality of Life-
improved in
95% of patients

Mortality
89% reduction in
5-year mortality

CCF
©2005

Fig. 3. (*A*) Body systems impacted by obesity in females. (*B*) Body systems impacted by obesity in males. (Copyright © The Cleveland Clinic Foundation 2014.)

B

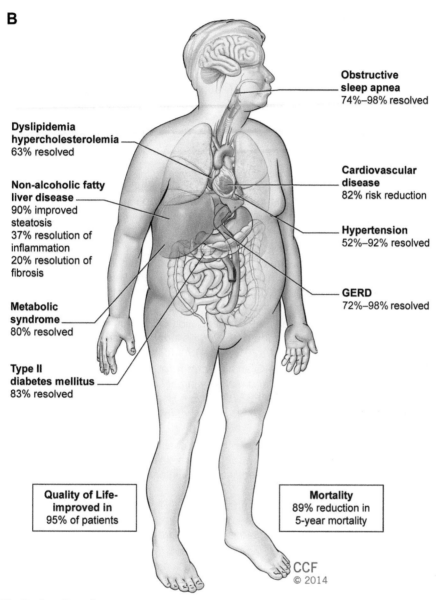

**Obstructive
sleep apnea**
74%–98% resolved

**Dyslipidemia
hypercholesterolemia**
63% resolved

**Cardiovascular
disease**
82% risk reduction

**Non-alcoholic fatty
liver disease**
90% improved
steatosis
37% resolution of
inflammation
20% resolution of
fibrosis

Hypertension
52%–92% resolved

GERD
72%–98% resolved

**Metabolic
syndrome**
80% resolved

**Type II
diabetes mellitus**
83% resolved

**Quality of Life-
improved in**
95% of patients

Mortality
89% reduction in
5-year mortality

CCF
© 2014

Fig. 3. *(continued)*

SUMMARY

Obesity and its impact on overall mortality is a significant public health burden in both the United States and world populations. Obesity has been identified as a leading modifiable risk factor for death attributed to cardiovascular disease, cancer, and stroke. Multiple studies have demonstrated the protective effect of bariatric surgery on reducing mortality. Studies have been primarily conducted in young women; however, the results were reproducible in older, obese men enrolled in VA medical centers.

In addition to increased mortality, obesity is linked to increased incidence of obesity-related comorbidities. Multiple studies have demonstrated improvement/resolution of weight-related comorbidities (ie, cardiovascular disease, diabetes, cancer, metabolic syndrome) after bariatric surgery. Some researchers have demonstrated a level of recalcitrance in remission of diabetes, particularly in patients with long-standing disease. More studies are needed to identify subgroups of patients that are at risk for nonresponsiveness to bariatric surgery. However, overall results are supportive of surgical cure of obesity as a treatment of weight-related comorbidities and mortality risk reduction.

REFERENCES

1. WHO obesity and overweight. WHO n.d.Available at: http://www.who.int/mediacentre/factsheets/fs311/en/. Accessed November 1, 2015.
2. Yoon PW, Bastian B, Anderson RN, et al. Potentially preventable deaths from the five leading causes of death–United States, 2008-2010. MMWR Morb Mortal Wkly Rep 2014;63(17):369–74.
3. Danaei G, Ding EL, Mozaffarian D, et al. The preventable causes of death in the United States: comparative risk assessment of dietary, lifestyle, and metabolic risk factors. Plos Med 2009;6(4):e1000058 [Erratum appears in PLoS Med 2011;8(1)].
4. Flegal KM, Kit BK, Orpana H, et al. Association of all-cause mortality with overweight and obesity using standard body mass index categories: a systematic review and meta-analysis. JAMA 2013;309(1):71–82.
5. Oreopoulos A, McAlister FA, Kalantar-Zadeh K, et al. The relationship between body mass index, treatment, and mortality in patients with established coronary artery disease: a report from APPROACH. Eur Heart J 2009;30(21):2584–92.
6. Chang VW, Asch DA, Werner RM. Quality of care among obese patients. JAMA 2010;303(13):1274–81.
7. Schenkeveld L, Magro M, Oemrawsingh RM, et al. The influence of optimal medical treatment on the 'obesity paradox', body mass index and long-term mortality in patients treated with percutaneous coronary intervention: a prospective cohort study. BMJ Open 2012;2:e00535.
8. Steinberg BA, Cannon CP, Hernandez AF, et al. Medical therapies and invasive treatments for coronary artery disease by body mass: the "obesity paradox" in the Get With The Guidelines database. Am J Cardiol 2007;100(9):1331–5.
9. Hastie CE, Padmanabhan S, Slack R, et al. Obesity paradox in a cohort of 4880 consecutive patients undergoing percutaneous coronary intervention. Eur Heart J 2010;31(2):222–6.
10. Auyeung TW, Lee JS, Leung J, et al. Survival in older men may benefit from being slightly overweight and centrally obese–a 5-year follow-up study in 4,000 older adults using DXA. J Gerontol A Biol Sci Med Sci 2010;65(1):99–104.
11. Doehner W, Clark A, Anker SD. The obesity paradox: weighing the benefit. Eur Heart J 2010;31(2):146–8.
12. The Downey Obesity Report. Available at: http://www.downeyobesityreport.com/2009/09/fact-sheet-2-quick-facts/.
13. N C H S – Health E Stats – Prevalence overweight, obesity and extreme obesity among adults: United States trends 1960-62 through 2005-2006. Available at: http://www.cdc.gov/nchs/data/hestat/overweight/overweight_adult.htm. Accessed November 15, 2015.

14. Arterburn DE, Olsen MK, Smith VA, et al. Association between bariatric surgery and long-term survival. JAMA 2015;313(1):62–70.
15. Adams TD, Mehta TS, Davidson LE, et al. All-cause and cause-specific mortality associated with bariatric surgery: a review. Curr Atheroscler Rep 2015;17(12):74.
16. Flum DR, Dellinger EP. Impact of gastric bypass operation on survival: a population-based analysis. J Am Coll Surg 2004;199(4):543–51.
17. Christou NV, Sampalis JS, Liberman M, et al. Surgery decreases long-term mortality, morbidity, and health care use in morbidly obese patients. Ann Surg 2004; 240(3):416–23 [discussion: 423–4].
18. Sjöström L, Narbro K, Sjöström CD, et al. Effects of bariatric surgery on mortality in Swedish obese subjects. N Engl J Med 2007;357(8):741–52.
19. Adams TD, Gress RE, Smith SC, et al. Long-term mortality after gastric bypass surgery. N Engl J Med 2007;357(8):753–61.
20. Maciejewski ML, Livingston EH, et al. Survival Among High-Risk Patients After Bariatric Surgery. JAMA 2011;305(23):2419–26.
21. Longitudinal Assessment of Bariatric Surgery (LABS) Consortium, Flum DR, Belle SH, et al. Perioperative safety in the longitudinal assessment of bariatric surgery. N Engl J Med 2009;361(5):445–54.
22. Telem DA, Talamini M, Laurie Shroyer A, et al. Long-term mortality rates (>8-year) improve as compared to the general and obese population following bariatric surgery. Surg Endosc 2015;29(3):529–36.
23. Sjöström L, Larsson B, Backman L, et al. Swedish Obese Subjects (SOS). Recruitment for an intervention study and a selected description of the obese state. Int J Obes Relat Metab Disord 1992;16(6):465–79.
24. Sjöström L, Peltonen M, Jacobson P, et al. Bariatric surgery and long-term cardiovascular events. JAMA 2012;307(1):56–65.
25. Vest AR, Heneghan HM, Agarwal S, et al. Bariatric surgery and cardiovascular outcomes: a systematic review. Heart 2012;98(24):1763–77.
26. Gloy VL, Briel M, Bhatt DL, et al. Bariatric surgery versus non-surgical treatment for obesity: a systematic review and meta-analysis of randomised controlled trials. BMJ 2013;347:f5934.
27. Kwok CS, Pradhan A, Khan MA, et al. Bariatric surgery and its impact on cardiovascular disease and mortality: a systematic review and meta-analysis. Int J Cardiol 2014;173(1):20–8.
28. American Diabetes Association. Data from the National Diabetes Statistics Report, 2014. Available at: http://www.diabetes.org/diabetes-basics/statistics/. Accessed June 10, 2014.
29. Dixon JB, Zimmet P, Alberti KG, et al. International Diabetes Federation taskforce on epidemiology and prevention. Bariatric surgery: an IDF statement for obese type 2 diabetes [review]. Arq Bras Endocrinol Metabol 2011;55(6):367–82.
30. Rubino F, Kaplan LM, Schauer PR, et al. The Diabetes Surgery Summit consensus conference: recommendations for the evaluation and use of gastrointestinal surgery to treat type 2 diabetes mellitus. Ann Surg 2010;251(3):399–405.
31. Arterburn DE, Bogart A, Sherwood NE, et al. A multisite study of long-term remission and relapse of type 2 diabetes mellitus following gastric bypass. Obes Surg 2013;23(1):93–102.
32. Mingrone G, Panunzi S, De Gaetano A, et al. Bariatric surgery versus conventional medical therapy for type 2 diabetes. N Engl J Med 2012;366(17):1577–85.
33. Schauer PR, Bhatt DL, Kirwan JP, et al. Bariatric surgery versus intensive medical therapy for diabetes–3-year outcomes. N Engl J Med 2014;370(21):2002–13.

34. Sjöström L, Peltonen M, Jacobson P, et al. Association of bariatric surgery with long-term remission of type 2 diabetes and with microvascular and macrovascular complications. JAMA 2014;311(22):2297–304.
35. Schauer DP, Arterburn DE, Livingston EH, et al. Impact of bariatric surgery on life expectancy in severely obese patients with diabetes: a decision analysis. Ann Surg 2015;261(5):914–9.
36. Cancer facts and figures 2015. Available at: http://www.cancer.org/acs/groups/content/@editorial/documents/document/acspc-044552.pdf. Accessed November 15, 2015.
37. Does body weight affect cancer risk? Available at: http://www.cancer.org/cancer/cancercauses/dietandphysicalactivity/bodyweightandcancerrisk/body-weight-and-cancer-risk-effects. Accessed April 24, 2015.
38. Ashrafian H, Ahmed K, Rowland SP, et al. Metabolic surgery and cancer: protective effects of bariatric procedures. Cancer 2011;117(9):1788–99.
39. Sjöström L. Review of the key results from the Swedish Obese Subjects (SOS) trial - a prospective controlled intervention study of bariatric surgery [review]. J Intern Med 2013;273(3):219–34.
40. Tee MC, Cao Y, Warnock GL, et al. Effect of bariatric surgery on oncologic outcomes: a systematic review and meta-analysis. Surg Endosc 2013;27(12):4449–56.
41. Casagrande DS, Rosa DD, Umpierre D, et al. Incidence of cancer following bariatric surgery: systematic review and meta-analysis. Obes Surg 2014;24(9):1499–509.
42. Hensrud DD, Klein S. Extreme obesity: a new medical crisis in the United States. Mayo Clin Proc 2006;81(Suppl 10):S5–10.
43. Zhang W, Mason EE, Renquist KE, et al. Factors influencing survival following surgical treatment of obesity. Obes Surg 2005;15(1):43–50.
44. Marsk R, Freedman J, Tynelius P, et al. Antiobesity surgery in Sweden from 1980 to 2005: a population-based study with a focus on mortality. Ann Surg 2008;248(5):777–81.
45. Perry CD, Hutter MM, Smith DB, et al. Survival and changes in comorbidities after bariatric surgery. Ann Surg 2008;247(1):21–7.

Patient Safety and Quality Improvement Initiatives in Contemporary Metabolic and Bariatric Surgical Practice

Dan E. Azagury, MD, John Magaña Morton, MD, MPH*

KEYWORDS

- Bariatric surgery • Patient safety • Quality improvement • Outcomes

KEY POINTS

- Patient safety and quality improvement have been part of bariatric surgery since its inception.
- A strong accreditation program exists in bariatric surgery (Metabolic and Bariatric Surgery Accreditation and Quality Improvement Program [MBSAQIP]), as a result of the merger of the American Society for Metabolic and Bariatric Surgery (ASMBS) and American College of Surgeons (ACS)-led programs.
- Accreditation has been shown to have a favorable impact on outcomes of bariatric surgery, including, morbidity, mortality, length of stay, failure to rescue, and costs.
- Bariatric surgery lends itself well to improvements in processes and use of perioperative protocols, such as ulcer and thromboembolic prophylaxis prevention or gallstone prevention and management.
- With a comprehensive data reporting requirement, MBSAQIP provides a strong platform for quality improvement initiatives, such as the decrease in readmissions project from ASMBS.

INTRODUCTION

Quality improvement has been a core aspect of surgery for more than a century. In 1910, Ernest A. Codman, envisioned that poor outcomes could be linked to the absence of adequate patient records and resultant lack of feedback on patient's ultimate outcomes. When the ACS was founded 3 years later, Dr Codman was appointed to chair a committee on hospital standardization. This led to the 1919 minimum standard document.[1] This short document already describes the necessity for

The authors have nothing to disclose.
Section of Bariatric and Minimally Invasive Surgery, Stanford University School of Medicine, Stanford University, 300 Pasteur Drive, H3680A, Stanford, CA 94305-5655, USA
* Corresponding author.
E-mail address: morton@stanford.edu

"accurate and complete records be written for all patients and filled in in an accessible manner in the hospital." This document ultimately led to the creation of the Joint Commission on Accreditation of Hospitals in 1951 and the Joint Commission on Accreditation of Healthcare Organizations in 1987. But beyond this, the idea he developed of adequately documenting outcomes to learn from them is the cornerstone concept behind the ACS National Surgery Quality Improvement Program. This program takes the concept one step further, however, allowing obtaining standardized data on a larger scale to better analyze outcomes and benchmark current results to population means. As surgical outcomes have improved, the amount and detail of data necessary to detect improvements and outcomes are constantly increasing. In 1999, the Institute of Medicine published a report, "To Err is Human."[2] This research on medical errors in the United States highlighted the fact that preventable medical errors in hospitals exceeded the number of deaths from motor vehicle accidents or breast cancer. This report served as a wakeup call, leading to multiple initiatives ranging from government to nonprofit organizations and to health care providers.

PATIENT SAFETY AND QUALITY IMPROVEMENT IN BARIATRIC SURGERY

As discussed previously, the first and necessary step to improving quality is to have a means of accurately measuring outcomes. As a young specialty, bariatric surgery was born in the era of quality improvement and patient safety and rapidly adopted its own programs: the ACS and the ASMBS created 2 parallel accreditation programs for bariatric surgery in 2004 and 2005. These programs have now merged their accreditation systems to create the MBSAQIP in 2013.[3] More than 800 centers currently participate in MBSAQIP and more than 650 bariatric surgery centers are accredited throughout the United States. This program, however, is not limited to a database. If the reporting of outcomes is a cornerstone of this program, it also focuses on quality improvement: it emphasizes surgeon leadership and multidisciplinary teams and defines and monitors the current bariatric center accreditation process. These features relate back to the principles defined by Avedis Donabedian, whereby quality of health care can be assessed by measuring aspects of structure, processes, and outcomes.

Bariatric surgery outcomes have followed a significant improvement in mortality and morbidity over the past 15 years. Between 1998 and 2004, the number of cases performed increase practically 10-fold whereas inpatient mortality decreased by nearly the same amount (0.2% to 0.03%).[4] Since then, the implementation of center accreditation as led to further improvements. The different aspects of quality improvement in bariatric surgery are described.

ACCREDITATION

Accreditation is a core feature of quality in surgery. It addresses all 3 aspects: structure, processes, and outcomes. Accreditation has also been topical in bariatric surgery for more than a decade. The Centers for Medicare and Medicaid Services (CMS) had initially made accreditation a prerequisite for reimbursement of bariatric surgery procedures. This policy has recently been reverted by CMS; however, all major insurers require bariatric surgery center accreditation and the preponderance of evidence clearly supports accreditation. Furthermore, without a requirement for accreditation, hospitals would be reluctant to provide resources to maintain data collection.

To be an accredited MBSAQIP center, all programs must report their outcomes to a centralized database. These should include all bariatric surgeries performed and require a minimum 90-day follow-up. All potential adverse events are clearly predefined, such as superficial versus deep surgical site infections, blood transfusions, and reoperations. In addition, data are collected by members independent of the care team.

The centers also need to meet core standard requirements. These requirements are different depending on the level of the center, defined as low-acuity centers versus comprehensive centers. Low-acuity centers are accredited to perform bariatric surgery, but the revisional procedures or high-risk patients are reserved for comprehensive centers. The fundamental difference between the 2 types of centers is focused on minimal annual volumes of procedures performed as well as resources available. If low-acuity centers must perform a minimum of 25 bariatric procedures every year procedures every year, comprehensive centers must perform a minimum of 50 cases annually to be accredited as such. High-risk patients are defined for this purpose as adults over the age of 65, men with a body mass index greater than 55 kg/m^2, women with body mass index greater than 60 kg/m^2, transplant patients, or patients with organ failure. Case volume constitutes the first of 7 core standards defined for accreditation. The other standards are commitment to quality of care, appropriate equipment and instruments, 24/7 critical care support, continuum of care, data collection, and continuous quality improvement process (**Table 1**). The rationale for case volume has also been settled law but has long been a debated topic in the surgical literature. A recent systematic review did show a positive association between high-volume centers and high-volume surgeons and patient outcomes.[5] Some modest discrepancy existed, however, among the studies cited, with 5 of the 24 studies failing to show association.[6–10] Prior minimum annual case requirements for bariatric surgery centers of excellence were higher (100 cases per 24 month/surgeon and more than 125 cases per institution/year). These cases did not differentiate, however, between a Roux-en-Y gastric bypass and a gastric band placement, for example. A more recent study, using the most recent MBSAQIP volume cutoff numbers, supports these new requirements by demonstrating a 2.5-times decrease in mortality in higher-volume centers.[11] Furthermore, the increased mortality appears to be more significant in higher-risk patients, supporting the requirement for these patients to undergo surgery at comprehensive centers. In a historical study by Flum and colleagues[12] the mortality rates for patients greater than 65 years old was 9% at 30 days and 21% at 1 year if volume was less than 15 cases/y, compared with 2.2% and 5.0% in patients younger than 65 years. This is compared with higher procedures performed in higher-volume centers with mortality rates of 1.1% and 3.6% in patients over 65% and 1.2% and 3.1% in the younger patients.

Impact of Accreditation

Multiple studies have established the impact of accreditation on bariatric surgery outcomes. Five of them have shown a reduction in mortality compared with nonaccredited centers, reductions ranging between 2.26-fold and 3.5-fold.[11,13–16] Regarding complications, only 1 study showed an increase in serious morbidity (odds ratio 0.84) in accredited centers.[11] However, 6 other recent studies have demonstrated a reduction in morbidities when bariatric surgery is performed in an accredited center. These studies encompass data for more than 430,000 patients with odds ratios ranging from 1.09 to 1.39.[14,15,17–20] Studies comparing accredited and nonaccredited centers also demonstrated an improvement in other outcomes: reduction in reoperation from 3.2% to 2.1%[21]; reduced readmission rates: 19.9% to 15.4%[21]; payments ($24,363 to $19,746)[21]; and length of stay: 3.5 versus 3.1 days.[19]

Another concept increasingly taken into consideration is "failure to rescue." This metric is tracked and defined by the Agency for Healthcare Research and Quality

Table 1
Metabolic and Bariatric Surgery Accreditation and Quality Improvement Program core standard requirements

Standards	Requirements				
Case Volume	Depends on center designation (see text)				
Commitment to quality care	Bariatric committee, including a director/surgeon, a coordinator, a clinical reviewer	Facility accreditation (Joint Commission)	Surgeons • Credentialed in bariatric surgery • Undergo annual verification • Cover a bariatric call schedule	Clinic and inpatient • Designated area available • Trained nursing staff	Multidisciplinary specialized team, including • Nursing staff • Registered dieticians • Psychologists/psychiatrists • Physical therapists
Appropriate equipment and instruments	Extremely detailed and includes every aspect of care: operating room tables, imaging equipment, blood pressure cuffs, adequate bedding, showers, toilets, etc.				
Critical care support	Stabilization and transfer capabilities	Presence of Advanced Cardiovascular Life Support qualified provider	Established protocols and availability for bariatric patient management • Anesthesia • 24/7 Critical/intensive care unit • Endoscopy • Diagnostic and interventional radiology	Written transfer agreement to transfer patients to a facility providing services, such as interventional radiology if not available on site	
Continuum of care	Use of clinical education and perioperative protocols	Long-term follow-up and available support groups			
Data collection	See text.				
Continuous quality improvement process	Maintain a collaborative between all bariatric surgeons in the institution	Minimum of 1 quality improvement initiative per year	Continuous monitoring of safety and outcomes		

and takes into account the mortality rate in patients having experienced a serious complication, such as pulmonary embolism, sepsis, or acute bleeding.[22] This metric has a potential for increased sensitivity to detect adverse events compared with complications alone for example. The authors' group has previously demonstrated a reduction of approximately 50% of failure to rescue bariatric surgery patients in accredited versus nonaccredited centers.[15]

PROCESSES AND QUALITY IMPROVEMENT

Many of the processes commonly used in bariatric surgery are part of the accreditation requirements, notably the need for multidisciplinary teams and patient assessment. Also, the preoperative patient evaluation and patient selection are discussed in another article in this issue (See Guerron Cruz AD, Portenier DD: Patient Selection and Surgical Management of High Risk Patients with Morbid Obesity, in this issue). It is, however, important that the difference between the 2 tiers of accreditation (ie, comprehensive and low-acuity centers) revolves around the ability to manage high-risk patients. It is, therefore, important to carefully evaluate patients preoperatively to determine the risk status and ensure they are treated in the facility most adequate to their risk profile.

As discussed later in the paragraph about decreasing remissions, the nature of bariatric surgery lends itself well to standardization of perioperative management. Some aspects of these processes are highlighted.

Deep Venous Thromboembolism Prevention

Pulmonary embolism (PE) remains one of the leading causes of postbariatric surgery mortality.[23] According to the Rogers score,[24] all laparoscopic sleeve gastrectomy or Roux-en-Y gastric bypass patients are considered medium risk for venous thromboembolism (VTE). This score uses preoperative factors to determine VTE/PE risk, with 7 points medium risk and 10 representing a high risk for deep venous thrombosis/PE. A procedure with a relative value unit greater than 17, gastrointestinal surgery, and a clean/contaminated wound is sufficient to add up to a score of 8, which constitutes an intermediate risk. This risk is often higher in the authors' patient population because an American Society of Anesthesiologists (ASA) score of 2 is an extra point, an ASA score of 3 or more is 2 points, and female gender adds 1 point. These risk factors common occurrences and these patients are considered high risk based on this score. Based on this evaluation and others,[25] VTE prophylaxis is, therefore, warranted for all patients undergoing a Roux-en-Y gastric bypass or a sleeve gastrectomy. The type of prophylaxis however is still somewhat debated. The most recent guidelines[26,27] recommend that all bariatric patients receive at least mechanical prophylaxis (intermittent pneumatic compression) and early ambulation. All high-risk patients (defined by 1 of the previous scores) should, in addition, receive chemoprophylaxis in the form of low-molecular-weight or unfractioned heparin. This includes, for example, an ASA 2 female patient.

Ulcer Prophylaxis

In patients undergoing Roux-en-Y gastric bypass, an additional risk exists regarding the development of marginal ulcers at the gastrojejunostomy site. The reported incidence of this pathology ranges from 0.6% to 25%.[28] The pathogenesis is still unclear, but acid exposure as well as mucosal ischemia in the pouch are likely causes of marginal ulcer development. Multiple recent studies have tried to identify risk factors for the development of these ulcers: diabetes and smoking or nonsteroidal anti-inflammatory drugs seem the most commonly reported risk factors, but other risk factors include history of peptic ulcers, use of nonabsorbable sutures, corticosteroids, *Helicobacter pylori*, and hypertension.[28–35] Even if the pathophysiology and risk factors are debated, the literature regarding the use of postoperative prophylactic proton pump inhibitors is rather unanimous.[36–40] This has also resulted in a wide adoption of proton pump inhibitor prophylaxis after Roux-en-Y gastric bypass: a recent international survey showed that approximately 90% of bariatric surgeons prescribe prophylaxis for 30 to 90 days postoperatively.[41] The authors currently systematically prescribe 6 months of proton pump inhibitors to all bariatric surgery patients.

Gallstone Prophylaxis

Contrary to ulcer prophylaxis, the management of gallstone prophylaxis is significantly debated and varies significantly. The increased risk of gallstone formation with rapid weight loss after bariatric surgery is not disputed. Prevention strategies vary, however, and can be summarized as follows: chemoprophylaxis alone, selective cholecystectomy at the time of bariatric surgery (based on the presence of gallstones on systematic preoperative ultrasound), or systematic cholecystectomy in all bariatric surgery patients. The discussion regarding prophylactic cholecystectomy is outside of the realm of this article. A large retrospective study, however, of more than 20,000 cholecystectomies in bariatric surgery patients, recently advocated for systematic cholecystectomy[42] whereas a recent meta-analysis on more than 6000 patients showed a cholecystectomy rate of 6.8% after gastric bypass, with 0% mortality and 1.8% morbidity.[43] Common bile duct pathologies occurred in 0.2% of cases for common bile duct stones and 0.2% for biliary pancreatitis. The impetus for some form of gallstone prophylaxis is, therefore, not contested. From quality and process perspectives, it is important to have a systematic protocol in place for the management of this issue: if cholecystectomy is not performed at time of gastric bypass surgery, chemoprophylaxis in the form of ursodiol should be systematically used. Ursodiol has been demonstrated to significantly reduce the incidence of symptomatic/gallstone formation, from 32% to 2%, and a recent meta-analysis also showed a significant reduction, with 8.8% of patients on prophylaxis developing gallstones compared with 27.7% for placebo.[44–46]

PROCESS IMPROVEMENT: DECREASING READMISSIONS THROUGH OPPORTUNITIES PROVIDED

In the past decade, the field of bariatric surgery has made significant gains in improving quality. Since the advent of hospital and center-based accreditation in 2007, both mortality and serious complications have decreased substantially. Currently, individual serious complications, such as anastomotic leak, small bowel obstruction, venous-thrombotic events, and myocardial infarction, all are less than 1%, according to the 2014 MBSAQIP data registry.

An area for potential quality improvement for metabolic and bariatric surgery is 30-day readmissions after principal operative surgical procedures. This particular outcome has become an outcome of interest for payers, including the CMS and others.

Additionally, all-cause 30-day readmissions are a metaoutcome, incorporating multiple elements of care, including complications, cost, and physician and patient satisfaction. At this time, the MBSAQIP data registry reports that all-cause 30-day readmissions are at approximately 5%, indicating an opportunity for improvement. Furthermore, the new MBSAQIP standards call for each center to actively participate in a quality improvement project, and the Decreasing Readmissions through

Opportunities Provided (DROP) project is in alignment with this (see "Standard 7: Continuous Quality Improvement Process" from *Resources for the Optimal Care of the Metabolic and Bariatric Surgery Patient 2014*).[47]

Several metabolic and bariatric surgery programs have demonstrated improvement in 30-day readmissions through better coordination of care, as indicated in the 2013 Obesity Week readmissions symposium. For example, the Stanford Bariatric Surgery Program reported a 69% decline in 30-day readmissions after implementing a readmission bundle. In the 2013 Obesity Week forum, current best practices were identified. The coordination of care incorporates the 3 phases of operative care: preoperative, inpatient, and postoperative. The DROP program provides a specific toolkit and standardization, which address 30-day readmissions in all phases of operative care, which include

DROP readmission bundle for metabolic and bariatric surgery patients
- Preoperative
  - Education video modules (surgeon, nurse, nutrition, psychologist, pharmacy)
  - Postoperative prescription given
  - Postoperative visit scheduled
  - On-call and clinic phone numbers given
- Inpatient
  - Clinical roadmap implementation
  - Discharge checklist completed
  - Nutritional consult
- Postoperative
  - Follow-up phone call completed
  - Postoperative visit with surgeon and nutritionist completed
  - Primary care provider letter sent
  - Monthly readmissions review

The goal of the project is to decrease 30-day all-cause readmissions for primary bariatric procedures by 20% nationally.

Program inclusion criteria:
- Participation in a comprehensive accredited MBSAQIP program
- Agreement to participate in complete hospital survey and monthly webinars and provide hospital specific and collaborative data to complete the project
- Complete custom fields in the MBSAQIP Data Registry for the readmission bundle

The completion of DROP is anticipated in March 2016, with full analysis completed in September 2016. In addition to demonstrating reduction of readmissions, it is anticipated that patient satisfaction may increase based on the higher level of coordination of care provided by DROP centers.

REFERENCES

1. The 1919 Minimum Standard Document. Available at: https://www.facs.org/about%20acs/archives/pasthighlights/minimumhighlight. Accessed November 20, 2015.
2. Kohn LT, Corrigan JM, Donaldson MS. To Err Is Human:: Building a Safer Health System - Committee on Quality of Health Care in America, Institute of Medicine - Google Books. Washington, DC: National Academy Press; 2000.
3. Mbsaqip.org. Available at: http://www.mbsaqip.org. Accessed September 12, 2014.

4. AHRQ Bariatric Surgery Utilization and Outcomes. Available at: http://www.hcup-us.ahrq.gov/reports/statbriefs/sb23.jsp. Accessed November 23, 2015.
5. Zevin B, Aggarwal R, Grantcharov TP. Volume-outcome association in bariatric surgery: a systematic review. Ann Surg 2012;256(1):60–71.
6. Alami RS, Morton JM, Sanchez BR, et al. Laparoscopic Roux-en-Y gastric bypass at a Veterans Affairs and high-volume academic facilities: a comparison of institutional outcomes. Am J Surg 2005;190(5):821–5.
7. Livingston EH. Bariatric surgery outcomes at designated centers of excellence vs nondesignated programs. Arch Surg 2009;144(4):319–25 [discussion: 325].
8. Carbonell AM, Lincourt AE, Matthews BD, et al. National study of the effect of patient and hospital characteristics on bariatric surgery outcomes. Am Surg 2005; 71(4):308–14.
9. O'Rourke RW, Andrus J, Diggs BS, et al. Perioperative morbidity associated with bariatric surgery: an academic center experience. Arch Surg 2006;141(3):262–8.
10. Voitk A, Voitk J Jr, Joffe J. Impartial long-term review of vertical banded gastroplasty in a low volume community hospital practice. Obes Surg 2001;11(5): 546–50.
11. Jafari MD, Jafari F, Young MT, et al. Volume and outcome relationship in bariatric surgery in the laparoscopic era. Surg Endosc 2013;27(12):4539–46.
12. Flum DR, Salem L, Elrod JAB, et al. Early mortality among Medicare beneficiaries undergoing bariatric surgical procedures. JAMA 2005;294(15):1903–8.
13. Gebhart A, Young M, Phelan M, et al. Impact of accreditation in bariatric surgery. Surg Obes Relat Dis 2014;10(5):767–73.
14. Young MT, Jafari MD, Gebhart A, et al. A decade analysis of trends and outcomes of bariatric surgery in medicare beneficiaries. J Am Coll Surg 2014;219(3):480–8.
15. Morton JM, Garg T, Nguyen N. Does hospital accreditation impact bariatric surgery safety? Ann Surg 2014;260(3):504–9.
16. Nguyen NT, Nguyen B, Nguyen VQ, et al. Outcomes of bariatric surgery performed at accredited vs nonaccredited centers. J Am Coll Surg 2012;215(4): 467–74.
17. Telem DA, Talamini M, Altieri M, et al. The effect of national hospital accreditation in bariatric surgery on perioperative outcomes and long-term mortality. Surg Obes Relat Dis 2015;11(4):749–57.
18. Kwon S, Wang B, Wong E, et al. The impact of accreditation on safety and cost of bariatric surgery. Surg Obes Relat Dis 2013;9(5):617–22.
19. Nguyen NT, Hohmann S, Slone J, et al. Improved bariatric surgery outcomes for Medicare beneficiaries after implementation of the medicare national coverage determination. Arch Surg 2010;145(1):72–8.
20. Kohn GP, Galanko JA, Overby DW, et al. High Case Volumes and Surgical Fellowships Are associated with improved outcomes for bariatric surgery patients: a justification of current credentialing initiatives for practice and training. J Am Coll Surg 2010;210(6):909–18.
21. Flum DR, Kwon S, MacLeod K, et al. The use, safety and cost of bariatric surgery before and after medicare's national coverage decision. Ann Surg 2011;254(6): 860–5.
22. AHRQ Failure to Rescue. Availabe at: http://www.qualityindicators.ahrq.gov/Downloads/Modules/PSI/V50-ICD10/TechSpecs/PSI_04_Death_among_Surgical_Inpatients.pdf. Accessed November 29, 2015.
23. Sapala JA, Wood MH, Schuhknecht MP, et al. Fatal pulmonary embolism after bariatric operations for morbid obesity: a 24-year retrospective analysis. Obes Surg 2003;13(6):819–25.

24. Rogers SOJ, Kilaru RK, Hosokawa P, et al. Multivariable predictors of postoperative venous thromboembolic events after general and vascular surgery: results from the patient safety in surgery study. J Am Coll Surg 2007;204(6):1211–21.
25. Caprini JA. Thrombosis risk assessment as a guide to quality patient care. Dis Mon 2005;51(2–3):70–8.
26. Gould MK, Garcia DA, Wren SM, et al. Prevention of VTE in nonorthopedic surgical patients: antithrombotic therapy and prevention of thrombosis, 9th ed: American College of Chest Physicians Evidence-Based Clinical Practice Guidelines. Chest 2012;141(2 Suppl):e227S–77S.
27. American Society for Metabolic and Bariatric Surgery Clinical Issues Committee. ASMBS updated position statement on prophylactic measures to reduce the risk of venous thromboembolism in bariatric surgery patients. Surg Obes Relat Dis 2013;9(4):493–7.
28. Coblijn UK, Goucham AB, Lagarde SM, et al. Development of ulcer disease after Roux-en-Y gastric bypass, incidence, risk factors, and patient presentation: a systematic review. Obes Surg 2014;24(2):299–309.
29. Coblijn UK, Lagarde SM, de Castro SMM, et al. Symptomatic marginal ulcer disease after Roux-en-Y gastric bypass: incidence, risk factors and management. Obes Surg 2015;25(5):805–11.
30. Sverdén E, Mattsson F, Sondén A, et al. Risk factors for marginal ulcer after gastric bypass surgery for obesity: a population-based cohort study. Ann Surg 2016;263(4):733–7.
31. Vasquez JC, Wayne Overby D, Farrell TM. Fewer gastrojejunostomy strictures and marginal ulcers with absorbable suture. Surg Endosc 2008;23(9):2011–5.
32. Bhayani NH, Oyetunji TA, Chang DC, et al. Predictors of marginal ulcers after laparoscopic Roux-en-Y gastric bypass. J Surg Res 2012;177(2):224–7.
33. Ben-Meir A, Sonpal I, Patterson L, et al. Cigarette smoking, but not NSAID or alcohol use or comorbidities, is associated with anastomotic ulcers in Roux-en-Y Gastric Bypass (RYGB) patients. Surg Obes Relat Dis 2005;1(3):263–4.
34. Azagury DE, Abu Dayyeh BK, Greenwalt IT, et al. Marginal ulceration after Roux-en-Y gastric bypass surgery: characteristics, risk factors, treatment, and outcomes. Endoscopy 2011;43(11):950–4.
35. Rasmussen JJ, Fuller W, Ali MR. Marginal ulceration after laparoscopic gastric bypass: an analysis of predisposing factors in 260 patients. Surg Endosc 2007;21(7):1090–4.
36. Moon RC, Teixeira AF, Goldbach M, et al. Management and treatment outcomes of marginal ulcers after Roux-en-Y gastric bypass at a single high volume bariatric center. Surg Obes Relat Dis 2014;10(2):229–34.
37. Garrido AB Jr, Rossi M, Lima SE Jr, et al. Early marginal ulcer following Roux-en-Y gastric bypass under proton pump inhibitor treatment: prospective multicentric study. Arq Gastroenterol 2010;47(2):130–4. Available at: http://eutils.ncbi.nlm.nih.gov/entrez/eutils/elink.fcgi?dbfrom=pubmed&id=20721455&retmode=ref&cmd=prlinks.
38. Coblijn UK, Lagarde SM, de Castro SMM, et al. The influence of prophylactic proton pump inhibitor treatment on the development of symptomatic marginal ulceration in Roux-en-Y gastric bypass patients: a historic cohort study. Surg Obes Relat Dis 2015. http://dx.doi.org/10.1016/j.soard.2015.04.022.
39. Ying VWC, Kim SHH, Khan KJ, et al. Prophylactic PPI help reduce marginal ulcers after gastric bypass surgery: a systematic review and meta-analysis of cohort studies. Surg Endosc 2015;29(5):1018–23.

40. André D'Hondt M, Pottel H, Devriendt D, et al. Can a Short course of prophylactic low-dose proton pump inhibitor therapy prevent stomal ulceration after laparoscopic roux-en-y gastric bypass? Obes Surg 2010;20(5):595–9.

41. Steinemann DC, Bueter M, Schiesser M, et al. Management of Anastomotic ulcers after roux-en-Y gastric bypass: results of an international survey. Obes Surg 2013; 24:741–6.

42. Weiss AC, Inui T, Parina R, et al. Concomitant cholecystectomy should be routinely performed with laparoscopic Roux-en-Y gastric bypass. Surg Endosc 2015;29:1–6.

43. Warschkow R, Tarantino I, Ukegjini K, et al. Concomitant cholecystectomy during laparoscopic Roux-en-Y gastric bypass in obese patients is not justified: a meta-analysis. Obes Surg 2013;23(3):397–407.

44. Sugerman HJ, Brewer WH, Shiffman ML, et al. A multicenter, placebo-controlled, randomized, double-blind, prospective trial of prophylactic ursodiol for the prevention of gallstone formation following gastric-bypass-induced rapid weight loss. Am J Surg 1995;169(1):91–6 [discussion: 96–7]. Available at: http://eutils.ncbi.nlm.nih.gov/entrez/eutils/elink.fcgi?dbfrom=pubmed&id=7818005&retmode=ref&cmd=prlinks.

45. Stokes CS, Gluud LL, Casper M, et al. Ursodeoxycholic acid and diets higher in fat prevent gallbladder stones during weight loss: a meta-analysis of randomized controlled trials. Clin Gastroenterol Hepatol 2014;12(7):1090–100.e2 [quiz: 61].

46. Morton J. The first metabolic and bariatric surgery accreditation and quality improvement program quality initiative: decreasing readmissions through opportunities provided. Surg Obes Relat Dis 2014;10(3):377–8.

47. Available at: http://www.mbsaqip.org/docs/Resources%20for%20Optimal%20Care%20of%20the%20MBS%20Patient.pdf.

Patient Selection and Surgical Management of High-Risk Patients with Morbid Obesity

A. Daniel Guerron, MD, Dana D. Portenier, MD*

KEYWORDS

- Risk factors • High risk • End organ failure

KEY POINTS

- Bariatric surgery is the most effective way to improve comorbidities related to obesity.
- Since the introduction of minimally invasive laparoscopic surgery in the bariatric surgery techniques, the number of procedures has increased substantially; advances in techniques and the transition from open to minimally invasive procedures have decreased morbidity and mortality.
- Improvement in techniques and training programs have made it possible for patients who were previously at unacceptable high risk to now be candidates for bariatric surgery.
- Knowledge of the preoperative factors that predict for greater mortality could aid surgeons in surgical decision-making and help inform patients of their risks with bariatric surgery.
- Multidisciplinary teams in charge of the operative planning, surgical act, and postoperative recovery are determinant in the success of the management of high-risk bariatric patients; careful identification and preoperative management of these higher-risk patients is crucial in decreasing complications after weight loss surgery.

INTRODUCTION

The prevalence of obesity as of 2011 to 2012 was reported at 36.5% among US adults.[1] Bariatric surgery is the most effective way to improve comorbidities related to obesity.[2–4] The surgical treatment of the morbidly obese with significant medical conditions remains a challenge. Since the introduction of minimally invasive laparoscopic surgery in the bariatric surgery techniques, the number of procedures has increased substantially. Advances in techniques and transition from open to minimally invasive procedures have decreased the morbidity and mortality. Improvement in techniques and training programs has made it possible for patients who were

Department of General Surgery, Duke University Health System, 407 Crutchfield Street, Durham, NC 27704, USA
* Corresponding author.
E-mail address: dana.portenier@duke.edu

Surg Clin N Am 96 (2016) 743–762
http://dx.doi.org/10.1016/j.suc.2016.03.009
0039-6109/16/$ – see front matter © 2016 Elsevier Inc. All rights reserved.
surgical.theclinics.com

previously at unacceptably high risk to now be candidates for bariatric surgery. These advancements have made it possible for bariatric surgery to expand into even higher-risk patients, such as the increasing subset of patients with end-organ failure. Access to organ transplantation and other complex surgical procedures is affected by obesity and the high-risk profile. Knowledge of the preoperative factors that predict for greater mortality could aid surgeons in surgical decision-making and help inform patients of their risks with bariatric surgery. Multidisciplinary teams in charge of the operative planning, surgical act, and postoperative recovery are determinant in the success of the management of high-risk bariatric patients. Careful identification and preoperative management of these higher-risk patients is crucial in decreasing complications after weight loss surgery.

High volume and near ubiquitous utilization of a minimally invasive approach, combined with advancement in perioperative care, have further mitigated postoperative morbidity in such high-risk patients. Bariatric surgery candidates usually have an extensive range of potential medical, surgical, and psychological comorbidities. These individuals should be carefully selected, extensively evaluated, and optimized so as to achieve best outcomes following an elective surgery. Therefore, a comprehensive multidisciplinary preoperative assessment is of great importance, especially in high-risk patients.

IDENTIFICATION OF HIGH-RISK FACTORS
Age

In the United States, 42.5% of women and 38.1% of men are obese in the range of 60 to 69 years, whereas among those 70 and 79 years, 31.9% of women and 28.9% of men are in this condition.[5–7] Both overweight and obesity in the elderly are linked to physical disability.[5,8] The increased life expectancy and higher prevalence of obesity have forced the number of elderly patients who need bariatric surgery to increase.[6] Aside from the extensively reported comorbidity amelioration, the aim of the operation in the elderly is to increase disability-free survival and improve quality of life.[6] In the elderly, age-related changes in body composition include a progressive increase in fat mass and a decline in lean mass and bone. Body fat redistribution occurs with an increment in visceral abdominal fat and a decrease in subcutaneous abdominal fat.[9]

Advanced age increases postoperative morbidity and mortality for any surgery. Patients older than 50 have higher rates of morbidity and mortality.[10,11] Adverse event rates progressively increased with age, exhibiting a sharp increase at older than 60 years. Beyond the age of 65 years, the adverse event rate exceeded 20% and mortality was 3.2%.[12] Livingston and Langert[12] in 2006 demonstrated that advanced age ($\geq$65 years) was an independent risk factor for adverse outcomes, as defined as length of hospital stay greater than 95th percentile, being discharged to a long-term care facility, or having died during the hospital admission for weight loss surgery. Nguyen and colleagues[13] found that age older than than 60 was a significant factor for in-hospital mortality. Because of lower physiological reserve and tolerance for complications, in this group of patients a rigorous verification of health status is implemented.

This increased risk profile has led some institutions to implement age restrictions. At Duke, no such restrictions exist, patients are evaluated on a case-by-case basis. Increased time is spent educating elderly patients of the relative unproven possibility that they may have aged out of lengthened survival. However, elderly patients seem to be interested in maintaining their lifestyle and independence (functional status), which worsening obesity tends to erode as people age.

Gender

The prevalence of extreme obesity (body mass index [BMI] ≥40) in 2003 to 2004 was 2.8% in men and 6.9% in women.[7] Typically, approximately 15% to 20% of participants in bariatric surgery studies are men.[14,15] Men who seek bariatric surgery are generally older and have a higher BMI and more obesity-related comorbidities compared with women.[14–17]

Male gender is an independent risk factor for perioperative complications, and a predictor of adverse outcomes and adverse events after bariatric surgery.[10,15,18] Nguyen and colleagues[13] suggested that even more than advanced age, male gender was associated with greater mortality after bariatric surgery.

Body Mass Index

Approximately 6.3% of the US adult population is severely obese.[19,20] The prevalence of severe obesity (BMI 40) increased 50%, and the prevalence of superobesity (BMI 50) increased 75%.[21–23] As the BMI increases, the physiology of the patient deteriorates. High BMI present challenges for the patient's overall health due to higher incidence of cardiopulmonary insufficiency, pulmonary hypertension, obstructive sleep apnea, and obesity-related hypoventilation syndrome. For greater BMI, technical challenges encountered during the operation are attributed to a thickened abdominal wall, enlarged liver, increased intraperitoneal fat, and limited working space after insufflation. These obstacles may lengthen the duration of surgery, increasing the preoperative risk. Several studies have correlated the increment of BMI and the surgical risk. DeMaria and colleagues[24] showed that BMI greater than 50 represents a significant risk factor. With the continuous increment of BMI, surgical groups are performing surgery in heavier patients. Reports denote the safety of the procedure,[25,26] but the risk of complications remains elevated.

At Duke, since 2009 we have performed surgery on 25 patients over 500 lb with BMI ranging from 64 to 112. Patients in this weight range present several unique challenges, including immobility and deep vein thrombosis/pulmonary embolism (DVT/PE) concerns, weight often exceeds the maximum capacity of diagnostic radiograph equipment that can be used in the postoperative period, high-risk airways, thick stiff abdominal walls, excessive intra-abdominal fat, and challenging psychosocial situations.

Our protocol has been to admit many of these patients and work to reduce risk with inpatient preoperative weight loss. Up to this point, we have used liquid diet, but will certainly consider utilization of gastric balloons in the future. Attempts should be made to get the patient to a weight that can be accommodated by diagnostic radiographic equipment, such as computed tomography scanners that may be needed postoperatively. Many of these patients have large extracellular space fluid burdens in their legs, which respond well to albumin and Lasix. In several cases, we have reduced the patient's weight by several hundred pounds in a month or two. In several patients, we have used preoperative Greenfield filters and tracheostomy. Typically, cardiac examinations are so limited by body habitus that they are often obtained but rarely helpful. Special intraoperative attention must be paid to patient positioning, which may require 2 operative beds or creative table extensions. Additional trocars should be used liberally because a very thick abdominal wall creates excessive torque limiting range of motion. You should anticipate need for more than one liver retractor as a possibility. Attempts should be made to minimize and monitor for the real risk of rhabdomyolysis in these patients. One patient operated on at 700 lb developed post sleeve gastrectomy rhabdomyolysis with subsequent renal failure and hemodialysis. At the time, there were no available outpatient dialysis options for patients above 400 lb, necessitating a 1-year hospital stay until 400 lb was obtained.

From a psychosocial standpoint, many of these patients have underlying psychological disorders at an incidence similar to our typical patient. However, what sets them apart is the strong possibility of an individual in their life who enables poor food choices helping these patients achieve super morbid obesity status. We have found these to be everyone from caretakers, spouses, and family who become upset when their historic care patterns are disrupted. In one case we had to have security remove this individual who was continually sneaking the patient's "favorite" foods into the hospital.

Deep Vein Thrombosis

Obese individuals have chronically elevated intra-abdominal pressure and decreased blood velocity in the common femoral vein, resulting in venous stasis and ultimately contributing to increased risk for deep venous thrombus formation. The incidence of venous thromboembolism (VTE), presenting as DVT or PE, after bariatric surgery has been reported at between 0.5% and 2.0%.[27–29] PE is the leading cause of mortality in bariatric surgery centers.[30] Several groups used DVT/PE as an important factor in the calculation or risk stratification before bariatric surgery. DeMaria and colleagues[24] found that the combination or presence of previous VTE event, previous inferior vena cava filter placement, history of right heart failure or pulmonary hypertension, history of physical findings of venous stasis, including brawny edema or typical ulcerations, was highly statistically significant as a predictor of postoperative mortality. At our institution, Lovenox (enoxaparin) is typically given the day of surgery and a prophylaxis continued based on BMI. Also, patients with a BMI greater than 55, previous DVT/PE event, known hypercoagulable state, or impaired mobility are also given 2 to 4 weeks of extended prophylaxis after hospital discharge.

Cardiovascular Risk

The challenge for the clinician before surgery is to identify the severely obese patient who is at higher perioperative cardiovascular risk. Physical examination often underestimates cardiac dysfunction in severely obese patients. Cardiac symptoms, such as exertional dyspnea and lower-extremity edema, are nonspecific in obesity, and the severely obese patient with poor functional capacity should receive careful clinical evaluation. The prevalence of myocardial infarction, angina pectoris, percutaneous coronary intervention, and coronary artery bypass graft may be as high as 11.5% in morbidly obese women (BMI > 40).[31,32] Rates of cardiac arrest and annualized mortality were 1.6% and 1.5%, respectively, among patients undergoing bariatric procedures.[12,32] Severely obese patients with 3 or more coronary heart disease risk factors or diagnosed coronary heart disease may require additional noninvasive testing if the clinician believes that the results will change management.[32]

Diagnosed or occult coronary heart disease increases surgical risk. The prevalence of diagnosed coronary heart disease was not reported in a population-based analysis of 25,428 patients undergoing bariatric surgery, but the event rate for cardiac complications was 6.8 to 15.3 per 1000 patients.[12] Thus, it is easy to understand that patients with higher BMIs are at a higher risk for perioperative events.[31] The obtainment of a 12-lead electrocardiogram and a chest radiograph is reasonable in all severely obese patients under consideration for surgery.

Obstructive Sleep Apnea

In the bariatric surgery population, the prevalence of obstructive sleep apnea (OSA) has been found to be greater than 70%.[33,34] The incidence of OSA increases significantly as obesity increases to almost 50% of hospitalized patients with a BMI greater than 50 kg/m^2.[35] Studies have demonstrated that surgical patients with sleep apnea are at increased risk of having perioperative complications, including hypoxemia, pneumonia, difficult intubation, myocardial infarction, PE, atelectasis, cardiac arrhythmias, and unanticipated admission to the intensive care unit.[36]

We use a low threshold for preoperative screening. Also, patients with known sleep apnea on continuous positive airway pressure (CPAP) who have had a significant weight gain since last titration are sent in for CPAP titration before surgery. Patients are warned before surgery that we will not proceed on the day of surgery if they do not bring their own CPAP machine from home. On the floor, all CPAP patients are on telemetry and continuous pulse oximetry in the postoperative period.

Diabetes Mellitus

Ninety percent of all patients with type 2 diabetes are overweight or obese.[37] Hyperglycemia causes delay in healing and prolongs electrolyte and fluid shifts in the body. Uncontrolled diabetes leads to macrovascular and microvascular complications, including myocardial infarction, stroke, blindness, neuropathy, and renal failure in many patients.[38] Patients with poorly controlled or brittle diabetes are seen by our in-house endocrinologist for optimization and immediate postoperative planning. In the hospital, we have a dedicated diabetes team to tackle the rapid medication changes required in these difficult patients with diabetes.

Functional Status

Weight gain and fat accumulation interfere with an individual's functional capacity. The ability to walk is an important component of quality of life, because it reflects the capacity to undertake day-to-day activities. Walking difficulties become a functional limitation. DeSouza and colleagues[39] documented dynamic aspects of gait in severely obese subjects. Variables included speed, cadence, stride, support base, and foot angle, which were compared with reference values for the Brazilian population. All variables were significantly lower in the obese patients, except for support base, which was increased. These findings are consistent with poor skeletal muscle performance, high metabolic expenditure, and constant physical exhaustion. Functional status worsens with increasing BMI[40] and bariatric surgery results in substantial improvements in functional status.[39,41,42] The lack of activity has a negative impact on several organ systems and raises the risk profile of any patient with bariatric surgery. The patient with poor functional capacity presents a particular challenge, because it is important to distinguish between deconditioning with some expected dyspnea and underlying cardiac disease.[32] Obvious functional impairment when patients present to the office in a wheelchair displays significant risk. Patients with difficult mobility can be evaluated with the 6-minute walk test (6MWT). This test is a well-known instrument for assessing the functional capacity of a variety of groups, including the obese.[42] Nonambulatory status is a predisposing factor to DVT/PE, sarcopenia, decrement of muscle mass, and diabetes. Measures, such as extended DVT prophylaxis, is a strategy used in our center to avoid complications. Attention should be paid not only to the metabolic management but also to the physical rehabilitation required in cases of advanced obesity.[39]

Surgical Factors

As described earlier, patients with a larger BMI present greater technical difficulties for the surgeon. These difficulties tend to be more troublesome in laparoscopic procedures because of the need to work within a limited and tightly sealed abdominal compartment distended with gas. When visualization disappears in laparoscopic procedures, the margin of safety similarly evaporates.[43] Technical challenges in doing the procedure include greater thickness of the abdominal wall, greater amounts of perivisceral fat in the abdominal compartment, and fatty infiltration of the liver, which can increase its size tremendously.

Prior upper abdominal surgery can cause adhesions that can make exposure difficult. Adhesions may require tedious and often lengthy lysis of adhesions before enough small bowel is released to measure and create the jejunojejunostomy or releasing a fused stomach and the liver before the formation of the pouch, sleeve, and so forth.

Occasionally weight loss surgery is required in patients who have received transplanted organs. These group presents additional challenges due to adhesions and tissue quality due to immunosuppressants.

Revisional bariatric surgery is beyond the scope of this article. However, is worth analyzing revisional surgery with regard to risk. Nesset and colleagues[44] evaluated 218 patients who underwent open revisional bariatric surgery and they reported a 0.9% mortality rate and a 26% serious operative morbidity rate (wound infection in 13%, leak in 3%, PE in 2%, anemia/hemorrhage in 2%, pneumonia/prolonged ventilation in 2%, and other in 4%), Coakley and colleagues,[45] in a 10-year retrospective review of revisional bariatric surgery for failed vertical-banded gastroplasty and laparoscopic Roux-en-Y gastric bypass (LRYGB), reported a major morbidity rate of 17%, with no mortality. Obtaining previous operative notes can help prepare the surgeon for the environment that he or she is about to discover. Advanced endoscopic and laparoscopic skills are desirable to repair any surgical misadventures that may be encountered.

Estimating the Risk

Several groups have tried to determine the risk stratification using scoring systems.

DeMaria and colleagues[24] proposed the obesity surgery mortality risk score (OS-MRS). The OS-MRS is a simple, clinically relevant scoring system that stratifies mortality risk into low (Class A), intermediate (Class B), and high (Class C) risk groups. The group prospectively collected data from 2075 consecutive patients undergoing LRYGB. Multivariate analysis showed BMI of 50 kg/m^2 or higher, male gender, hypertension, and PE risk, and patient age of 45 years or older as variables that correlated with mortality. A scoring system was developed by arbitrarily scoring the presence of each independent variable as equal to 1 point, resulting in an overall score of 0 to 5 points. Class A consisted of patients with 0 or 1 comorbidity, class B consisted of patients with 2 to 3 comorbidities, and class C consisted of patients with 4 to 5 comorbidities. Each class was correlated with a mortality rate of 0.31%, 1.90%, and 7.56%, respectively. To date, it is the most widely used system to categorize or score the risk of bariatric surgery. OS-MRS fails to separate open and laparoscopic cases and is restricted to gastric bypass surgery.

Nguyen and colleagues,[13] during the 8-year period, analyzed 105,287 patients to assess the preoperative factors that might predict in-hospital mortality after bariatric surgery. The investigators identified 6 factors significantly associated with greater mortality after bariatric surgery: age older than 60 years, male gender, the presence of diabetes, an open surgical technique, Medicare payer, and LRYGB. Factors were classified in major and minor and a score devised by assigning 1 point or 0.5 point, respectively. The mortality rate was 0.10% for class I patients, 0.15% for class II, 0.33% for class III, and 0.70% for class IV. Limitations of this database included the lack of the BMI.

Turner and colleagues[46] reviewed patient factors and patient outcomes for those who had undergone bariatric surgical procedures to determine relationships and developed a nomogram to calculate individualized patient risk. Using the American College of Surgeons National Surgical Quality Improvement Program (ACS-NSQIP) database, 32,426 bariatric surgery patients were identified. The greatest impacts on the estimated probability of morbidity/mortality were determined to be age, BMI, serum albumin, and functional status. Gender and diabetes mellitus were omitted due to the small impact on the predicted probability arising from this logistic model. The investigators concluded the nomogram may prove useful in patient preoperative counseling on postoperative complication risk.

Gupta and colleagues[47] proposed that the estimation of postoperative morbidity might be helpful in the choice of surgical procedure and consent, as well as targeting and reducing specific factors that can increase the risks associated with this surgery. Using the 2007 ACS-NSQIP dataset, the group reviewed 11,023 patients. Risk factors associated with increased risk of postoperative morbidity included recent myocardial infarction/angina, dependent functional status, stroke, bleeding disorder, hypertension, BMI, and type of bariatric surgery. The study excluded laparoscopic sleeve gastrectomy (LSG) due to coding issues. The morbidity risk calculator mean age was 44.6 years, 20% were men, 77% were white, and mean BMI was 48.9. Thirty-day morbidity and mortality were 4.2% and 0.2%, respectively. The morbidity risk calculator is available online at http://www.surgicalriskcalculator.com.

In 2012, a group from Nebraska using 21,891 patients undergoing bariatric operations (11,846 LRYGB) from the ACS-NSQIP dataset reported 7 independent predictors of mortality: peripheral vascular disease, dyspnea, previous percutaneous coronary intervention, age, BMI, chronic corticosteroid use, and type of bariatric surgery. Overall, death within 30 days was 0.14% and overall morbidity 5.5%. The group did not include sleep apnea and history of VTE as risk factors.[48]

The Edmonton obesity staging system, is a 5-point ordinal classification system that considers comorbidity and functional status.[49] This staging system does not directly or indirectly measure adiposity, rather the system is intended to complete anthropometric indices and provide incremental clinically relevant prognostic information. The major incremental contribution is the direct measurement of the presence and severity of underlying obesity-related comorbidities, which enables a more comprehensive and individual assessment of risk.[50,51]

Khan and colleagues[52] aimed to evaluate the factors capable of predicting perioperative mortality based on preoperative characteristics with a national patient sample from the ACS-NSQIP database. Most of the procedures performed included LRYGB (54%). Independent predictors associated with significantly increased mortality included age older than 45 years, male gender, BMI of 50 kg/m^2 or higher, open bariatric procedures, functional status of total dependency before surgery, prior coronary intervention, dyspnea at preoperative evaluation, more than 10% unintentional weight loss in 6 months, and bleeding disorders. Risk stratification based on the number of preoperative comorbid factors showed an exponential increase in mortality as follows: 0 to 1 comorbidities (0.03%), 2 to 3 comorbidities (0.16%), and 4 comorbidities or more (7.4%). Notably, baseline functional status before surgery is the single most powerful predictor of perioperative survival.

Aminian and colleagues[53] reviewed cases of primary LSG using the ACS-NSQIP. Thirty-day postoperative mortality and composite adverse events rates were 0.05% and 2.4%, respectively. Early reoperation was observed in 1.4%. A user-friendly version of the risk calculator is accessible at http://www.r-calc.

In our institution, all patients deemed to be medically high risk initially undergo a thorough medical assessment. Based on this assessment, the patient is referred for additional investigations or consultation with other specialties as indicated. We believe thorough risk stratification and risk factor optimization, as well as postoperative medical expertise and management, for these high-risk patients are essential.

SPECIAL HIGH-RISK POPULATIONS
Patients with Severe End-Organ Disease

As the rate of obesity increases in the general population, so does the incidence of obesity-related diseases such as hypertension, diabetes, hyperlipidemia, nonalcoholic fatty liver disease (NAFLD)/nonalcoholic steatohepatitis (NASH), which in turn can lead to severe end-organ failure that can lead to organ transplantation. Diet, exercise, and medication in general are not reliable weight loss options for patients with end-organ disease; hence, bariatric surgery should be considered.[54] Many centers exclude obese patients from transplantation programs. Obesity with its associated comorbid conditions may lead to early graft failure and poor outcome, including death after transplantation.[55] Considerations on which is the best bariatric procedure and timing of the procedure are the current debate. As the epidemic progresses and less invasive treatments for metabolic surgery evolve, we are likely to see more patients lose weight before transplantation.[56] Additional details, such immunosuppression and absorption, should be taken into account in this high-risk population.

Cardiac Failure

Most patients with obesity cardiomyopathy have diastolic dysfunction. Data suggest that excess weight is likely an independent risk factor for cardiomyopathy and subsequent heart failure because of its effects on cardiac physiology and structure.[57] As this epidemic expands, physicians will continue to see an increasing number of obese patients with severe heart failure, some of whom will eventually progress to a point at which an orthotopic heart transplant may be the only means of long-term survival. Unfortunately, attaining successful weight loss in patients with significant heart failure using medical therapy alone can prove to be extremely difficult. Concomitant heart failure, multiple comorbidities, and limited exercise tolerance, results in high likelihood of the patients increasing their weight, worsening heart failure, and further limiting functional status. Patients with BMI greater than 35 kg/m^2 are 46% less likely to receive a heart transplant than normal-weight patients.[58] In the setting of patients who progress to needing a cardiac transplant, adequate weight loss after bariatric surgery will allow them to be considered as optimal cardiac graft recipients. Bariatric surgery, especially with the decreased risks associated with minimally invasive techniques, may be the only effective and durable treatment option for these patients. With adequate weight loss, some of these patients may become appropriate transplant recipients or delay or alleviate the need for transplantation.[57,59–64]

Data are not clear regarding the weight loss goal at which point it is safe to perform cardiac transplantation. Expert recommendation suggests weight loss to achieve a BMI of less than 30 kg/m^2 target before listing for cardiac transplantation (Level of Evidence: C),[65] most centers prefer to transplant patients with mild obesity (35 kg/m^2) due to long-term survival. Komoda and colleagues[66] reported that patients classified as overweight had a higher 1-year survival than both the normal-weight and obese individuals (74% vs 62% and 50.6%, respectively) a phenomenon described as the "obesity paradox."[67]

When selecting an optimal bariatric operation for a potential cardiac allograft recipient, one needs to consider how the procedure will affect absorption of immunosuppressive medication. LSG is a purely restrictive procedure and should not cause significant malabsorption of those vital medications. Operative times for LSG are considerably shorter than times seen while performing LRYGB and, therefore, make it an attractive option in this patient population.[63] During the immediate perioperative period, the patients should be managed by an anesthesiology team with experience in management of high-risk cardiac patients to ensure adequate heart function throughout the procedure. Postoperatively, these patients will also require a multidisciplinary approach, including intensive cardiac care, and access to a cardiologist and cardiac surgeons, as well as to bariatric specialists. Thus, routine operations on these patients can be safely performed only at tertiary centers with appropriate amenities. At our center, we have used several approaches to the obese patient with cardiac failure: concomitant bariatric surgery at the time of Left Ventricular Assist Device (LVAD) placement, LVAD for stabilization of cardiomyopathy followed by bariatric surgery to get on the transplant list, and finally post cardiac transplant to avoid the risks associated with excessive weight gain.

Lung Failure

According to International Society of Heart and Lung Transplantation criteria, high BMI of 30 kg/m^2 or higher is a relative contraindication for lung transplantation.[68] Because of the increased mortality and decreased graft function seen in obese transplant patients, several published guidelines for lung transplantation have included obesity (BMI >25–30 kg/m^2) as a contraindication to lung transplantation.[69–71] Kanasky and colleagues[71] analyzed 85 lung transplant recipients and found that a pretransplant BMI of greater than 30 kg/m^2 was the strongest independent predictor of posttransplant mortality, with a threefold increase in risk.

Mathier and colleagues[72] report a case of a morbidly obese patient with severe pulmonary arterial hypertension (PAH) and functional impairment who underwent LRYGB. A 3-drug combination regimen consisting of oral bosentan and sildenafil and inhaled iloprost produced sufficient hemodynamic improvement to allow for the performance of bariatric surgery. BMI was 49.9 kg/m^2, and he walked a distance of 257 m during the 6MWT. Over the first 7 months following surgery, the patient had a substantial decrease in weight (to 106.8 kg) and BMI (to 33.7 kg/m^2). Over the subsequent 7 months, body weight, oxygen requirement, functional class, and 6-minute walk distance all improved dramatically despite the persistence of PAH. Although such surgery is typically denied to patients with PAH, we suggest that aggressive medical therapy for patients with PAH may allow for its safe performance, and that the clinical improvement resulting from the subsequent weight loss may be quite dramatic.

A case report of an obese patient with end-stage rheumatoid interstitial lung disease and severe pulmonary hypertension was determined to be nearing the requirement for lung transplantation but was excluded from consideration because of her obesity. She achieved a BMI of less than 30 kg/m^2 at 5 months after surgery and was accepted as a lung transplant candidate after LRYGB. Her marked improvement in functional status has delayed her need for a lung transplantation by 2 years or longer. The investigators suggested the creation of specialized "high-risk" bariatric surgical services.[73]

Liver Failure

Parallel to the epidemic of obesity, a major increase in NAFLD has been recorded in Western countries. Leonard and colleagues[74] noted that between 1990 and 2003, the percentage of liver transplant candidates obese at the time of transplantation increased from 15% to 25%, and later, Kim and colleagues[75] reported that, by 2011, 34.4% of liver transplant candidates were obese.[76] Perez-Protto and colleagues[77] showed no significant association between obesity and any other long-term adverse outcomes and recommended that morbid obesity per se should not exclude patients from consideration for transplantation; however, obesity still remains a contraindication for the American Association for the Study of Liver Diseases and obese patients suffer from a limited access to liver transplantation.[78] There are no data to support an absolute cutoff for BMI and liver transplantation, although patients with a BMI greater than 40 kg/m^2 are likely to have an increased postoperative and long-term mortality.[79,80]

Laparoscopic adjustable gastric banding (LAGB) and LSG seem to be feasible and effective for weight loss in strictly selected patients. Nevertheless, complication rates are 3 to 4 times higher than in the general population, with a staple line leak rate of 14.3% and a reoperation rate of 12.5%. LSG is the most common technique used.[81] This technique has been preferred because it does not modify the endoscopic access to the biliary tract and, theoretically, does not include any intestinal bypass; thus, it does not affect the absorption of immunosuppressive medications.

Endoscopic access to the biliary tree after LRYGB remains a real issue. Biliary complications are not infrequent after liver transplantation, as they have been reported in up to 17% of patients after deceased donor liver transplantation.[82] Bile leaks usually occur in the early postoperative period, and strictures can occur even several years later.[83] However, this may not be a true limitation, as biliary complications can be managed by interventional radiology by the transhepatic route[84] or by surgical access to the remnant stomach.[85–87]

All possibilities have been explored regarding the timing of bariatric surgery and liver transplantation. It seems logical to reduce weight in transplant candidates, but this approach has some limitations, as operating on transplant candidates comes down to operating on cirrhotic and often malnourished patients. Limitations to this approach are secondary to the fact that one-third of transplant recipients develop a de novo obesity and metabolic syndrome in the years following liver transplantation.[81] Bariatric surgery before liver transplantation probably improves the outcome of liver transplantation; its real impact on the natural history of obesity (and its comorbidities) in liver recipients seems to be limited.

In the 2 studies on bariatric surgery before liver transplantation, mortality was nil and reoperation rates were 5.0% and 16.6%.[88–90] Endoscopic procedures have been performed as a first step preceding liver transplantation. Balloon was performed in a patient on the waitlist for liver transplantation with a BMI of 47 kg/m^2. The patient lost 18 kg with a reduction of almost 6 points of BMI (41.3 kg/m^2). Liver transplantation took place more than 2 years later and was complicated by a biliary stenosis. As endoscopic treatment happened to be unsatisfactory, a surgical repair was planned, and a Roux-en-Y biliary diversion was performed at the same time. Choundary and colleagues[91] reported intragastric balloon placement before liver transplantation. Weight loss was consistent: BMI reduced up to 9.2 kg/m^2. 5 out of 8 patients underwent successful liver transplantation.

Bariatric surgery concomitant to liver transplantation could be an interesting option, as it would reduce the number of major surgeries. Patients undergo 2 major surgeries while still in a poor nutritional status and receive an intensive immunosuppression therapy, yet have a new functional liver. Combined liver transplantation with LAGB[92] and LSG[93] has been reported with variable degrees of success.

The third possibility is bariatric surgery after liver transplantation. The clear advantage of this approach is the selection of patients surviving liver transplantation and developing (or maintaining) obesity in the following years. Intervention is reported as technically challenging and has been performed directly by an open approach.[81] Morbidity is higher than in the general population and a reoperation rate of 33% has been reported.[90] Al-Nowaylati and colleagues[94] observed that with open Roux-en-Y gastric bypass after liver transplantation there was a therapeutic weight loss, improved glycemic control, and improved high-density lipoprotein levels in the presence of continued dyslipidemia. Duchini and Brunson[95] successfully performed an LRYGB on 2 morbidly obese patients who received liver transplantation and achieved resolution of their marked steatohepatitis and other metabolic abnormalities.

Lin and colleagues,[90] in a report of 9 morbidly obese patients with prior liver transplants, concluded LSG is technically feasible after liver transplantation and resulted in weight loss without adversely affecting graft function and immunosuppression. Three complications were reported. Calcineurin inhibitor levels and hepatic and renal functions remained stable with no episodes of graft rejection. Patients undergoing bariatric surgery years after liver transplantation have lower doses of immunosuppressing drugs and are usually in a better nutritional status. However, data on liver function and immunosuppression therapy after bariatric surgery are still lacking.

Recommendations on optimal timing of bariatric surgery and liver transplantation are limited to the number of studies reported. In view of the complexity of patients, we consider the mortality and morbidity rates are acceptable; nevertheless, they should be interpreted with caution because of the heterogeneity in the bariatric procedures used, the incompleteness of the data, and the presence of case reports that may represent a selection bias.

Cirrhosis

A few studies have been published on cirrhosis and bariatric surgery.[48–51] In most of those cases, cirrhosis was unknown before the bariatric procedure and when the Child-Pugh classification was used, almost all patients were Child A. Complications rated up to 34.8% have been reported, with a leak rate of up to 12.5%.[48] Mortality was also higher than in the general population.[52,53] In single-center studies, 1 death occurred in the early postoperative time of 61 patients.[48–50] Nevertheless, in a national survey, surgeons responding to the questionnaire reported a mortality rate for patients with cirrhosis after bariatric surgery of 4%.[50] Similarly, a register study, based on the National Income Sample, reported a 1.2% mortality for this specific population.[51]

Kidney Failure

In 2006, of all patients starting dialysis, 34.6% had a BMI higher than 30, compared with only 19.1% in 1995[96]; by 2009, this proportion had risen to 37.9%. Obese patients with end-stage renal disease (ESRD) who receive a kidney transplant experience greater rates of posttransplantation diabetes, delayed graft function,[97] and local wound complications. Ahmadi and colleagues[98] meta-analyses indicated that compared to normal BMI, underweight, overweight, and obese levels of BMI were associated with higher mortality. Jamal and colleagues[96] retrospectively reviewed 21 dialysis patients. Eighteen patients underwent LRYGB, 2 patients underwent LSG, and 1 patient LAGB. Early major complications (<30 days of surgery) occurred in 2 patients (1 anastomotic leak and 1 anastomotic stricture). Four patients had a late complication. There was 1 death in this cohort, at 45 days after LRYGB, that was unrelated to a surgery. The group concluded chronic renal failure requiring dialysis should not be considered a contraindication to bariatric surgery.

Modanlou and colleagues[99] examined Medicare billing claims within US Renal Data System registry data (1991–2004). Of 188 bariatric surgery cases, 72 were performed prelisting, 29 on the wait list, and 87 posttransplant. LRYGB was the most common procedure. Thirty-day mortality after bariatric surgery performed on the wait list and posttransplant was 3.5%, and 1 transplant recipient lost the graft within 30 days after bariatric surgery. Nearly 70% of the candidates who underwent bariatric surgery while on the wait list were ultimately transplanted.

In a study of 19 patients with chronic renal failure at the time of LRYGB, 8 had transplantation followed by LRYGB, and 3 had LRYGB and then transplantation. Eight patients, with a mean age of 38.4 ± 4.2 years at time of transplantation, became morbidly obese after transplantation and developed secondary complications related to being overweight. Seven of these patients were on steroids at the time of LRYGB. The mean time to LRYGB was 5.6 ± 0.6 years. The mean BMI at the time of LRYGB was 48.9 ± 2.3, and the reduction in excess BMI at 1, 2, and 3 years was 70.9%, 76.5%, and 69.7%, respectively. In patients with LRYGB and then transplantation, the average time to transplantation was 1.7 ± 0.0 years, and the average BMI at time of transplantation was 32 ± 3.8.[100]

More recently, laparoscopic LSG has gained acceptance as an effective weight-loss procedure.[89,101,102] Golomb and colleagues[103] published the most recent series of 10 cases of LSG that occurred on average 6 years after transplantation. The median decrease in BMI was −13 kg/m^2 with an average % EBWL of 75% at 1 year. One patient failed weight control with sleeve gastrectomy and required conversion to biliopancreatic diversion at 14 months. Contrary to an LRYGB, there is no malabsorption and no intestinal anastomoses. The decreased complexity of the operation makes it an attractive option in high-risk patients.

LRYGB, on the other hand, has been shown to have excellent lifelong results,[102,104–107] relative risk reduction in mortality, and no effects on posttransplant dosing regimens.[102] Takata and colleagues[88] in a retrospective review of the 15 patients to evaluate the safety and efficacy of LRYGB in patients with ESRD and laparoscopic LSG in patients with cirrhosis or end-stage lung disease determined obesity-associated comorbidities improved or resolved in all patients. No mortality was reported and only 2 patients developed complications (both with cirrhosis). Of 15 patients, 93% reached the BMI limit for transplantation. Unfortunately, these 2 series had heterogeneous populations mixing liver, lung, and kidney patients, making generalizations to the renal failure population difficult.[108]

Koshy and colleagues[54] reported 3 patients who underwent LAGB which enabled sufficient weight loss to gain eligibility for kidney transplantation. All these patients subsequently underwent successful uncomplicated kidney transplantations.

Considering the malabsorptive sequelae of the LRYGB, there was a concern for altered absorption of micronutrients and immunosuppressants. A study of mycophenolic acid, tacrolimus, and sirolimus after LRYGB indicated that dosing levels would likely need to be higher, to account for the differences in pharmacokinetics, than in the nonbypass population.[109] Aside from steroids, however, current immunosuppressants may be effectively monitored using routine blood levels; however, it has been reported that the absorption of immune suppressors was not altered.[102,107]

In considering the balance of benefit and risk, the surgeon needs to compare the sum of the operative risks of bariatric surgery in the patient with chronic renal failure and the potentially improved risks of kidney transplantation in a less-obese recipient versus the combined risks of kidney transplantation in an obese candidate and the risks of bariatric surgery in an immunosuppressed patient.[108]

Pancreas

A report of 4 patients who underwent bariatric surgery before successful pancreas transplantation concluded LRYGB and LAGB present as equivalent alternatives for weight reduction in the population of morbidly obese diabetic patients who are possible candidates for pancreas transplantation. The investigators favored LAGB placement as a more suitable procedure.[110]

Immunosuppressed Patients

Given the rise in the incidence of severe obesity worldwide, more patients on chronic immunosuppressants are being referred for and are undergoing bariatric surgery, especially in the transplant-recipient or candidate population that is severely obese.[99] However, the literature on the postoperative outcomes in patients on chronic steroid or other immunosuppressants following primary bariatric surgery is limited.[111,112] Immunocompromised patients are at high risk of medical complications. Gagne and colleagues[111] reported in their retrospective review of 61 patients, a total of 26 complications in 20 patients; 49 patients no longer required immunosuppressive medications owing to improvement of their underlying disease. The group concluded that immunocompromised patients can safely undergo bariatric surgery with good weight loss results and improvement in comorbidities. Andalib and colleagues[112] using the ACS-NSQIP database found that the 30-day postoperative mortality rate among patients who are dependent on chronic use of steroids/immunosuppressants after primary bariatric surgery was near sevenfold higher than that for nondependent patients. The occurrences of major morbidity in the 30-day postoperative period were also more than twofold higher in the steroid/immunosuppressant-dependent patient compared with the nondependent patients. The investigators concluded LRYGB did not pose a higher risk than LSG in terms of 30-day postoperative morbidity.

Aside from steroids, however, current immunosuppressants may be effectively monitored using routine blood levels; however, it has been reported that the absorption of immune suppressors was not altered.[102,107] It was shown that the absorption of tacrolimus and sirolimus occurs mainly in the proximal duodenum. This site of absorption is practically excluded in the LRYGB transplant patients. Therefore, substantially higher dosing of the immunosuppression is needed to achieve therapeutic levels of these drugs.[109] Other comorbidities and complications represent a challenge in the management of immunosuppressed patients. Although an uncommon complication, leaks could be more complicated to manage in a patient on immunosuppressive medication.[108]

Intraoperative Conduct

In an effort to minimize the associated morbidity and mortality in patients with high BMI, several surgeons have advocated a 2-stage approach. The conduct in the operating room is to minimize operative time while ensuring integrity of the anastomoses. Regan and colleagues[113] described the 2-stage operation, which consists of an LSG (first stage) to be followed by an LRYGB or duodenal switch (second stage). Aminian and colleagues[25] suggested LSG as a durable procedure with less morbidity and mortality, such as LSG is more appropriate and can also be devised into a 2-step surgical approach, which could reduce the early operative mortality and improve the comorbidity profile. The rationale is that the first-stage operation, LSG, is comparatively simple (no anastomosis) and quick. The LSG is a lower-risk option in these high-risk patients compared with LRYGB, but it is probably less effective in terms of maximal weight loss. Initial weight loss with the stage 1 procedure is effective in reducing operative risk. The second stage, which involves the gastrojejunostomy and jejunoje-junostomy and is the more technically challenging aspect of the LRYGB, is performed in a much lower-risk patient who is technically much less challenging because of the weight loss from stage 1.[43]

Postoperative Management

High volume and near-ubiquitous utilization of a minimally invasive approach, combined with advancement in perioperative care, have further mitigated postoperative morbidity in high-risk bariatric patients. Risk factors identified during preoperative work up should direct postoperative care using a multidisciplinary approach. Close attention to detail promotes optimal outcomes. Judicious fluid management is key to avoid dehydration or fluid overload. Laboratory data monitors post operative complications, commonly bleeding, AKI or rhabdomyolysis. Prompt imaging in suspected complications is effective in diagnosing and triggering early interventions. DVT/PE prophylaxis and early ambulation with dedicated team of physical therapist provides the patient with an advantage to avoid undesired events. A comprehensive multidisciplinary preoperative assessment is of great importance In the special organ failure high-risk populations, active comanagement with the organ expert and the transplant team is essential for good patient outcomes. Immunosuppressive medication levels need to be followed closely in the perioperative period.

REFERENCES

1. Ogden CL, Carroll MD, Kit BK, et al. Prevalence of childhood and adult obesity in the United States, 2011-2012. JAMA 2014;311(8):806–14.
2. Buchwald H, Avidor Y, Braunwald E, et al. Bariatric surgery: a systematic review and meta-analysis. JAMA 2004;292(14):1724–37.
3. Brethauer SA, Aminian A, Romero-Talamás H, et al. Can diabetes be surgically cured? Long-term metabolic effects of bariatric surgery in obese patients with type 2 diabetes mellitus. Ann Surg 2013;258(4):628–36 [discussion: 636–7].
4. Schauer PR, Bhatt DL, Kirwan JP, et al. Bariatric surgery versus intensive medical therapy for diabetes–3-year outcomes. N Engl J Med 2014;370(21):2002–13.
5. Zamboni M, Mazzali G. Obesity in the elderly: an emerging health issue. Int J Obes (Lond) 2012;36(9):1151–2.
6. Nassif PA, Malafaia O, Ribas-Filho JM, et al. When and why operate elderly obese. Arq Bras Cir Dig 2015;28(Suppl 1):84–5.
7. Ogden CL, Carroll MD, Curtin LR, et al. Prevalence of overweight and obesity in the United States, 1999-2004. JAMA 2006;295(13):1549–55.
8. Villareal DT, Apovian CM, Kushner RF, et al. Obesity in older adults: technical review and position statement of the American Society for Nutrition and NAASO, the obesity society. Am J Clin Nutr 2005;82(5):923–34.
9. Zamboni M, Mazzali G, Zoico E, et al. Health consequences of obesity in the elderly: a review of four unresolved questions. Int J Obes (Lond) 2005;29(9):1011–29.
10. Livingston EH, Huerta S, Arthur D, et al. Male gender is a predictor of morbidity and age a predictor of mortality for patients undergoing gastric bypass surgery. Ann Surg 2002;236(5):576–82.
11. Sosa JL, Pombo H, Pallavicini H, et al. Laparoscopic gastric bypass beyond age 60. Obes Surg 2004;14(10):1398–401.
12. Livingston EH, Langert J. The impact of age and Medicare status on bariatric surgical outcomes. Arch Surg 2006;141(11):1115–20 [discussion: 1121].

13. Nguyen NT, Nguyen B, Smith B, et al. Proposal for a bariatric mortality risk classification system for patients undergoing bariatric surgery. Surg Obes Relat Dis 2013;9(2):239–46.
14. Farinholt GN, Carr AD, Chang EJ, et al. A call to arms: obese men with more severe comorbid disease and underutilization of bariatric operations. Surg Endosc 2013;27(12):4556–63.
15. Natvik E, Gjengedal E, Moltu C, et al. Translating weight loss into agency: men's experiences 5 years after bariatric surgery. Int J Qual Stud Health Well-being 2015;10:27729.
16. Maciejewski ML, Winegar DA, Farley JF, et al. Risk stratification of serious adverse events after gastric bypass in the bariatric outcomes longitudinal database. Surg Obes Relat Dis 2012;8(6):671–7.
17. Arterburn D, Livingston EH, Schifftner T, et al. Predictors of long-term mortality after bariatric surgery performed in Veterans Affairs medical centers. Arch Surg 2009;144(10):914–20.
18. Zhang W, Mason EE, Renquist KE, et al. Factors influencing survival following surgical treatment of obesity. Obes Surg 2005;15(1):43–50.
19. Flegal KM, Carroll MD, Kit BK, et al. Prevalence of obesity and trends in the distribution of body mass index among US adults, 1999-2010. JAMA 2012;307(5): 491–7.
20. Arterburn DE, Courcoulas AP. Bariatric surgery for obesity and metabolic conditions in adults. BMJ 2014;349:g3961.
21. Maciejewski ML, Livingston EH, Smith VA, et al. Survival among high-risk patients after bariatric surgery. JAMA 2011;305(23):2419–26.
22. Flegal KM, Carroll MD, Ogden CL, et al. Prevalence and trends in obesity among US adults, 1999-2008. JAMA 2010;303(3):235–41.
23. Sturm R. Increases in morbid obesity in the USA: 2000-2005. Public Health 2007;121(7):492–6.
24. DeMaria EJ, Portenier D, Wolfe L. Obesity surgery mortality risk score: proposal for a clinically useful score to predict mortality risk in patients undergoing gastric bypass. Surg Obes Relat Dis 2007;3(2):134–40.
25. Aminian A, Jamal MH, Andalib A, et al. Is laparoscopic bariatric surgery a safe option in extremely high-risk morbidly obese patients? J Laparoendosc Adv Surg Tech A 2015;25(9):707–11.
26. Daigle CR, Andalib A, Corcelles R, et al. Bariatric and metabolic outcomes in the super-obese elderly. Surg Obes Relat Dis 2015;12:132–7.
27. Winegar DA, Sherif B, Pate V, et al. Venous thromboembolism after bariatric surgery performed by Bariatric Surgery Center of Excellence Participants: analysis of the Bariatric Outcomes Longitudinal Database. Surg Obes Relat Dis 2011; 7(2):181–8.
28. Longitudinal Assessment of Bariatric Surgery (LABS) Consortium, Flum DR, Belle SH, et al. Perioperative safety in the longitudinal assessment of bariatric surgery. N Engl J Med 2009;361(5):445–54.
29. Parker SG, McGlone ER, Knight WR, et al. Enoxaparin venous thromboembolism prophylaxis in bariatric surgery: a best evidence topic. Int J Surg 2015; 23(Pt A):52–6.
30. Mechanick JI, Kushner RF, Sugerman HJ, et al. American Association of Clinical Endocrinologists, the Obesity Society, and American Society for Metabolic & Bariatric Surgery medical guidelines for clinical practice for the perioperative nutritional, metabolic, and nonsurgical support of the bariatric surgery patient. Endocr Pract 2008;14(Suppl 1):1–83.

31. McTigue K, Larson JC, Valoski A, et al. Mortality and cardiac and vascular outcomes in extremely obese women. JAMA 2006;296(1):79–86.

32. Poirier P, Alpert MA, Fleisher LA, et al. Cardiovascular evaluation and management of severely obese patients undergoing surgery: a science advisory from the American Heart Association. Circulation 2009;120(1):86–95.

33. Frey WC, Pilcher J. Obstructive sleep-related breathing disorders in patients evaluated for bariatric surgery. Obes Surg 2003;13(5):676–83.

34. O'Keeffe T, Patterson EJ. Evidence supporting routine polysomnography before bariatric surgery. Obes Surg 2004;14(1):23–6.

35. Piper AJ, Grunstein RR. Obesity hypoventilation syndrome: mechanisms and management. Am J Respir Crit Care Med 2011;183(3):292–8.

36. Vasu TS, Grewal R, Doghramji K. Obstructive sleep apnea syndrome and perioperative complications: a systematic review of the literature. J Clin Sleep Med 2012;8(2):199–207.

37. Buchwald H, Estok R, Fahrbach K, et al. Weight and type 2 diabetes after bariatric surgery: systematic review and meta-analysis. Am J Med 2009;122(3): 248–56.e5.

38. Schauer PR, Kashyap SR, Wolski K, et al. Bariatric surgery versus intensive medical therapy in obese patients with diabetes. N Engl J Med 2012;366(17): 1567–76.

39. de Souza SA, Faintuch J, Fabris SM, et al. Six-minute walk test: functional capacity of severely obese before and after bariatric surgery. Surg Obes Relat Dis 2009;5(5):540–3.

40. Fontaine KR, Barofsky I. Obesity and health-related quality of life. Obes Rev 2001;2(3):173–82.

41. Melissas J, Kontakis G, Volakakis E, et al. The effect of surgical weight reduction on functional status in morbidly obese patients with low back pain. Obes Surg 2005;15(3):378–81.

42. Maniscalco M, Zedda A, Giardiello C, et al. Effect of bariatric surgery on the six-minute walk test in severe uncomplicated obesity. Obes Surg 2006;16(7): 836–41.

43. DeMaria EJ, Schauer P, Patterson E, et al. The optimal surgical management of the super-obese patient: the debate. Presented at the annual meeting of the Society of American Gastrointestinal and Endoscopic Surgeons, Hollywood, Florida, USA, April 13-16, 2005. Surg Innov 2005;12(2):107–21.

44. Nesset EM, Kendrick ML, Houghton SG, et al. A two-decade spectrum of revisional bariatric surgery at a tertiary referral center. Surg Obes Relat Dis 2007; 3(1):25–30 [discussion: 30].

45. Coakley BA, Deveney CW, Spight DH, et al. Revisional bariatric surgery for failed restrictive procedures. Surg Obes Relat Dis 2008;4(5):581–6.

46. Turner PL, Saager L, Dalton J, et al. A nomogram for predicting surgical complications in bariatric surgery patients. Obes Surg 2011;21(5):655–62.

47. Gupta PK, Franck C, Miller WJ, et al. Development and validation of a bariatric surgery morbidity risk calculator using the prospective, multicenter NSQIP dataset. J Am Coll Surg 2011;212(3):301–9.

48. Ramanan B, Gupta PK, Gupta H, et al. Development and validation of a bariatric surgery mortality risk calculator. J Am Coll Surg 2012;214(6):892–900.

49. Sharma AM, Kushner RF. A proposed clinical staging system for obesity. Int J Obes (Lond) 2009;33(3):289–95.

50. Padwal RS, Pajewski NM, Allison DB, et al. Using the Edmonton obesity staging system to predict mortality in a population-representative cohort of people with overweight and obesity. CMAJ 2011;183(14):E1059–66.

51. De Cos AI, Cardenas JJ, Pelegrina B, et al. Obesity associated risk using Edmonton staging in bariatric surgery. Nutr Hosp 2015;31(1):196–202 [in Spanish].

52. Khan MA, Grinberg R, Johnson S, et al. Perioperative risk factors for 30-day mortality after bariatric surgery: is functional status important? Surg Endosc 2013;27(5):1772–7.

53. Aminian A, Brethauer SA, Sharafkhah M, et al. Development of a sleeve gastrectomy risk calculator. Surg Obes Relat Dis 2015;11(4):758–64.

54. Koshy AN, Coombes JS, Wilkinson S, et al. Laparoscopic gastric banding surgery performed in obese dialysis patients prior to kidney transplantation. Am J Kidney Dis 2008;52(4):e15–7.

55. Udgiri NR, Kashyap R, Minz M. The impact of body mass index on renal transplant outcomes: a significant independent risk factor for graft failure and patient death. Transplantation 2003;75(2):249.

56. Killackey M, Zhang R, Sparks K, et al. Challenges of abdominal organ transplant in obesity. South Med J 2010;103(6):532–40.

57. McCloskey CA, Ramani GV, Mathier MA, et al. Bariatric surgery improves cardiac function in morbidly obese patients with severe cardiomyopathy. Surg Obes Relat Dis 2007;3(5):503–7.

58. Weiss ES, Allen JG, Russell SD, et al. Impact of recipient body mass index on organ allocation and mortality in orthotopic heart transplantation. J Heart Lung Transplant 2009;28(11):1150–7.

59. Ristow B, Rabkin J, Haeusslein E. Improvement in dilated cardiomyopathy after bariatric surgery. J Card Fail 2008;14(3):198–202.

60. Ramani GV, McCloskey C, Ramanathan RC, et al. Safety and efficacy of bariatric surgery in morbidly obese patients with severe systolic heart failure. Clin Cardiol 2008;31(11):516–20.

61. Samaras K, Connolly SM, Lord RV, et al. Take heart: bariatric surgery in obese patients with severe heart failure. Two case reports. Heart Lung Circ 2012; 21(12):847–9.

62. Gill RS, Karmali S, Nagandran J, et al. Combined ventricular assist device placement with adjustable gastric band (VAD-BAND): a promising new technique for morbidly obese patients awaiting potential cardiac transplantation. J Clin Med Res 2012;4(2):127–9.

63. Wikiel KJ, McCloskey CA, Ramanathan RC. Bariatric surgery: a safe and effective conduit to cardiac transplantation. Surg Obes Relat Dis 2014;10(3):479–84.

64. Chaudhry UI, Kanji A, Sai-Sudhakar CB, et al. Laparoscopic sleeve gastrectomy in morbidly obese patients with end-stage heart failure and left ventricular assist device: medium-term results. Surg Obes Relat Dis 2015;11(1):88–93.

65. Mehra MR, Kobashigawa J, Starling R, et al. Listing criteria for heart transplantation: International Society for Heart and Lung Transplantation guidelines for the care of cardiac transplant candidates–2006. J Heart Lung Transplant 2006;25(9):1024–42.

66. Komoda T, Drews T, Hetzer R, et al. Overweight is advantageous for heart-transplant candidates to survive the period of critically ill status. ASAIO J 2012;58(4):390–5.

67. Chrysant SG, Chrysant GS. New insights into the true nature of the obesity paradox and the lower cardiovascular risk. J Am Soc Hypertens 2013;7(1): 85–94.

68. Ruttens D, Verleden SE, Vandermeulen E, et al. Body mass index in lung transplant candidates: a contra-indication to transplant or not? Transplant Proc 2014; 46(5):1506–10.
69. Glanville AR, Estenne M. Indications, patient selection and timing of referral for lung transplantation. Eur Respir J 2003;22(5):845–52.
70. Orens JB, Estenne M, Arcasoy S, et al. International guidelines for the selection of lung transplant candidates: 2006 update–a consensus report from the Pulmonary Scientific Council of the International Society for Heart and Lung Transplantation. J Heart Lung Transplant 2006;25(7):745–55.
71. Kanasky WF Jr, Anton SD, Rodrigue JR, et al. Impact of body weight on long-term survival after lung transplantation. Chest 2002;121(2):401–6.
72. Mathier MA, Zhang J, Ramanathan RC. Dramatic functional improvement following bariatric surgery in a patient with pulmonary arterial hypertension and morbid obesity. Chest 2008;133(3):789–92.
73. Martin MJ, Bennett S. Pretransplant bariatric surgery: a new indication? Surg Obes Relat Dis 2007;3(6):648–51.
74. Leonard J, Heimbach JK, Malinchoc M, et al. The impact of obesity on long-term outcomes in liver transplant recipients—results of the NIDDK liver transplant database. Am J Transplant 2008;8(3):667–72.
75. Kim WR, Stock PG, Smith JM, et al. OPTN/SRTR 2011 annual data report: liver. Am J Transplant 2013;13(Suppl 1):73–102.
76. Beckmann S, Ivanović N, Drent G, et al. Weight gain, overweight and obesity in solid organ transplantation–a study protocol for a systematic literature review. Syst Rev 2015;4:2.
77. Perez-Protto SE, Quintini C, Reynolds LF, et al. Comparable graft and patient survival in lean and obese liver transplant recipients. Liver Transpl 2013;19(8): 907–15.
78. Murray KF, Carithers RL Jr, AASLD. AASLD practice guidelines: evaluation of the patient for liver transplantation. Hepatology 2005;41(6):1407–32.
79. Newsome PN, Allison ME, Andrews PA, et al. Guidelines for liver transplantation for patients with non-alcoholic steatohepatitis. Gut 2012;61(4):484–500.
80. Saab S, Lalezari D, Pruthi P, et al. The impact of obesity on patient survival in liver transplant recipients: a meta-analysis. Liver Int 2015;35(1):164–70.
81. Lazzati A, Iannelli A, Schneck AS, et al. Bariatric surgery and liver transplantation: a systematic review a new frontier for bariatric surgery. Obes Surg 2015; 25(1):134–42.
82. Duailibi DF, Ribeiro MA Jr. Biliary complications following deceased and living donor liver transplantation: a review. Transplant Proc 2010;42(2):517–20.
83. Verdonk RC, Buis CI, Porte RJ, et al. Anastomotic biliary strictures after liver transplantation: causes and consequences. Liver Transpl 2006;12(5):726–35.
84. Lastovickova J, Peregrin J. Biliary strictures after orthotopic liver transplantation: long-term results of percutaneous treatment in patients with nonfeasible endoscopic therapy. Transplant Proc 2012;44(5):1379–84.
85. Patel JA, Patel NA, Shinde T, et al. Endoscopic retrograde cholangiopancreatography after laparoscopic Roux-en-Y gastric bypass: a case series and review of the literature. Am Surg 2008;74(8):689–93 [discussion: 693–4].
86. Ceppa FA, Gagné DJ, Papasavas PK, et al. Laparoscopic transgastric endoscopy after Roux-en-Y gastric bypass. Surg Obes Relat Dis 2007;3(1):21–4.
87. Richardson JF, Lee JG, Smith BR, et al. Laparoscopic transgastric endoscopy after Roux-en-Y gastric bypass: case series and review of the literature. Am Surg 2012;78(10):1182–6.

88. Takata MC, Campos GM, Ciovica R, et al. Laparoscopic bariatric surgery improves candidacy in morbidly obese patients awaiting transplantation. Surg Obes Relat Dis 2008;4(2):159–64 [discussion: 164–5].

89. Lin MY, Tavakol MM, Sarin A, et al. Laparoscopic sleeve gastrectomy is safe and efficacious for pretransplant candidates. Surg Obes Relat Dis 2013;9(5):653–8.

90. Lin MY, Tavakol MM, Sarin A, et al. Safety and feasibility of sleeve gastrectomy in morbidly obese patients following liver transplantation. Surg Endosc 2013; 27(1):81–5.

91. Choudhary NS, Puri R, Saraf N, et al. Intragastric balloon as a novel modality for weight loss in patients with cirrhosis and morbid obesity awaiting liver transplantation. Indian J Gastroenterol 2016;35(2):113–6.

92. Campsen J, Zimmerman M, Shoen J, et al. Adjustable gastric banding in a morbidly obese patient during liver transplantation. Obes Surg 2008;18(12):1625–7.

93. Heimbach JK, Watt KD, Poterucha JJ, et al. Combined liver transplantation and gastric sleeve resection for patients with medically complicated obesity and end-stage liver disease. Am J Transplant 2013;13(2):363–8.

94. Al-Nowaylati AR, Al-Haddad BJ, Dorman RB, et al. Gastric bypass after liver transplantation. Liver Transpl 2013;19(12):1324–9.

95. Duchini A, Brunson ME. Roux-en-Y gastric bypass for recurrent nonalcoholic steatohepatitis in liver transplant recipients with morbid obesity. Transplantation 2001;72(1):156–9.

96. Jamal MH, Corcelles R, Daigle CR, et al. Safety and effectiveness of bariatric surgery in dialysis patients and kidney transplantation candidates. Surg Obes Relat Dis 2015;11(2):419–23.

97. Nicoletto BB, Fonseca NK, Manfro RC, et al. Effects of obesity on kidney transplantation outcomes: a systematic review and meta-analysis. Transplantation 2014;98(2):167–76.

98. Ahmadi SF, Zahmatkesh G, Streja E, et al. Body mass index and mortality in kidney transplant recipients: a systematic review and meta-analysis. Am J Nephrol 2014;40(4):315–24.

99. Modanlou KA, Muthyala U, Xiao H, et al. Bariatric surgery among kidney transplant candidates and recipients: analysis of the United States renal data system and literature review. Transplantation 2009;87(8):1167–73.

100. Alexander JW, Goodman HR, Gersin K, et al. Gastric bypass in morbidly obese patients with chronic renal failure and kidney transplant. Transplantation 2004; 78(3):469–74.

101. MacLaughlin HL, Hall WL, Patel AG, et al. Laparoscopic sleeve gastrectomy is a novel and effective treatment for obesity in patients with chronic kidney disease. Obes Surg 2012;22(1):119–23.

102. Szomstein S, Rojas R, Rosenthal RJ. Outcomes of laparoscopic bariatric surgery after renal transplant. Obes Surg 2010;20(3):383–5.

103. Golomb I, Winkler J, Ben-Yakov A, et al. Laparoscopic sleeve gastrectomy as a weight reduction strategy in obese patients after kidney transplantation. Am J Transplant 2014;14(10):2384–90.

104. Freeman CM, Woodle ES, Shi J, et al. Addressing morbid obesity as a barrier to renal transplantation with laparoscopic sleeve gastrectomy. Am J Transplant 2015;15(5):1360–8.

105. Tariq N, Moore LW, Sherman V. Bariatric surgery and end-stage organ failure. Surg Clin North Am 2013;93(6):1359–71.

106. Oberholzer J, Giulianotti P, Danielson KK, et al. Minimally invasive robotic kidney transplantation for obese patients previously denied access to transplantation. Am J Transplant 2013;13(3):721–8.
107. Arias RH, Mesa L, Posada JG, et al. Kidney transplantation and gastric bypass: a better control of comorbidities. Obes Surg 2010;20(7):851–4.
108. Chan G, Garneau P, Hajjar R. The impact and treatment of obesity in kidney transplant candidates and recipients. Can J Kidney Health Dis 2015;2:26.
109. Rogers CC, Alloway RR, Alexander JW, et al. Pharmacokinetics of mycophenolic acid, tacrolimus and sirolimus after gastric bypass surgery in end-stage renal disease and transplant patients: a pilot study. Clin Transplant 2008;22(3): 281–91.
110. Porubsky M, Powelson JA, Selzer DJ, et al. Pancreas transplantation after bariatric surgery. Clin Transplant 2012;26(1):E1–6.
111. Gagne DJ, Papasavas PK, Dovec EA, et al. Effect of immunosuppression on patients undergoing bariatric surgery. Surg Obes Relat Dis 2009;5(3):339–45.
112. Andalib A, Aminian A, Khorgami Z, et al. Early postoperative outcomes of primary bariatric surgery in patients on chronic steroid or immunosuppressive therapy. Obes Surg 2015. [Epub ahead of print].
113. Regan JP, Inabnet WB, Gagner M, et al. Early experience with two-stage laparoscopic Roux-en-Y gastric bypass as an alternative in the super-super obese patient. Obes Surg 2003;13(6):861–4.

Laparoscopic Sleeve Gastrectomy

Surgical Technique and Perioperative Care

Kellen Hayes, MD[a], George Eid, MD[a,b,c],*

KEYWORDS

- Laparoscopic sleeve gastrectomy • Bariatric surgical technique • Perioperative care

KEY POINTS

- Laparoscopic sleeve gastrectomy (LSG) has demonstrated durable long-term weight loss and metabolic improvements in obese patients.
- It has proved a safe procedure with a low complication rate in appropriately selected patients.
- Adherence to key surgical tenets is critical for safe and effective patient outcomes.

 Video content accompanies this article at http://www.surgical.theclinics.com

INTRODUCTION

Bariatric surgery has continued to evolve over the past several decades in terms of technique and indication not only for weight loss but also as an effective treatment of type 2 diabetes mellitus and metabolic syndrome abnormalities in general.[1] The STAMPEDE (The Surgical Therapy and Medications Potentially Eradicate Diabetes Efficiently) trial demonstrated bariatric surgery as superior to the best aggressive medical treatment in terms of durable weight loss and improvement of diabetes.[2] Although LSG is largely viewed as a restrictive procedure created for weight loss in patients with morbid obesity, it also has been beneficial in treating metabolic derangements. It has evolved into an increasingly popular procedure compared with the Roux-en-Y gastric bypass and adjustable gastric banding due to its less complex surgical technique and comparable outcomes to Roux-en-Y gastric bypass with regard to durable weight loss and improvement in metabolic syndrome abnormalities. A laparoscopic adaptation of

Disclosures: The authors have nothing to disclose.
[a] Bariatric and Metabolic Institute, Allegheny Health Network, Suite 314, 320 East North Ave, Pittsburgh, PA 15212, USA; [b] Biomedical Engineering, Carnegie Mellon University, Pittsburgh, PA, USA; [c] Temple University, Philadelphia, PA, USA
* Corresponding author. Bariatric and Metabolic Institute, Allegheny Health Network, Suite 314, 320 East North Ave, Pittsburgh, PA 15212.
E-mail address: geid@wpahs.org

Surg Clin N Am 96 (2016) 763–771
http://dx.doi.org/10.1016/j.suc.2016.03.015   surgical.theclinics.com
0039-6109/16/$ – see front matter © 2016 Elsevier Inc. All rights reserved.

the Magenstrasse and Mill procedure, LSG was initially created as the first step in a 2-part procedure (biliopancreatic diversion with duodenal switch) for supermorbid obese patients in whom traditional bypass surgery was thought too high risk based on their associated comorbidities. The same 2-stage approach has also been studied for Roux-en-Y gastric bypass.[3,4] The goal was to initiate surgical weight loss, thereby improving the patient candidacy for a more complex bypass procedure in the future. The surgery consisted of restrictive gastrectomy, removing up to 80% of the stomach along the greater curvature, with subsequent revision to duodenal switch or Roux-en-Y anatomy after appropriate weight loss had occurred to reduce surgical risk.[5] The sleeve gastrectomy has since been found to have comparable results to other weight loss procedures, including the Roux-en-Y gastric bypass, and has become an increasingly popular option among both surgeons and patients. Advantages of laparoscopic sleeve gastrectomy over the roux-en-Y gastric bypass includes acceptable use in patients with inflammatory bowel disease, patients who are transplant candidates (liver and kidney), and patients with complex prior abdominal surgery or complex abdominal wall hernias. It is also a pylorus-sparing procedure that eliminates the risk of dumping syndrome. Finally, there is no increased risk of marginal ulceration or internal hernias compared with traditional bypass surgery. It is not, however, considered an antireflux procedure. Therefore, Barrett esophagus may be a contraindication. The American Society of Metabolic and Bariatric Surgery has published position statements regarding the use of sleeve gastrectomy as a bariatric procedure, establishing its safety, efficacy, and durability.[6]

An expert consensus statement published in 2012 by Rosenthal and colleagues[7] addressed the key components of surgical technique, indications for surgery, and postoperative management as well as management of complications. This article describes surgical technique for LSG as well as the preoperative work-up and perioperative management of patients undergoing the procedure at the authors' institution.

PREOPERATIVE PLANNING

The preoperative work-up for bariatric surgery typically begins several months prior to the procedure. Most patients in need of bariatric surgery have multiple obesity-related comorbidities, which require cardiopulmonary work-up and clearances, including psychological, nutritional, and sleep study evaluation.

All patients receive extensive preoperative education from a multidisciplinary team specializing in bariatric surgical patients, including bariatric nurse coordinators, dieticians, nutritionists, and exercise physiologists. Standard biochemical blood work is obtained, including complete blood cell count, chemistry panel, liver and thyroid panels, and evaluation for any vitamin deficiencies.

Preoperative dietary modifications with evidence of discipline and the ability to sustain moderate weight loss are essential. For some high-risk patients, it is the authors' preference to place patients on a liquid low-calorie diet prior to surgery to enhance weight loss.[8] Preoperative weight loss not only improves obesity-related comorbidities but also improves visualization during surgery by decreasing intra-abdominal adipose tissue and decreasing liver volume. The authors previously described a significant reduction in both visceral and subcutaneous adipose tissue as well as reduction of liver volume after an average of 9 weeks on a low-calorie liquid diet.[9] To foster dietary compliance prior to surgery, patients are counseled in monthly dietary sessions with a certified dietician.

Cardiopulmonary work-up includes an adenosine stress test on patients older than 40 years with a history significant for coronary artery disease and associated risk factors. Patients with congestive heart failure are evaluated with an echocardiogram if no recent study is available. Routine chest radiograph is performed on all patients. Those at high risk for pulmonary complications receive a sleep study and pulmonary function tests and are optimized accordingly with bronchodilators and/or positive pressure airway devices. Perhaps most important are education and insistence on smoking cessation prior to surgery and the continuation of abstinence from nicotine products postoperatively given the significantly increased complication rate associated with smoking.[10]

There is controversy surrounding the necessity for preoperative esophagogastroduodenoscopy (EGD) prior to bariatric surgery. When performed routinely, gastric and esophageal pathology can be found in a significant number of patients, with gastritis, Barrett esophagitis, and hiatal hernias the most common findings.[11] In some patients, especially those undergoing revisional cases, medical and/or surgical therapy may be modified based on EGD findings; therefore, routine preoperative EGD is used.

SURGICAL TECHNIQUE

Many variations exist regarding surgical technique; however, the basic tenets of LSG should be stringently followed. These include pyloric preservation with gastrectomy beginning 2 cm to 6 cm proximal to the pylorus, mobilization of the entire greater curvature with exposure and identification of the left crus and base of the right crus, avoidance of stricture at the gastric incisura, and proper apposition of the anterior and posterior aspects of the stomach when stapling to prevent a corkscrewing effect of the sleeve and avoid a large retained fundic pouch.

The following describes the technique used at the authors' institution. Preoperative antibiotics are administered in accordance with Surgical Care Improvement Project guidelines. A prophylactic dose of subcutaneous heparin is also administered preoperatively. Patients are placed on an operating table in supine position with arms abducted. Sequential compression devices are placed and confirmed to be functioning. All pressure points are padded to prevent deep tissue injury. A footboard is placed under the patients' feet and firmly secured to the bed. The legs and hips are secured with safety straps to prevent bowing or buckling of the knees or ankles. A urinary catheter is placed after induction of general anesthesia.

Pneumoperitoneum to a pressure of 15 mm Hg is achieved through Veress needle technique at Palmer point in the left upper quadrant. The incision is made large enough for placement of a 5-mm port. A laparoscopic camera is introduced and the remainder of the abdomen is inspected for any anatomic abnormalities or iatrogenic injury. Adhesiolysis is performed as necessary. The remaining ports are placed in the following positions: a 12-mm periumbilical port located approximately 15 cm to 17 cm from the xiphoid process; two 5-mm ports placed in the right subcostal position; and a 15-mm port placed in the right upper quadrant. Finally, it is the authors' preference to retract the falciform ligament using a suture passed percutaneously and secured at skin level with a small clamp to better visualize the operative field. A liver retractor is then placed through the most lateral 5 mm right subcostal port and secured to a malleable hands-free device attached to the operating table. Liver retractors may also be placed through a subxiphoid incision; however, caution must be taken to avoid injury to the pericardium, which lies in close proximity.

Once all ports are placed and adequate visualization of the anatomy is achieved, an orogastric tube is placed and the stomach is deflated under direct visualization. The orogastric tube is then removed along with any other foreign devices (esophageal temperature probes and esophageal stethescope). The patient is then placed in steep reverse Trendelenburg position, allowing the transverse colon and small intestine to fall in a caudal direction. Because the stomach is large and extends from foregut to midabdomen, different degrees of Trendelenburg positioning may be used to facilitate better exposure in a large abdomen.

The dissection is begun by identifying the pylorus and taking down any associated adhesions with an advanced vessel sealing device. The entire greater curvature is then mobilized proximal to the pylorus, taking down the lesser omentum and freeing any attachments to the transverse colon and its mesentery. The greater curvature is mobilized to the angle of His. Great care must be taken when dissecting and sealing the short gastric arteries because they are high risk for intraoperative and postoperative bleeding. The splenic artery should be identified and preserved before proceeding with the dissection.

Dissection of the greater curvature is complete when the left crus can be readily identified and exposed where it meets the base of the right crus. Any hiatal hernias should be addressed at this time and repaired in a posterior fashion.[12] Bioabsorbable mesh is used to reinforce repair of large hiatal hernias. All attachments to the posterior stomach are then taken down. It is critical to identify and preserve the left gastric artery (or any large vessels) to the lesser curvature, because they are the only blood supply to the remaining stomach.

Once dissection is complete, a 36-French blunt-tipped bougie tube is placed and slowly advanced under direct visualization to the level of the pylorus. Non–blunt-tipped bougie tubes should not be used because they are at risk for stapling across the tapered distal aspect, during creation of the sleeve. Controversy exists regarding the proper size of the bougie tube and its relation to durable weight-loss outcomes. The use of a small-caliber tube may increase the risk of stricture, whereas a large tube may not provide an adequate restrictive sensation. The authors caution against the use of any bougie tube smaller than 32 French[13,14] due to increased risk of complications, which include making the sleeve too tight, potentially leading to obstruction especially at the gastric incisura.

Creation of the sleeve begins 3 cm proximal to the pylorus. A consensus article published by Rosenthal and colleagues[7] endorses the first staple load to start between 2 cm and 6 cm proximal to the pylorus. Before firing the stapler, the bougie tube must be visualized passing distal to the stapler along the lesser curvature. The largest available staple height should be used for the initial firing. The staple height may then be decreased for subsequent firings based on the thickness of the gastric tissue, which may vary between patients. If using buttressing material for the staple line, it may be beneficial to use a larger staple height to compensate for the added thickness of the buttressing material. It is critical to expose the stomach such that the anterior and posterior aspects are properly opposed using lateral traction. This prevents a corkscrewing effect of the sleeve as well as avoiding leaving a large posterior fundus. In addition, great care must be taken not to narrow the incisura angularis, leaving at least 2 cm of width to prevent obstruction. The staple line is created cephalad to the angle of His, taking care to avoid injury to the underlying pancreas or any critical vascular structures, such as the left gastric and splenic arteries. It is important to avoid stapling too close to the gastroesophageal junction because it is a vascular watershed area and damage could lead to ischemia and a higher leak rate.

Feared postoperative complications include bleeding and leakage of the staple line; therefore, it is preferred that staple-line reinforcement of some type be used. Controversy exists regarding the method of reinforcement. It is the authors' preference to create a running, inverting Lembert suture the entire length of the staple line. Other methods include a simple oversewing encompassing the staple line and the use of a staple buttressing material at the time of stapler firing. There does not seem to be superiority of any method, but consensus remains that some type of staple-line reinforcement should be used because it confers a lower incidence of bleeding.[7,15–19]

Once the sleeve is created, a leak test is preferable. It may be used by flooding the surgical field with irrigant and insufflating the remaining stomach. Resulting air bubbles denote the presence of a leak and should be addressed appropriately. Methylene blue may also be placed in the stomach and any spillage of blue contents into the peritoneal cavity assess. The authors' preference is to affix the greater curvature mesentery to the sleeve using a running locking suture for further fixation. The excluded stomach is then removed through the 15-mm port site under direct visualization to ensure no gross spillage of gastric contents. Surgical drains are not necessary unless there is high concern for bleeding or leak postoperatively. Drains may be more beneficial when performing revisional surgery, which expectedly has a higher risk of complications. The 15-mm and 12-mm port sites are then closed laparoscopically using a suture passing device under direct visualization. The liver retractor and all remaining ports are then removed and pneumoperitoneum is released.

In summary, there are multiple variations of surgical technique for creation of a gastric sleeve. Certain key aspects of the procedure are critical, however, for safe outcomes and durable weight loss. These include complete mobilization of the greater curvature and posterior stomach, visual identification of the left crus and the base of the right crus, avoidance of vascular compromise to the lesser curvature and gastroesophageal junction, proper apposition of the anterior and posterior aspects of the stomach while stapling to avoid corkscrewing and leaving a large posterior fundic pouch, avoidance of narrowing of the incisura angularis, and utilization of staple-line reinforcement.

See **Fig. 1** and Videos 1–14 for a demonstration of the key surgical procedures for creation of a gastric sleeve.

IMMEDIATE POSTOPERATIVE CARE

Consistent and reliable postoperative care with support staff familiar with bariatric patients is essential. Patients are initially kept nothing by mouth after surgery. On postoperative day 1, sips of water are initiated with a goal rate of 30 mL every 30 minutes. If patients can tolerate this diet, they are advanced to a low-sugar phase 1 bariatric diet, as desired, consisting of clear noncarbonated liquids. The oral intake goal is at least 64 mL of fluid per day.

Perhaps the most common postoperative complaint of sleeve gastrectomy patients is severe nausea. Therefore, antiemetics play an important role in the immediate

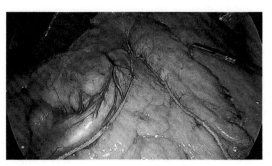

Fig. 1. LSG. (*Courtesy of* Dr Adrian Dan, Akron, Ohio.)

postoperative period to avoid undue stress on the staple line associated with retching and vomiting. It is the authors' preference to schedule 2 alternating antiemetics so that a patient receives 1 agent every 3 hours.

Routine deep vein thrombosis prophylaxis consists of sequential compression device placement and subcutaneous heparin. Maintenance intravenous fluids are administered and adequate urine output is closely monitored. Deep breathing and early ambulation are encouraged. The urinary catheter remains in place the night of surgery and is typically removed on postoperative day 1. Patient-controlled intravenous narcotics are used for pain management. These are discontinued on postoperative day 1 and transitioned to oral narcotic medication. If patients have obstructive sleep apnea and use a continuous positive airway device at home, they may use their machine the night of surgery and thereafter. Patients are typically discharged on postoperative day 2.

After discharge from the hospital, patients are continued on a phase 1 bariatric clear liquid diet for the first 7 days. This is advanced to a bariatric phase 2 pureed high-protein liquid diet for 4 weeks and then finally transitioned to a diet of soft foods. Patients are contacted at home several days after discharge for encouragement, diet reinforcement, and reminders to maintain hydration.

Postoperative patients require regular and frequent follow-up in clinic. They are seen at 1 week, 1 month, 3 months, 6 months, 12 months, 24 months, and then annually after the first year. Clinic visits consist of weight and nutritional monitoring as well as dietary counseling and psychology referral as needed. The importance of long-term follow-up with a surgeon is highly stressed. Ancillary avenues, such as support groups and social media, are also encouraged. Further rehabilitation and recovery consist of aerobic and anaerobic exercise starting 2 weeks postoperatively.

LONG-TERM OUTCOMES

Long-term follow-up has demonstrated durable weight loss and metabolic benefits comparable with Roux-en-Y gastric bypass.[20–23] Type 2 diabetes mellitus and diabetes-associated complications have been shown more effectively treated by bariatric surgery compared with the best medical therapy. The only significant predictor of long-term improvement of type 2 diabetes mellitus was a decrease in body mass index.[2] In addition, survival benefit has been demonstrated among obese patients undergoing bariatric surgery compared with those without surgical intervention. A retrospective cohort study showed a decrease in all-cause mortality at 5 years and 10 years in patients receiving bariatric surgery.[24]

The LSG has continued to gain popularity among both patients and surgeons due to its perceived technical simplicity compared with other bariatric surgical procedures. As data regarding patient outcomes after this procedure continue to accrue among institutions, promising results are being published more than 5 years out from surgery. Most publications report a mean percent excess weight loss of 55% or more over this time period.[21,25–29] The authors have published data from 6 years to 8 years postoperatively that demonstrate durable excess weight loss of 46% at 96 months.[30] LSG compares favorably to long-term weight loss data for laparoscopic Roux-en-Y gastric bypass over the same time frame. Improvements of type 2 diabetes mellitus and metabolic syndrome abnormalities are also similar compared with gastric bypass. Data pertaining to the improvement of gastroesophageal reflux disease or new onset of gastroesophageal reflux disease after sleeve gastrectomy continue to evolve, and dedicated objective studies are needed to better delineate this potential outcome.[31] Regarding the most feared complication, overall leak rates are reported between

0.7% and 3.7%, and a majority of these occur at the proximal third of the stomach staple line near the gastroesophageal junction.[32]

SUMMARY

LSG evolved from a staged procedure as part of the biliopancreatic diversion and duodenal switch and has emerged as a sole procedure for sustained weight loss and improvement of metabolic derangements. The surgery continues to gain popularity due to its perceived technical simplicity coupled with promising short-term and long-term data, which suggest results comparable to more established bariatric procedures. Certain key surgical tenets of the LSG are described in this article that are essential for safe and effective outcomes. The sleeve gastrectomy has clearly established itself as a successful stand-alone procedure for the effective treatment of obesity and related diseases.

SUPPLEMENTARY DATA

Supplementary data related to this article are found at http://dx.doi.org/10.1016/j.suc.2016.03.015.

REFERENCES

1. Mattar S, Velcu L, Schauer P. Surgically-induced weight loss significantly improves nonalcholoic fatty liver disease and the metabolic syndrome. Ann Surg 2005;242(4):610–7.

2. Schauer P, Bhatt DL, Kirwan JP, STAMPEDE Investigators. Bariatric surgery versus intensive medical therapy for diabetes - 3 year outcomes. N Engl J Med 2014;370(21):2002–13.

3. Johnston D, Dachtler J, Martin IG. The Magenstrasse and Mill operation for morbid obesity. Obes Surg 2003;13(1):10–6.

4. Cottam D, Qureshi FG, Mattar SG, et al. Laparoscopic sleeve gastrectomy as an initial weight-loss procedure for high-risk patients with morbid obesity. Surg Endosc 2006;20:859–63.

5. Regan JP, Inabnet W, Gagner M, et al. Early experience with two-stage laparoscopic Roux-en-Y gastric bypass as an alternative in the super obese patient. Obes Surg 2003;13(6):861–4.

6. ASMBS Clinical Issues Committee. Updated position statement on sleeve gastrectomy as a bariatric procedure. Surg Obes Relat Dis 2012;8(3):21–6.

7. Rosenthal R, International Sleeve Gastrectomy Expert Panel. International Sleeve Gastrectomy Expert Panel Consensus Statement: best practice guidelines based on experience of >12,000 cases. Surg Obes Relat Dis 2012;8(1):8–19.

8. Edholm D, Kullberg J, Sundbom M. Preoperative 4-Week Low-Calorie Diet Reduces Liver Volume and Intrahepatic Fat, and Facilitates Laparoscopic Gastric Bypass in Morbidly Obese. Obes Surg 2011;21(3):345–50.

9. Collins J, McCloskey C, Eid G. Preoperative weight loss in high-risk superobese bariatric patients: a computed-tomography based analysis. Surg Obes Relat Dis 2011;7(4):480–5.

10. Haskins IN, Amdur R, Vaziri K. The effect of smoking on bariatric surgical outcomes. Surg Endosc 2014;28(11):3074–80.

11. Schigt A, Coblijn U, van Wagensveld B. Is esophagogastroduodenoscopy before Roux-en-Y gastric bypass or sleeve gastrectomy mandatory? Surg Obes Relat Dis 2014;10(3):411–7.

12. Boules M, Corcelles R, Kroh M. The incidence of hiatal hernia and technical feasibility of repair during bariatric surgery. Surgery 2015;158(4):911–8.

13. Cal P, Deluca L, Fernandez E. Laparoscopic sleeve gastrectomy with 27 versus 39 Fr bougie calibration: a randomized controlled trial. Surg Endosc 2016;30(5): 1812–5.

14. Parikh M, Gagner M, Pomp A. Laparoscopic sleeve gastrectomy: does bougie size affect mean %EWL? Short-term outcomes. Surg Obes Relat Dis 2008;4(4): 528–33.

15. Rogula T, Khorgami Z, Schauer P. Comparison of Reinforcement Techniques Using Suture on Staple-Line in Sleeve Gastrectomy. Obes Surg 2015;25(11): 2219–24.

16. Aydin M, Aras O, Memisoglu K. Staple line reinforcement methods in laparoscopic sleeve gastrectomy: comparison of burst pressures and leaks. JSLS 2015;19(3) [pii:e2015.00040].

17. Chen B, Kiriakopoulos A, Frezza EE. Reinforcement does not necessarily reduce the rate of staple line leaks after sleeve gastrectomy. A review of the literature and clinical experiences. Obes Surg 2009;19(2):166–72.

18. Lauti M, Gormack S, MacCormick A. What does the excised stomach from sleeve gastrectomy tell us? Obes Surg 2015;26(4):839–42.

19. Galloro G, Ruggiero S, Manta R. Staple-line leak after sleeve gastrectomy in obese patients: a hot topic in bariatric surgery. World J Gastrointest Surg 2015; 7(9):843–6.

20. Vidal J, Ibarzabal A, Romero F, et al. Type 2 diabetes mellitus and the metabolic syndrome following sleeve gastrectomy in severely obese subjects. Obes Surg 2008;18:1077–82.

21. Bohdjalian A, Langer FB, Prager G. Sleeve gastrectomy as sole and definitive bariatric procedure: 5-year results for weight loss and ghrelin. Obes Surg 2010;20(5):535–40.

22. Fischer L, Hildebrandt C, Muller-Stich B. Excessive weight loss after sleeve gastrectomy: a systematic review. Obes Surg 2012;22(5):721–31.

23. Adams TD, Gress RE, Hunt SC. Long-term mortality after gastric bypass surgery. N Engl J Med 2007;57(8):753–61.

24. Arterburn D, Olsen M, Smith V, et al. Association between bariatric surgery and long-term survival. JAMA 2015;313(1):62–70.

25. Hauser D, Titchner R, Wilson M, et al. Long-term outcomes of laparoscopic Roux-en-Y gastric bypass in US Veterans. Obes Surg 2010;20(3):283–9.

26. Sarela A, Dexter S, McMahon M. Long-term follow-up after laparoscopic sleeve gastrectomy: 8-9 year results. Surg Obes Relat Dis 2012;8(6):679–84.

27. Himpens J. Adjustable gastric banding, sleeve gastrectomy and Roux-en-Y gastric bypass by laparoscopy: long term outcomes and laparoscopic solutions in case of failure (doctoral dissertation). 2013. Retrieved from Maastricht University database.

28. Baltasar A, Serra C, Ferri L. Laparoscopic sleeve gastrectomy: a multi-purpose bariatric operation. Obes Surg 2005;15(8):1124–8.

29. Himpens J, Dobbeleir J, Peeters G. Long-term results of laparoscopic sleeve gastrectomy for obesity. Ann Surg 2010;252:319–24.

30. Eid G, Brethauer S, Mattar SG, et al. Laparoscopic Sleeve Gastrectomy for Super Obese Patients Forty-eight Percent Excess Weight Loss After 6 to 8 Years With 93% Follow-Up. Ann Surg 2012;256(2):262–5.
31. Chiu S, Birch DW, Shi X, et al. Effect of sleeve gastrectomy on gastroesophageal reflux disease: a systematic review. Surg Obes Relat Dis 2011;7:510–5.
32. Marquez M, Ayza M, Poujoulet R. Gastric leak after laparoscopic sleeve gastrectomy. Obes Surg 2010;20(9):1306–11.

Laparoscopic Roux-en-Y Gastric Bypass

Surgical Technique and Perioperative Care

Lindsay Berbiglia, DO[a], John G. Zografakis, MD[a,b],
Adrian G. Dan, MD[a,b],*

KEYWORDS

- Obesity • Comorbid conditions • Laparoscopic Roux-en-Y gastric bypass

KEY POINTS

- Obesity is a global epidemic with the number of effected individuals steadily increasing.
- Surgical procedures have been developed to alter the gastrointestinal tract to combat obesity and its associated comorbid conditions.
- Laparoscopic Roux-en-Y gastric bypass is highly effective at reducing excess body weight with substantial efficacy against comorbid conditions and a favorable overall side effect profile.
- There are various techniques for performing the laparoscopic Roux-en-Y gastric bypass.
- Standardized preoperative and postoperative protocols derived from evidence-based recommendations are essential to long-term success.

 Video content accompanies this article at http://www.surgical.theclinics.com.

INTRODUCTION

The obesity epidemic, and the prevalence of associated comorbid conditions, is a problem of global proportions sparing no geographic, cultural, or demographic subset. Over the past 60 years, a host of surgical procedures have been developed and refined to anatomically and physiologically alter the gastrointestinal tract to combat obesity. Surgical interventions have proven to be among the most effective therapeutic options in the battle against obesity.

The minimally invasive and bariatric surgery fellowship is supported by The Foundation for Surgical Fellowships.
The authors have no conflicts of interest or disclosures.
[a] Bariatric Care Center, Akron City Hospital, Summa Health System, Akron, OH, USA;
[b] Northeast Ohio Medical University, Rootstown, OH, USA
* Corresponding author. 95 Arch Street, Suite 620, Akron, OH 44304.
E-mail address: dana@summahealth.org

The gastric bypass procedure was first introduced by Mason in 1967 as a variation of the Bilroth II reconstruction used after antrectomy in the treatment of peptic ulcer disease.[1] Over one-half of a century, numerous modifications led to the elegant minimally invasive procedures we perform today. The most noteworthy include the adoption of the Roux-en-Y configuration reported and advocated by Griffin in 1977[2] and the introduction of the laparoscopic Roux-en-Y gastric bypass (LRYGB) by Wittgrove and associates in 1993.[3]

Over the past 2 decades, the LRYGB has proven to be a highly effective operation against obesity and its associated comorbid conditions, and has a favorable metabolic side effect profile when compared with the more radical biliopancreatic diversion with duodenal switch. Numerous high-quality studies have demonstrated the efficacy and safety of the procedure. It has since become and remains the gold standard operation in the battle against the obesity epidemic.

Several technical variations exist with regard to the formation of the pouch and reconstruction of gastrointestinal continuity. These variations, as well as the evidence based recommendations for the preoperative and postoperative care of patients undergoing this procedure, are the focus of this article.

SURGICAL TECHNIQUE
Preoperative Planning

As with all surgical interventions, a detailed history should be obtained to avoid potential pitfalls. Certain subsets of patients may not be best suited for the LRYGB procedure, including those with a suspected hostile abdomen, multiple comorbid conditions for whom a lengthy operation may be detrimental, and conditions treated with psychotropic medications whose absorption is not amenable to LRYGB. The introduction of the laparoscopic sleeve gastrectomy offers a viable alternative for these patients.

Preoperative patient education is imperative, including a discussion of the risks and benefits, as well as knowledge of the procedure and expected postoperative lifestyle changes. The patient should be counseled on pregnancy avoidance for 12 to 18 months postoperatively, avoidance of nonsteroidal antiinflammatory drugs, smoking cessation indefinitely, and limited alcohol use. The patient should undergo psychosocial–behavioral and registered dietitian evaluation and clearance.[4] Preoperative weight management should be individualized and at the discretion of the surgeon.[5]

Preoperative testing should include blood glucose, lipid panel, comprehensive metabolic panel, hemogram, blood type, and when clinically indicated, endocrine and nutrient deficiency laboratory workup. All patients should have an electrocardiogram and chest radiography performed.[4] Obstructive sleep apnea (OSA) is prevalent in patients suffering from morbid obesity and can lead to cardiovascular disease and death. Testing for OSA and initiation of continuous positive airway pressure therapy should be considered in all patients.[6] Any significant gastrointestinal symptoms should be evaluated by imaging studies, upper gastrointestinal series or esophagogastroduodenoscopy before surgery.[4] In patients with symptomatic gallstones or history of cholecystitis, cholecystectomy is recommended. Concurrent laparoscopic cholecystectomy is acceptable and safe[7–10]; however, it should be kept in mind that treatment of choledocholithiasis is complicated by the anatomic changes associated with the gastric bypass procedure. Helicobacter pylori testing should be considered routinely and may be accomplished with esophagogastroduodenoscopy or stool testing.[4] Medical clearance from the patient's primary care physician, and cardiopulmonary or other specialists when indicated, should be obtained.[4]

Preparation and Patient Positioning

Most bariatric patients receive preoperative dosing with low-molecular-weight heparin and intravenous antibiotic prophylaxis.[4] It is ensured that the operating room table used can support adequate weight in the steep reverse Trendelenburg position and that it is equipped with right angle foot boards. After induction of general anesthesia, a Foley catheter is placed. Appropriately sized pneumatic compression devices are placed on both lower extremities. Many bariatric surgeons use split leg positioning, allowing the surgeon to stand in between the patient's legs. A securing strap is placed on both upper legs or across the hips. Extremities are placed in neutral abduction with adequate padding to prevent pressure injuries. The table is positioned with minimal break to open the upper abdomen. Upper body heating blankets are often placed to prevent hypothermia. The abdomen is prepped and draped in standard fashion.

Surgical Approach

The standard surgical approach to bariatric Roux-en-Y gastric bypass today is laparoscopic, with primary open procedures being of historic interest only (**Fig. 1**). There are reports of the robotic approach being safe and feasible.[11]

SURGICAL PROCEDURE
Trocar Placement

Accessing the abdominal cavity in the morbidly obese patient can be challenging. Most bariatric surgeons use the established safe technique of placement of a

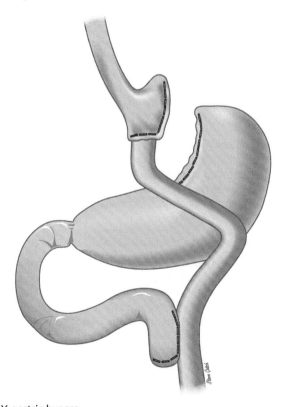

Fig. 1. Roux-en-Y gastric bypass.

bladeless optical view trocar with direct visualization by a 0° laparoscope at Palmer's point, in favor of the periumbilical access location. Pneumoperitoneum is established up to 18 mm Hg. A 30° laparoscope is used to perform a brief diagnostic laparoscopy noting presence or absence of hiatal hernia, adhesive disease, or other abnormalities. Abiding by minimally invasive surgical principles, the 4 remaining trocars are placed in an arc pattern. Minor variations in trocar size and location are determined by patient body habitus, surgical technique, and stapling device to be used.

Creation of the Gastric Pouch

The stomach is decompressed via placement of an orogastric tube, which is then removed along with any esophageal devices. Routine standardized communication with the anesthesia team should be established to ensure all tubes and devices are removed before gastric transection. There are varying modalities for determining pouch size, including placement of a sizing balloon, transection below the second lesser curve vascular bundle, and most commonly measurement from the gastroesophageal junction.[12] Regardless of technique, goal pouch size is 25 to 30 cm^3. The pouch vascular supply depends on the left gastric vessels. Depending on technique used, the pouch is created either vertically based on the lesser curvature, or horizontally based on the greater curvature. In vertical construction, the stomach is retracted caudally to expose the phrenoesophageal ligament and peritoneal reflection at the angle of His. This is incised, exposing the left diaphragmatic crus. Dissection is begun perigastric with sparing of the neurovascular bundle, or at the pars flacida with division of the lesser omentum by an energy device or by a stapling device with buttressing material to prevent bleeding. Access to the lesser sac and posterior stomach is obtained and the stomach is transected horizontally using a linear stapling device. The posterior wall of the stomach is examined and any adhesive attachments are divided. The fundus is retracted laterally to avoid redundancy, resulting in a large pouch. A retracting device is passed posteriorly, medial to the short gastric vessels, and deflected above the angle of His into the previously created space to allow for passage of the stapling device. Linear stapling devices are sequentially fired vertically. Care is taken to remain lateral to the esophageal fat pad to prevent esophageal transection or narrowing.

If a circular stapling device used, the anvil must be placed within the gastric pouch either transoral after pouch creation, or transgastric/abdominal before pouch completion. In transgastric/abdominal construction, the pouch can be created and the end opened to accommodate the anvil and refashioned[13] or, more commonly, a gastrotomy is made before pouch creation to allow passage of the anvil and the pouch is created around the anvil.[14]

Construction of the Roux and Biliopancreatic Limbs

The patient is returned to the supine position to facilitate cephalad retraction of the omentum and transverse colon to identify the ligament of Treitz. The ligament of Treitz is confirmed by identification of the adjacent inferior mesenteric vein. The bowel is run 30 to 50 cm distal to the ligament of Treitz, and transected using a linear stapling device. The proximal transected bowel becomes the biliopancreatic limb, and the distal bowel the Roux limb. The mesentery is further divided by use of an energy device or linear stapling device with buttressing material to allow for further mobility of the Roux limb and decreased tension on the gastrojejunostomy. The Roux limb is measured up to 150 cm distally and aligned with the biliopancreatic limb for creation of the jejuno-jejunostomy. Prospective randomized controlled trials have shown no weight loss benefit to longer Roux limbs in patients with a body mass index (BMI) of less than

50 kg/m^2 but improved control of diabetes mellitus type 2 and hyperlipidemia, and greater weight loss in BMI greater than 50 kg/m^2 is described.[15–17]

Creation of the Jejunojenostomy

The most common technique used for creation of the jejunojejunostomy anastomosis is a single fire of a linear stapler passed through antimesenteric enterotomies created on the parallel positioned biliopancreatic and Roux limbs with hand sewn closure of the common enterotomy.[12] Other techniques are the double staple, which uses a stapled closure of the common enterotomy, and triple staple involving both proximal and distal firing of the linear stapling device with stapled closure of the common enterotomy (**Figs. 2–7**). For stapled closure of the common enterotomy, sutures can be placed to aid proper positioning within the stapler and full-thickness closure. The triple staple technique was used to prevent stenosis or obstruction at the anastomosis noted with the double staple technique[18] and has been shown to be efficient and safe.[19,20] Completely hand sewn jejunojejunostomy is rarely performed.[12] An antiobstruction stitch, first described by Brolin,[21] is placed between the stapled end of the biliopancreatic limb and the adjacent limb, immediately distal to the anastomosis to prevent the stapled closure of the enteroenterostomy from folding on itself, causing pseudoobstruction. It is common to place a marking stitch and clips at the jejunojenostomy for later radiographic identification. The mesenteric defect is then closed with nonabsorbable suture in running or interrupted fashion.

Gastrojejunal Anastomosis

The most common configuration of the Roux limb is antecolic, antegastric.[12] Retrocolic orientation may reduce tension on the gastrojejunostomy anastomosis, but has been associated with a significant increase in the internal hernia rate.[22] A Penrose drain placed on the Roux limb can aid in retrocolic passage. The transverse colon mesentery, through which the Roux limb passes, is approximated using permanent suture incorporating the Roux limb, ligament of Treitz, and mesentery to prevent herniation. In antecolic passage, right-sided orientation of the Roux limb in the

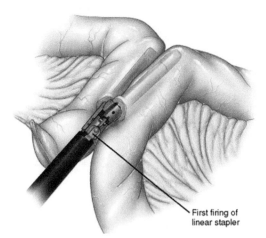

First firing of
linear stapler

Fig. 2. A white 2.5-mm staple load is used to join together the two loops of bowel. (*From* Zografakis JG, Frantzides CT. Laparoscopic Gastric Bypass with Roux-en-Y Gastrojejunostomy. In: Frantzides CT, Carlson MA, editors. Atlas of Minimally Invasive Surgery. Philadelphia: Elsevier Saunders; 2009. p. 53–66; with permission.)

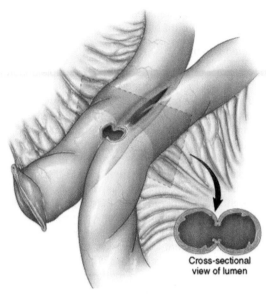

Fig. 3. Defect created after stapler removal. (*From* Zografakis JG, Frantzides CT. Laparoscopic Gastric Bypass with Roux-en-Y Gastrojejunostomy. In: Frantzides CT, Carlson MA, editors. Atlas of Minimally Invasive Surgery. Philadelphia: Elsevier Saunders; 2009. p. 53–66; with permission.)

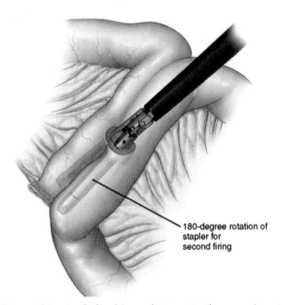

Fig. 4. Second 2.5-mm white staple load is used to create the opposing staple line for the triple-stapling technique. (*From* Zografakis JG, Frantzides CT. Laparoscopic Gastric Bypass with Roux-en-Y Gastrojejunostomy. In: Frantzides CT, Carlson MA, editors. Atlas of Minimally Invasive Surgery. Philadelphia: Elsevier Saunders; 2009. p. 53–66; with permission.)

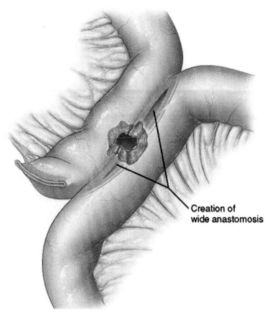

Fig. 5. A curved dissector is used to position the open enterotomy for the third and final firing of the linear stapler. (*From* Zografakis JG, Frantzides CT. Laparoscopic Gastric Bypass with Roux-en-Y Gastrojejunostomy. In: Frantzides CT, Carlson MA, editors. Atlas of Minimally Invasive Surgery. Philadelphia: Elsevier Saunders; 2009. p. 53–66; with permission.)

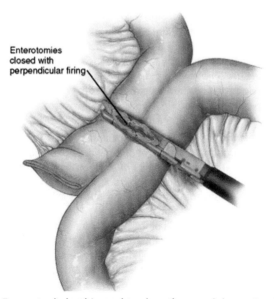

Fig. 6. A white 2.5-mm staple load is used to close the remaining enterotomy and restore bowel continuity. (*From* Zografakis JG, Frantzides CT. Laparoscopic Gastric Bypass with Roux-en-Y Gastrojejunostomy. In: Frantzides CT, Carlson MA, editors. Atlas of Minimally Invasive Surgery. Philadelphia: Elsevier Saunders; 2009. p. 53–66; with permission.)

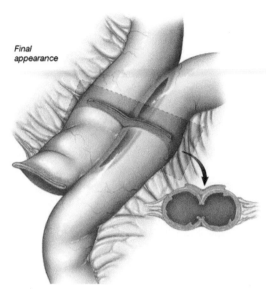

Final
appearance

Fig. 7. Perpendicular orientation of staple lines, and completed jejunojejunostomy utilizing the Frantzides-Madan triple-stapling technique. (*From* Zografakis JG, Frantzides CT. Laparoscopic Gastric Bypass with Roux-en-Y Gastrojejunostomy. In: Frantzides CT, Carlson MA, editors. Atlas of Minimally Invasive Surgery. Philadelphia: Elsevier Saunders; 2009. p. 53–66; with permission.)

jejejunojenostomy has been associated with a decreased rate of internal herniation of 0.5% when compared with a left-sided orientation, 9.0%.[23] If antecolic passage of the Roux limb is planned, it is helpful to divide the omentum using an energy device allowing the jejunojenunostomy to be brought anterior to the omentum to reduce tension on the gastrojejunal anastomosis. There are 3 main techniques used to fashion the gastrojejunal anastomosis, including circular stapler, linear stapler, and hand sewing. The most commonly used technique is the circular stapler.[12,24] Variations in each technique exist, but the common sequence is described below.

Gastrojejunal Anastomosis: Transoral Circular Stapler Technique

Transoral placement of the anvil is achieved via slow passage of an attached orogastric tube with direct laparoscopic visualization until the tip is oriented along the staple line of the gastric pouch at the intended site of anastomosis (Video 1). A small gastrotomy is made using ultrasonic scalpel, hook scissors, or hook cautery device. It is important to place the gastrotomy through the staple line to avoid creation of an ischemic tissue island and prevent subsequent leak. The orogastric tube is advanced out of the gastric pouch, grasped by a blunt instrument, and removed through a trocar with minimal force in coordination with the team member assisting oral passage of the attached anvil. Techniques that can facilitate passage of the anvil are deflation of the endotracheal tube, head flexion, and orienting the smooth part of the anvil toward the hard palate as the orogastric tube is removed from the abdomen pulling the anvil into the gastric pouch. A gentle "corkscrew" motion is used to ensure the anvil does not get caught on the patient's teeth or interfere with the endotracheal tube.[25] The securing suture is cut, allowing the orogastric tube to be removed and leaving the anvil in place within the gastric pouch, ready for anastomosis.

The Roux limb is brought up to the gastric pouch and run back to the jejunoje-nostomy to ensure proper mesenteric orientation and placement of the jejunoje-junostomy anterior to the omentum. This maneuver also reduces tension on the anastomosis. Other techniques used to further reduce tension on the gastrojejunos-tomy are division of the small bowel mesentery, omental division, pouch mobilization, creation of a vertical length pouch, and hitch suture placement at the gastrojejunal anastomosis.

The port site is enlarged to accommodate the end-to-end anastomosis (EEA) sta-pling device, which is fashioned with a dilating cone and sterile sleeve to decrease trauma and minimize wound infection. The stapling device is then passed into the abdominal cavity. The Roux limb staple line is opened to allow passage of the EEA sta-pling device. The post is advanced through the antimesenteric side of the jejunum and married to the anvil located in the gastric pouch (**Fig. 8**). The EEA device is closed and deployed. The sterile sleeve is retracted over the end of the device and it is removed from the abdomen. The anastomotic tissue rings are examined for completeness. The anastomosis is completed with closure of the Roux limb with a linear stapling device creating a very short blind or "candy cane" limb. The transected jejunum is placed into a sterile bag and removed. A minimum of 2 absorbable hitch sutures are placed to reinforce the anastomosis and minimize tension. An alternative to the end-to-side gastrojejunostomy described is an end-to-end configuration in which the EEA device is passed through a separate enterotomy created distally on the Roux limb, which is closed later.[26]

Gastrojejunal Anastomosis: Linear Stapler Technique

Linear stapler is the second most common technique for creation of the gastrojejunos-tomy (**Fig. 9**, Video 2).[12,24] This technique eliminates the need for port site dilation and

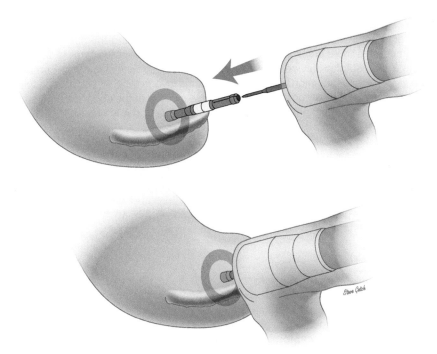

Fig. 8. Circular stapler.

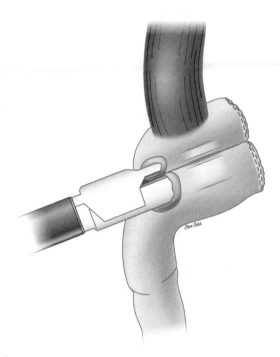

Fig. 9. Linear stapler.

split leg positioning. It is also associated with decreased operative times and stricture rates. The Roux limb is brought up to the gastric pouch as described previously. The Roux limb is approximated to the end or side of the adjacent gastric pouch using interrupted sutures. Enterotomies are created in the Roux limb and the gastric pouch to accommodate a linear stapling device. The common channel enterotomy is closed using the linear stapler device or hand sewing. Hand sewn closure is commonly completed in running fashion over a bougie, gastric lavage tube, or endoscope to prevent stenosis.[27,28] It is suggested that transverse closure of the common enterotomy, when compared with longitudinal closure, reduces anastomotic stricture.[27]

Gastrojejunal Anastomosis: Hand Sewn Technique

In the hand sewn technique, the Roux limb is approximated to the end or side of the gastric pouch using interrupted or running suture. Enterotomies are made on both the gastric pouch and roux limb to allow for anastomosis. The anastomosis is constructed in 2 layers, a running full-thickness absorbable suture and reinforcement anteriorly with interrupted permanent seromuscular sutures. A 34F to 36F tube is passed through the anastomosis before completion to prevent stenosis.

COMPLICATIONS

There are multiple complications associated with the LRYGB, including but not limited to bleeding, infection, small bowel obstruction secondary to internal or port site herniation, marginal ulceration, anastomotic leak, anastomotic stenosis or stricture, hypopharyngeal or esophageal injury, omental torsion or necrosis, pulmonary embolus, death, development of symptomatic cholelithiasis, inadequate weight loss, nutritional deficiencies, and symptomatic dumping syndrome. The incidence of specific complications can vary with the technique used.

Anastomotic leak is a dreaded complication most commonly occurring at the gastrojejunal anastomosis site.[29] Rates of anastomotic leak are similar (0.1%–8.3%)[16,30–33] regardless of the technique used, and significantly decreased in newer studies reporting only laparoscopic procedure rates (0%–3%).[26,34–40] Several methods to decrease leak have been attempted, including staple line oversewing, fibrin glue/sealant application, and staple line reinforcements,[41–45] but there is no prospective randomized evidence to suggest any method is effective. Most bariatric surgeons use a form of intraoperative leak testing that allows for immediate repair. Air insufflation via endoscope or orogastric tube and blue dye instillation are 2 commonly used techniques. If a leak is found, it should be repaired and the leak test repeated.[30] Routine drain placement at the gastrojejunal anastomosis is debated with proponents noting ability to diagnosis and control leak,[46,47] and opponents noting no benefit and potential increase in leak rate.[48,49]

Anastomotic stricture/stenosis is a widely studied complication that can occur with any gastrojejunostomy technique. Several large studies and 2 randomized control trials have shown stricture rates for hand sewn, linear stapler, and circular stapler techniques to be 4.1% to 7.7%, 0% to 10.1%, and 1.6% to 17.5%, respectively.[26,50–58] Two metaanalyses of comparative studies between linear stapler and circular stapler anastomoses have shown a statistically significant decreased risk of stricture associated with the linear technique.[59,60] There are 2 circular stapler sizes, 21 and 25 mm, which are associated with different diameters and cross-sectional areas, 12 and 113 mm versus 16 and 201 mm, respectively.[57] Several small comparative studies and 1 randomized control trial have noted an increased rate of symptomatic stenosis associated with use of the 21-mm stapling device when compared with the 25-mm device.[61–64] In patients who develop symptomatic stenosis, there are no differences in interval to stenosis (46–52 days) or number of interventions required between the 2 sizes.[61,62] Endoscopic balloon dilation is safe and effective treatment, and in 82% to 86% of patients only 1 dilation is required.[62,65] One study has shown that circular stapled anastomosis through the staple line versus the posterior gastric pouch decreases stenosis (0.8% vs 5.9%).[40] One randomized controlled trial noted the use of a circular stapler with a 3.5-mm staple height versus 4.8 mm also led to decreased stenosis (3.9% vs 16.0%).[52] Several studies have shown no difference in weight loss associated with the different anastomotic techniques, regardless of stricture occurence.[36,38,50,60–62,66]

Hypopharyngeal perforation and esophageal injury with transoral passage of the anvil are exceedingly rare in the literature, but have been reported.[14,67] The majority of difficulty is associated with passage through the upper esophageal sphincter and may be related to specific anvil characteristics.[28,68] Pretilted anvils for ease of passage and prevention of injury are widely available. A corkscrew action used during passage of the anvil and use of a 21-mm diameter stapler, versus the 25-mm stapler, may also ease placement.[25] Two large series specifically examining transoral passage have reported no injuries.[68,69]

An increased rate of wound infection from 3.6% to 23% has been described with the circular stapler technique, when compared with other techniques.[70]

Use of the circular stapling device requires port site dilation, resulting in trauma and necrosis of subcutaneous fat, as well as passage of the stapling device through the subcutaneous tissues, which can lead to the increased rate of infection. Methods created to combat these issues, including use of a cone-shaped stapler introduction device and sterile sleeve, preoperative chlorhexidine swish and swallow, wound irrigation, and loose wound closure with permanent monofilament suture, have resulted in reduced infection rates of 1%.[71,72]

Postoperative bowel obstructions can occur secondary to internal hernias, port site herniation, or pseudoobstruction of the biliopancreatic limb prevented by placement of the Brolin antiobstruction stitch previously described.

There are 3 common sites of internal herniation: the classic mesojejunal site, transmesocolic associated with retrocolic Roux limb passage, and in the potential space between the Roux limb and the transverse mesocolon, also known as Petersen's hernia. Closure of the mesenteric defect is routine for most surgeons performing gastric bypass today. Nonclosure and loss of mesenteric fat owing to postoperative weight loss[73] can lead to mesojejunal herniation, the most common type.[74] Internal hernias are a significant cause of late complications (0.4%–14.4%),[75] and the most frequent cause of late small bowel obstruction after LRYGB.[22,31,76] They often present with vague symptoms and computed tomography scanning has low sensitivity for diagnosis, but may show the classic finding of a "swirl sign" in the mesentery.[74] This finding can lead to delayed diagnosis, bowel strangulation, anastomotic dehiscence, gastric remnant dilation, and death.[77]

Port site herniation, including Richter's type hernia, can also present with vague symptoms leading to delays in diagnosis, bowel necrosis, and death. The incidence reported in most studies is less than 2%.[78,79] A cumulative review counterintuitively found a significantly increased incidence of herniation in LRYGB patients at sites where closure was attempted, from 0.36% to 1.1%.[78] The reason for this is unknown. There is currently no evidence to support routine fascial closure, but closure should be attempted at the umbilicus and at any enlarged or dilated sites, such as that created to accommodate the circular stapler. This is usually accomplished with an 0-absorbable suture and suture passing device under laparoscopic visualization.

IMMEDIATE POSTOPERATIVE CARE

Patients are transferred to the recovery area under observation of the operating surgeon and anesthesia team. Nursing staff should be trained in postoperative bariatric care and recognition of potential postoperative complications. Patients remain nil per os throughout postoperative day 0. Adequate hydration is ensured with intravenous crystalloid and monitoring of urine outputs. Most patients can be transferred to a surgical unit, but those with history of OSA, cardiac conditions, respiratory difficulties, or complicated cases will require telemetry monitoring or rarely intensive care.

Immediate postoperative laboratory studies should include blood counts and electrolyte levels, as well as a creatine phosphokinase level in any patient suffering from super morbid obesity (BMI >50 kg/m^3 or >400 lb) or with prolonged operating room times. Creatine phosphokinase levels should be reevaluated on postoperative day 1. Early identification of rhabdomyolysis allows for early intervention, decreasing renal damage.[80] Routine metabolic panels, magnesium level, and complete blood counts are obtained daily, unless increased frequency is indicated. Blood glucose level should be assessed immediately postoperatively and serially in all diabetic patients. Antidiabetic medications will require individualized adjustment postoperatively with glucose management with a short-acting insulin analogue while inpatient.[4]

Pain management is most commonly achieved with intravenous opioids while nil per os, with transition to oral opioids when diet is initiated and continuation of intravenous form for breakthrough pain. Intravenous acetaminophen and ketorolac may be considered in addition to narcotic management. Ice packs, abdominal binders, and nerve blockades may also assist in achieving adequate pain control. Inadequate pain control can lead to patient dissatisfaction, tachycardia, shallow respirations, immobility, increased complications, and increased duration of stay.

Aggressive postoperative pulmonary toilet can decrease complications and should be initiated immediately upon arrival to the floor.[81] This should include incentive spirometer use, deep breathing, coughing, and evaluation by a respiratory therapist. For patients diagnosed with OSA and preoperative use of continuous positive airway pressure, continuous positive airway pressure should be ordered postoperatively and the patient should bring their own mask to ensure proper fit.[6] Continuous pulse oximetry in OSA patients may reduce the risk of complications.[82]

The risk of venous thromboembolism and pulmonary embolus in average risk bariatric patients is less than 1%,[83–87] but risk continues for several weeks postoperatively[88,89] and remains a leading cause of preventable postoperative death.[90] Patients with a BMI of greater than 55 kg/m^2, immobility, venous stasis, pulmonary hypertension, obesity hypoventilation syndrome, hypercoagulable state, and history of venous thromboembolism, characteristics of most bariatric patients, are at high risk for venous thromboembolism.[91] Mechanical prophylaxis in combination with early ambulation alone may be sufficient[87,92] and is recommended for all patients.[4,91] Most bariatric programs use mechanical prophylaxis in combination with chemoprophylaxis initiated within 24 hours of surgery.[4,91] Based on available data, low-molecular-weight heparin is superior to unfractionated heparin for chemoprophylaxis.[84,91] Extended prophylaxis beyond the hospitalization period may be considered in high-risk patients. Inferior vena cava filters are associated with multiple complications, including death. Their use should only be considered when potential benefits outweigh these risks and always in conjunction with mechanical and chemoprophylaxis.[4,91]

Routine or selective upper gastrointestinal series soluble contrast study can be performed to evaluate the integrity and patency of both the gastrojejunostomy and jejunojejunostomy, identified by the surgically placed clips. Routine testing has been associated with a positive and negative predictive value for suspected leak of 67% and 99%, respectively,[93] and may lead to findings other than leak or stricture, such as dilation of the gastric remnant, trocar site hernia or internal hernia causing early postoperative obstruction, which may change postoperative care.[94] Despite these findings, there is increasing evidence to support selective testing.[95–98]

Postoperatively, a bariatric clear liquid diet, consisting of sugar-free liquids with minimal gastrointestinal residue and no carbonation or caffeine to avoid pouch irritation, is initiated. The use of straws is discouraged. Fluid intake recording is encouraged to ensure adequate hydration. Postoperative counseling on diet initiation and advancement, adequate hydration, and vitamin and mineral supplementation by a registered dietitian should be completed.[4]

Incisions and drains, when present, are examined daily while inpatient. Nursing staff and patients are educated on signs of wound infection and drain care.

Patients are generally discharged postoperative day 1 to 3. Patients and caretakers should be educated by the bariatric nurse case manager and registered dietitian on dietary and activity restrictions, wound and drain care if applicable, signs and symptoms of complications including anastomotic leak and venous thromboembolism, and home medications. They should be counseled on the avoidance of caffeine, nonsteroidal antiinflammatory drugs, alcohol, and nicotine exposure. Comorbid conditions may improve rapidly and patients are counseled to follow closely with their primary care physicians.

Recently, emphasis has been placed on adherence to Enhanced Recovery After Bariatric Surgery protocols. Enhanced Recovery After Bariatric Surgery interventions include shortened preoperative fasts, intraoperative humidification, early mobilization and feeding, avoidance of fluid overload, incentive spirometry, and use of prokinetics and laxatives. Short-term studies show Enhanced Recovery After Bariatric Surgery protocol adherence to be feasible and safe, and results in shortened duration of hospital stay and low 30-day readmission rates.[99]

LONG-TERM CARE AND FOLLOW-UP

The first patient follow-up is usually at 5 to 7 days postoperatively, which allows for drain removal if applicable; assessment of wounds, medications, and overall condition; and reinforcement of dietary progression, vitamin supplementation, and activity restrictions. Dietary progression generally proceeds from bariatric clear liquids to full liquids, pureed, and finally regular maintenance. Concentrated carbohydrates are eliminated to prevent dumping. Dietary protein intake should be 1.5 g/kg ideal body weight per day. Vitamin supplementation includes multivitamins plus minerals, calcium and vitamin D, thiamine, folic acid, iron, zinc, selenium, and copper as needed to maintain normal levels. Subsequent follow-up appointments should be scheduled at 1, 3, 6, and 12 months postoperatively and include weight loss and exercise monitoring, dietitian counseling/supplementation monitoring, evaluation of the need for support group participation or psychiatric follow-up, review of medications and comorbid conditions, and laboratory testing. Exercise is encouraged at 4 weeks postoperatively and should include aerobic activity and strength training 2 to 3 times per week.[100] It is currently recommended that a compete blood count and iron be checked at each visit, vitamin B_{12} every 3 to 6 months, lipids every 6 to 12 months, and calcium, folic acid, vitamin D, and intact parathyroid hormone be checked regularly. A 24-hour urinary calcium excretion test should be considered at 6 months. Copper, zinc, selenium, and thiamine levels should be checked if indicated clinically. Patients should be referred for bone density testing at 2 years postoperatively. Referral for body contouring surgery should be offered.[4]

Rapid weight loss after a gastric bypass procedure may lead to symptomatic gallstone formation that may require surgical intervention in 7% to 41% of patients.[101–103] This incidence may be reduced to 2% with the use of ursodiol 600 mg daily for 6 months postoperatively.[104] Marginal ulceration occurs with an incidence of 1% to 16%[105] and is more common in patients with H pylori infection.[106] The incidence is significantly reduced with prophylactic proton pump inhibitor therapy[105–108] with a suggested duration of 90 days[108] and preoperative H pylori eradication.

CLINICAL RESULTS IN THE LITERATURE

LRYGB performed at specialty centers by fellowship-trained bariatric surgeons has excellent outcomes with short durations of hospital stay and low readmission rates. The 30-day mortality rate is 0.3% and major complication rate is 4.3%.[109] The LRYGB is highly effective with regards to excess weight loss when compared with other contemporary procedures.[110,111] The average excess weight loss following LRYGB is 56% to 66% with average maintenance of 50% excess weight loss at 5 years.[112] Morbid obesity increases the risk of premature death[113,114] and the risk of morbid obesity outweighs the risks of bariatric surgery.[115,116] Furthermore, several studies show improvement in life expectancy after bariatric surgery.[115,117–119] Several randomized control trials, metaanalyses, and outcomes studies have shown improvement or resolution in type 2 diabetes, hypertension, hyperlipidemia, and OSA, as well as improved outcomes when compared with medical interventions.[110–112,119–122] Bariatric surgery, including LRYGB, is also associated with improvement of obesity-related cardiac dysfunction,[123] polycystic ovarian syndrome and resolution of associated infertility,[124] gastroesophageal reflux disease, and osteoarthritis. Outcomes are improved at centers with comprehensive programs including bariatricians, dietitians, psychologists, and bariatric nurse case managers, which facilitates long-term follow-up and support.

SUMMARY

The LRYGB is the gold standard metabolic/bariatric procedure used today to combat the growing morbid obesity epidemic. This procedure is highly effective at reducing excess body weight and has substantial efficacy against the multiple comorbid conditions associated with obesity. There are varying techniques for procedure performance, as described. The most common technique today is a circular stapled gastrojejunal anastomosis with antecolic Roux limb and stapled jejunojenostomy with hand sewn common enterotomy closure. Complications are associated to varying degrees with technique used. It is important to be aware of these complications and be prepared for expeditious management. Regardless of the technique used, the LRYGB performed at specialty centers by fellowship trained surgeons with adherence to evidence-based care protocols for perioperative care has excellent outcomes.

SUPPLEMENTARY DATA

Supplementary data related to this article can be found at http://dx.doi.org/10.1016/j.suc.2016.03.003.

REFERENCES

1. Mason E, Ito C. Gastric bypass in obesity. Surg Clin North Am 1967;47(6): 1345–51.
2. Griffen W Jr, Young V, Stevenson C. A prospective comparison of gastric and jejunoileal bypass procedures for morbid obesity. Ann Surg 1977;186(4):500–9.
3. Wittgrove AC, Clark GW, Tremblay LJ. Laparoscopic gastric bypass, Roux-en-Y: preliminary report of five cases. Obes Surg 1994;4:353–7.
4. Mechanick JI, Youdim A, Jones DB, et al. Clinical practice guidelines for the perioperative nutritional, metabolic, and nonsurgical support of the bariatric surgery patient – 2013 update: cosponsored by American Association of Clinical Endocrinologists, The Obesity Society, and American Society for Metabolic and Bariatric Surgery. Surg Obes Relat Dis 2013;9:159–91.
5. Wudel LJ Jr. Prevention of gallstone formation in morbidly obese patients undergoing rapid weight loss: results of a randomized controlled pilot study. J Surg Res 2002;102(1):50–6.
6. ASMBS Clinical Issues Committee. Peri-operative management of obstructive sleep apnea. Surg Obes Relat Dis 2012;8:27–32.
7. Nougou A, Suter M. Almost routine prophylactic cholecystectomy during laparoscopic gastric bypass is safe. Obes Surg 2008;18(5):535–9.
8. Sreenarasimhaiah J. Prevention or surgical treatment of gallstones in patients undergoing gastric bypass surgery for obesity. Curr Treat Options Gastroenterol 2004;7(2):99–104.
9. Fobi M, Lee H, Igwe D, et al. Prophylactic cholecystectomy with gastric bypass operation: incidence of gallbladder disease. Obes Surg 2002;12(3):350–3.
10. Hamad GG, Ikramuddin S, Gourash WF, et al. Elective cholecystectomy during laparoscopic Roux-en-Y gastric bypass: is it worth the wait? Obes Surg 2003; 13(1):76–81.

11. Sanchez BR, Mohr CJ, Morton JM, et al. Comparison of totally robotic laparoscopic Roux-en-Y gastric bypass and traditional laparoscopic Roux-en-Y gastric bypass. Surg Obes Relat Dis 2005;1(6):549–54.

12. Madan AK, Harper JL, Tichansky DS. Techniques of laparoscopic gastric bypass: on-line survey of American Society for Bariatric Surgery practicing surgeons. Surg Obes Relat Dis 2008;4:166–73.

13. Teixeira JA, Borno FJ, Thomas TA, et al. An alternative technique for creating the gastrojejunostomy in laparoscopic Roux-en-Y gastric bypass: experience with 28 consecutive patients. Obes Surg 2000;10:240–4.

14. Scott DJ, Provost DA, Jones DB. Laparoscopic Roux-en-Y gastric bypass: transoral or transgastric anvil placement? Obes Surg 2000;10:361–5.

15. Choban PS, Flancbaum L. The effect of Roux limb lengths on outcome after Roux-en-Y gastric bypass: a prospective randomized clinical trial. Obes Surg 2002;12:540–5.

16. Inabet WB, Quinn T, Gagner M, et al. Laparoscopic Roux-en-Y gastric bypass in patients with BMI <50: a prospective randomized trial comparing short and long limb lengths. Obes Surg 2005;15:51–7.

17. Pinheiro JS, Schiavon CA, Pereira PB, et al. Long-long limb Roux-en-Y gastric bypass is more efficacious in treatment of type 2 diabetes and lipid disorders in super-obese patients. Surg Obes Relat Dis 2008;4:521–5.

18. Nguyen NT, Neuhaus AM, Furdui GG, et al. A prospective evaluation of intracorporeal laparoscopic small bowel anastomosis during gastric bypass. Obes Surg 2001;11(2):196–9.

19. Franzides CT, Zeni TM, Madan AK, et al. Laparoscopic Roux-en-Y gastric bypass utilizing the triple stapling technique. JSLS 2006;10:176–9.

20. Madan AK, Frantzides CT. Triple staple technique of jejunostomy for laparoscopic gastric bypass. Arch Surg 2003;138:1029–32.

21. Brolin RE. The anti-obstruction stitch in stapled Roux-en-Y enteroenterostomy. Am J Surg 1995;169:355–7.

22. Rondelli F, Bugiantella W, Desio M, et al. Antecolic or retrocolic alimentary limb in laparoscopic Roux-en-Y gastric bypass? A meta-analysis. Obes Surg 2016; 26(1):182–95.

23. Quebbemann BB, Dallal RM. The orientation of the antecolic Roux limb markedly affects the incidence of internal hernias after laparoscopic gastric bypass. Obes Surg 2005;15(6):766–70.

24. Finks JF, Carlin A, Share D, et al. Effect of surgical techniques on clinical outcomes after laparoscopic gastric bypass – results from the Michigan Bariatric Surgery Collaborative. Surg Obes Relat Dis 2011;7:284–9.

25. Davis R, Davis GP. Ensuring safe passage of the OrVil anvil utilizing a corkscrew maneuver. Surg Obes Relat Dis 2013;9:329–30.

26. Wittgrove AC, Clark GW. Laparoscopic gastric bypass, Roux-en-Y – 500 patients: technique and results, with 3-60 month follow up. Obes Surg 2000;10: 233–9.

27. Mueller CL, Jackson TD, Swanson T, et al. Linear-stapled gastrojejunostomy with transverse hand-sewn enterotomy closure significantly reduces strictures for laparoscopic Roux-en-Y gastric bypass. Obes Surg 2013;23:1302–8.

28. Brethauer SA, Schauer PR, Schirmer BD. Minimally invasive bariatric surgery. 2nd edition. New York: Springer; 2015. p. 232–44.

29. Csendes A, Burgos AM, Braghetto I. Classification and management of leaks after gastric bypass for patients with morbid obesity: a prospective study of 60 patients. Obes Surg 2012;22(6):855–62.

30. Kim J, Azagury D, Eisenberg D, et al. ASMBS position statement on prevention, detection and treatment of gastrointestinal leak after gastric bypass and sleeve gastrectomy, including the roles of imaging, surgical exploration, and nonoperative management. Surg Obes Relat Dis 2015;11:739–48.

31. Podnos YD, Jimenez JC, Wilson SE, et al. Complications after laparoscopic gastric bypass. A review of 3464 cases. Arch Surg 2003;138(9):957–61.

32. Gonzalez R, Sarr MG, Smith CD, et al. Diagnosis and contemporary management of anastomotic leaks after gastric bypass for obesity. J Am Coll Surg 2007;204(1):47–55.

33. Champion JK, Williams MD. Prospective randomized comparison of linear staplers during laparoscopic Roux-en-Y gastric bypass. Obes Surg 2003;13(6): 855–9.

34. Hutter MM, Schirmer BD, Jones DB, et al. First report from the American College of Surgeons Bariatric Surgery Center Network: laparoscopic sleeve gastrectomy has morbidity and effectiveness positioned between the band and the bypass. Ann Surg 2011;254(3):410–20.

35. Murr MM, Gallagher SF. Technical considerations for transabdominal loading of the circular stapler in laparoscopic Roux-en-Y gastric bypass. Am J Surg 2003; 185:585–8.

36. Lois AW, Frelich MJ, Goldblatt MI, et al. Gastrojejunostomy technique and anastomotic complications in laparoscopic gastric bypass. Surg Obes Relat Dis 2015;11:808–13.

37. Gonzalez R, Lin E, Venkatesh KR, et al. Gastrojejunostomy during laparoscopic gastric bypass, analysis of three techniques. Arch Surg 2003;138:181–4.

38. Edholm D, Sundbom M. Comparison between circular and linear stapled gastrojejunostomy in laparoscopic Roux-en-Y gastric bypass – a cohort from the Scandinavian obesity registry. Surg Obes Relat Dis 2015;11(6):1233–6.

39. Stroh CE, Nesterov G, Weiner R, et al. Circular versus linear versus hand-sewn gastrojejunostomy in Roux-en-Y gastric bypass influence on weight loss and amelioration of comorbidities: data analysis from the quality assurance study of the surgical treatment of obesity in Germany. Front Surg 2014;1(23):1–5.

40. Suter M, Donadini A, Calmes JM, et al. Improved surgical technique for laparoscopic Roux-en-Y gastric bypass reduces complications at the gastrojejunostomy. Obes Surg 2010;20:841–5.

41. Silecchia G, Boru CE, Mouiel J, et al. Clinical evaluation of fibrin glue in the prevention of anastomosis leak and internal hernia after laparoscopic gastric bypass: preliminary results of a prospective randomized trial. Obes Surg 2006;16:125–31.

42. Miller KA, Pump A. Use of bioabsorbable staple reinforcement material in gastric bypass: a prospective randomized clinical trial. Surg Obes Relat Dis 2007;3(4):417–21.

43. Shikora SA. The use of staple-line reinforcement during laparoscopic gastric bypass. Obes Surg 2004;14(10):1313–20.

44. Sapala JA, Wood MH, Schuhknecht MP. Anastomotic leak prophylaxis using a vapor-heated fibrin sealant: report on 738 gastric bypass patients. Obes Surg 2004;14(1):35–42.

45. Nandakumar G, Richards BG, Trencheva K, et al. Surgical adhesive increases burst pressure and seals leaks in stapled gastrojejunostomy. Surg Obes Relat Dis 2010;6(5):498–501.

46. Chousleb E, Szomstein S, Podkameni D, et al. Routine abdominal drains after laparoscopic Roux-en-Y gastric bypass: a retrospective review of 593 patients. Obes Surg 2004;14(9):1203–7.

47. Liscia G, Scaringi S, Facchiano E, et al. The role of drainage after Roux-en-Y gastric bypass for morbid obesity: a systematic review. Surg Obes Relat Dis 2014;10(1):171–6.

48. Dallal RM, Bailey L, Nahmais N. Back to basics – clinical diagnosis in bariatric surgery. Routine drains and upper GI series are unnecessary. Surg Endosc 2007;21(12):2268–71.

49. Kavuturu S, Rogers AM, Haluck RS. Routine drain placement in Roux-en-Y gastric bypass: an expanded retrospective comparative study of 755 patients and review of the literature. Obes Surg 2012;22(1):177–81.

50. Awad S, Aguilo R, Agrawal S, et al. Outcomes of linear-stapled versus hand-sewn gastrojejunal anastomosis in laparoscopic Roux-en-Y gastric bypass. Surg Endosc 2015;29:2278–83.

51. Leyba JL, Llopis SN, Isaac J, et al. Laparoscopic gastric bypass for morbid obesity – a randomized controlled trial comparing two gastrojejunal anastomosis techniques. JSLS 2008;12(4):385–8.

52. Nguyen NT, Dakin G, Needleman B, et al. Effect of staple height on gastojejunostomy during laparoscopic gastric bypass: a multicenter prospective randomized trial. Surg Obes Relat Dis 2010;6:477–84.

53. Schauer PR, Ikramuddin S, Gourash W, et al. Outcomes after laparoscopic Roux-en-Y gastric bypass for morbid obesity. Ann Surg 2000;232:515–29.

54. Higa K, Ho T, Boone K. Laparoscopic Roux-en-Y gastric bypass; technique and 3-year follow up. J Laparoendosc Adv Surg Tech A 2001;11:377–82.

55. Wittgrove AC, Endres JE, Davis M, et al. Perioperative complications in single surgeon's experience with 1,000 consecutive laparoscopic Roux-en-Y gastric bypass operations for morbid obesity. Obes Surg 2002;12:457–8.

56. DeMaria EJ, Surgerman HJ, Kellum JM, et al. Results of 281 consecutive total laparoscopic Roux-en-Y gastric bypass in morbid obesity. Ann Surg 2002; 235:640–7.

57. Carrodeguas L, Szomstein S, Zundel N, et al. Gastrojejunal anastomotic strictures following laparoscopic Roux-en-Y gastric bypass surgery: analysis of 1291 patients. Surg Obes Relat Dis 2006;2(2):92–7.

58. Kravetz AJ, Reddy S, Murtaza G, et al. A comparative study of handsewn versus stapled gastrojejunal anastomosis in laparoscopic Roux-en-Y gastric bypass. Surg Endosc 2011;25(4):1287–92.

59. Penna M, Markar SR, Venkat-Raman V, et al. Linear-stapled versus circular-stapled laparoscopic gastrojejunal anastomosis in morbid obesity: meta-analysis. Surg Laparosc Endosc Percutan Tech 2012;22(2):95–101.

60. Giordano S, Salminen P, Biancari F, et al. Linear stapler technique may be safer than circular in gastrojejunal anastomosis for laparoscopic Roux-en-Y gastric bypass: a meta-analysis of comparative studies. Obes Surg 2011;21:1958–64.

61. Markar SR, Penna M, Venkat-Ramen V, et al. Influence of circular stapler diameter on postoperative stenosis after laparoscopic gastrojejunal anastomosis in morbid obesity. Surg Obes Relat Dis 2012;8:230–5.

62. Nguyen NT, Stevens CM, Wolfe BM. Incidence and outcome of anastomotic stricture after laparoscopic gastric bypass. J Gastrointest Surg 2003;7(8): 997–1003.

63. Baccaro LM, Vunnamadala K, Sakharpe A, et al. Stricture rate after laparoscopic Roux-en-Y gastric bypass with a 21-mm circular stapler versus a 25-mm linear stapler. Bariatr Surg Pract Patient Care 2015;10(1):33–7.
64. Fisher BL, Atkinson JD, Cottam D. Incidence of gastroenterostomy stenosis in laparoscopic Roux-en-Y gastric bypass using 21- or 25-mm circular stapler: a randomized prospective blinded study. Surg Obes Relat Dis 2007;3(2):176–9.
65. Alasfar F, Sabnis AA, Liu RC, et al. Stricture rate after laparoscopic Roux-en-Y gastric bypass with a 21-mm circular stapler: the Cleveland Clinic experience. Med Princ Pract 2009;18:364–7.
66. Cottam D, Fisher B, Sridhar V, et al. The effect of stoma size on weight loss after laparoscopic gastric bypass surgery: results of a blinded randomized controlled trial. Obes Surg 2009;19:13–7.
67. Nguyen NT, Wolfe BM. Hypopharyngeal perforation during laparoscopic Roux-en-Y gastric bypass. Obes Surg 2000;10(1):64–7.
68. Wittgrove AC, Clark GW. Laparoscopic gastric bypass: endostapler transoral or transabdominal anvil placement. Obes Surg 2000;10:376.
69. Wittgrove AC, Clark GW. Combined laparoscopic/endoscopic anvil placement for the performance of the gastroenterostomy. Obes Surg 2001;11:565–9.
70. Scandinavian Obesity Surgery Registry (SOReg). Annual report 2012. Available at: http://www.ucr.uu.se/soreg/.
71. Alasfar F, Sabnis A, Liu R, et al. Reduction of circular stapler-related in patients undergoing laparoscopic Roux-en-Y gastric bypass, the Cleveland Clinic technique. Obes Surg 2010;20(2):168–72.
72. Muller MK, Wildi S, Clavien PA, et al. New device for the introduction of circular stapler in laparoscopic gastric bypass surgery. Obes Surg 2006;16(12):1559–62.
73. Garrard CL, Clements RH, Nanney L, et al. Adhesion formation is reduced after laparoscopic surgery. Surg Endosc 1999;13(1):10–3.
74. Kawkabani MA, Denys A, Paroz A, et al. The four different types of internal hernia occurring after laparoscopic Roux-en-Y gastric bypass performed for morbid obesity: are there any multidetector computed tomography (MDCT) features permitting their distinction? Obes Surg 2011;21:506–16.
75. Delko T, Kraljevic M, Kostler T, et al. Primary non-closure of the mesenteric defects in laparoscopic Roux-en-Y gastric bypass: reoperations and intraoperative findings in 146 patients. Surg Endosc 2015. [Epub ahead of print].
76. Gunabushamam G, Shankar S, Czerniach DR, et al. Small bowel obstruction after laparoscopic Roux-en-Y gastric bypass surgery. J Comput Assist Tomogr 2009;33:369–75.
77. Higa KD, Ho T, Boone KB. Internal hernias after laparoscopic Roux-en-Y gastric bypass: incidence, treatment and prevention. Obes Surg 2003;13(3):350–4.
78. Phillips E, Santos D, Towfigh S. Working port site hernias: to close or not to close? Does it matter in the obese? Bariatric Times 2011;8(6):24–30.
79. Lancaster RT, Hutter MM. Bands and bypasses: 30-day morbidity and mortality of bariatric surgical procedures as assessed by prospective, multi-center, risk-adjusted ACS-NSQIP data. Surg Endosc 2008;22:2554–63.
80. Chakravartty S, Sarma DR, Patel AG. Rhabdomyolysis in bariatric surgery: a systematic review. Obes Surg 2013;23(8):1333–40.
81. Cassidy MR, Rosenkranz P, McCabe K, et al. I COUGH: reducing postoperative pulmonary complications with a multidisciplinary patient care program. JAMA Surg 2013;148(8):740–5.
82. Gross JB, Bachenberg KL, Benumof JL, et al. Practice guidelines for the perioperative management of patients with obstructive sleep apnea: a report by the

American society of anesthesiologists task force on perioperative management of patients with obstructive sleep apnea. Anesthesiology 2006;104:1081–93.

83. Becattini C, Agnelli G, Manina G, et al. Venous thromboembolism after laparoscopic bariatric surgery for morbid obesity: clinical burden and prevention. Surg Obes Relat Dis 2012;8:108–15.

84. Birkmeyer NJ, Finks JF, Carlin AM, et al. Comparative effectiveness of unfractionated and low-molecular-weight heparin for prevention of venous thromboembolism following bariatric surgery. Arch Surg 2012;147:994–8.

85. Finks JF, English WJ, Carlin AM, et al. Predicting risk for venous thromboembolism with bariatric surgery: results from the Michigan Bariatric Surgery Collaborative. Ann Surg 2012;255:1100–4.

86. Flum DR, Belle SH, King WC, et al. Perioperative safety in the longitudinal assessment of bariatric surgery. N Engl J Med 2009;361:445–54.

87. Clements RH, Yellumahanthi K, Ballem N, et al. Pharmacologic prophylaxis against venous thromboembolic complications is not mandatory for all laparoscopic Roux-en-Y gastric bypass procedures. J Am Coll Surg 2009;208:917–21.

88. Huber O, Bounameaux H, Borst F, et al. Postoperative pulmonary embolism after hospital discharge: an underestimated risk. Arch Surg 1992;127:310–3.

89. Steele KE, Schweitzer MA, Prokopowicz G, et al. The long-term risk of venous thromboembolism following bariatric surgery. Obes Surg 2011;21:1371–6.

90. Sapala JA, Wood MH, Schuhknecht MP, et al. Fatal pulmonary embolism after bariatric operations for morbid obesity: a 24-year retrospective analysis. Obes Surg 2003;13:819–25.

91. The ASMBS Clinical Issues Committee. ASMBS updated position statement on prophylactic measures to reduce the risk of venous thromboembolism in bariatric surgery patients. Surg Obes Relat Dis 2013;9:493–7.

92. Frantzides CT, Welle SN, Ruff TM, et al. Routine anticoagulation for venous thromboembolism prevention following laparoscopic gastric bypass. JSLS 2012;16: 33–7.

93. Madan AK, Stoecklein HH, Ternovits CA, et al. Predictive value of upper gastrointestinal studies versus clinical signs for gastrointestinal leaks after laparoscopic gastric bypass. Surg Endosc 2007;21:194–6.

94. Raman R, Raman B, Raman P, et al. Abnormal findings on routine upper GI series following laparoscopic Roux-en-Y gastric bypass. Obes Surg 2007;17(3): 311–6.

95. Kolakowski S, Kirkland ML, Schuricht AL. Routine postoperative upper gastrointestinal series after Roux-en-Y gastric bypass: determination of whether it is necessary. Arch Surg 2007;142(10):930–4.

96. Lee SD, Khouzam MN, Kellum JM, et al. Selective, versus routine, upper gastrointestinal series leads to equal morbidity and reduced hospital stay in laparoscopic gastric bypass patients. Surg Obes Relat Dis 2007;3(4):413–6.

97. Doraiswamy A, Rasmussen JJ, Pierce J, et al. The utility of routine postoperative upper GI series following laparoscopic gastric bypass. Surg Endosc 2007; 21(12):2159–62.

98. Brockmeyer JR, Simon TE, Jacob RK, et al. Upper gastrointestinal swallow study following bariatric surgery: institutional review and review of the literature. Obes Surg 2012;22:1039–43.

99. Awad S, Carter S, Purkayastha S, et al. Enhanced recovery after bariatric surgery (ERABS): clinical outcomes from a tertiary referral bariatric centre. Obes Surg 2014;24(5):753–8.

100. Pollock ML, Gaesser GA, Butcher JD, et al. ACSM position stand: the recommended quantity and quality of exercise for developing and maintaining cardiorespiratory and muscular fitness, and flexibility in healthy adults. Med Sci Sports Exerc 1998;30(6):975–91.
101. Villegas L, Schneider B, Provost D, et al. Is routine cholecystectomy required during laparoscopic gastric bypass? Obes Surg 2004;14:206–11.
102. Shiffman ML, Sugerman HJ, Kellum JM, et al. Gallstone formation after rapid weight loss: a prospective study in patients undergoing gastric bypass surgery for treatment of morbid obesity. Am J Gastroenterol 1991;86(8):1000–5.
103. Portenier DD, Grant JP, Blackwood HS, et al. Expectant management of the asymptomatic gallbladder at Roux-en-Y gastric bypass. Surg Obes Relat Dis 2007;3(4):476–9.
104. Sugerman HJ, Brewer WH, Shiffman ML, et al. A multicenter, placebo-controlled, randomized, double-blind, prospective trial of prophylactic ursodiol for the prevention of gallstone formation following gastric-bypass-induced rapid weight loss. Am J Surg 1995;169(1):91–6.
105. Ying VW, Kim SH, Khan KJ, et al. Prophylactic PPI help reduce marginal ulcers after gastric bypass surgery: a systematic review and meta-analysis of cohort studies. Surg Endosc 2015;29(5):1018–23.
106. D'Hondt MA, Pottel H, Devriendt D, et al. Can a short course of prophylactic low-dose proton pump inhibitor therapy prevent stomal ulceration after laparoscopic Roux-en-Y gastric bypass? Obes Surg 2010;20(5):595–9.
107. Coblijn UK, Lagarde SM, de Castro SM, et al. The influence of prophylactic proton pump inhibitor treatment on the development of marginal ulceration in Roux-en-Y gastric bypass patients: a historic cohort study. Surg Obes Relat Dis 2016;12(2):246–52.
108. Kang X, Zurita-Macias-Valadez L, Hong D, et al. A comparison of 30 versus 90 day proton pump inhibitor therapy in prevention of marginal ulcers after laparoscopic Roux-en-Y gastric bypass. Surg Obes Relat Dis 2015. [Epub ahead of print].
109. The Longitudinal Assessment of Bariatric Surgery (LABS) Consortium, Flum DR, Belle SH, et al. Perioperative safety in the longitudinal assessment of bariatric surgery. JAMA 2009;361(5):445–54.
110. Schauer PR, Bhatt DL, Kirwan JP, et al. Bariatric surgery versus intensive medical therapy for diabetes – 3-year outcomes. N Engl J Med 2014;370(21): 2002–13.
111. Mingrone MD, Panunzi S, DeGaetano A, et al. Bariatric surgery versus conventional medical therapy for type 2 diabetes. N Engl J Med 2012;366(17):1577–85.
112. Buchwald H, Avidor Y, Braunwald E, et al. Bariatric surgery: a systematic review and meta-analysis. JAMA 2004;292(14):1724–37.
113. U.S. Department of Health and Human Services Office of the Surgeon General. Overweight and obesity: health and consequences. 2007. Available at: http://www.surgeongeneral.gov/topics/obesity/calltoaction/fact_consequences.htm. Accessed December 2015.
114. Abdullah A, Wolfe R, Stoelwinder JU, et al. The number of years lived with obesity and the risk of all-cause and cause-specific mortality. Int J Epidemiol 2011;1:1–12.
115. Christou NV, Sampalis JS, Liberman M, et al. Surgery decreases long-term mortality, morbidity, and health care use in morbidly obese patients. Ann Surg 2004; 240(3):416–23.

116. Schauer DP, Arterburn DE, Livingston EH, et al. Decision modeling to estimate the impact of gastric bypass surgery on life expectancy for the treatment of morbid obesity. Arch Surg 2010;145(1):57–62.

117. Sjostrom L, Narbro K, Sjostrom D, et al. Effects of bariatric surgery on mortality in Swedish obese subjects. N Engl J Med 2007;357:741–52.

118. Adams TD, Gress RE, Smith SC, et al. Long-term mortality after gastric bypass surgery. N Engl J Med 2007;357:753–61.

119. Ikramuddin S, Korner J, Lee WJ, et al. Roux-en-Y gastric bypass versus intensive medical management for the control of type 2 diabetes, hypertension and hyperlipidemia: An international, multicenter, randomized trial. JAMA 2013;309(21):2240–9.

120. Courcoulas AP, Christian NJ, Belle SH, et al. Weight change and health outcomes at 3 years after bariatric surgery among individuals with severe obesity. JAMA 2013;310(22):2416–25.

121. Schauer PR, Burguera B, Ikramuddin S, et al. Effect of laparoscopic Roux-en-Y gastric bypass on type 2 diabetes mellitus. Ann Surg 2003;238(4):467–84.

122. Skroubis G, Anesidis S, Kehagias I, et al. Roux-en-Y gastric bypass versus a variant of biliopancreatic diversion in non-superobese population: prospective comparison of the efficacy and the incidence of metabolic deficiencies. Obes Surg 2006;16:488–95.

123. Aggarwal R, Harling L, Efthimiou E, et al. The effects of bariatric surgery on cardiac structure and function: a systematic review of cardiac imaging outcomes. Obes Surg 2015. [Epub ahead of print].

124. Jamal M, Capper A, Eid A, et al. Roux-en-Y bypass ameliorates polycystic ovary syndrome and dramatically improves conception rates: a 9-year analysis. Surg Obes Relat Dis 2012;8(4):440–4.

Update on Treatment of Morbid Obesity with Adjustable Gastric Banding

Emanuele Lo Menzo, MD, PhD, Samuel Szomstein, MD,
Raul Rosenthal, MD*

KEYWORDS

- Morbid obesity • Laparoscopic adjustable gastric banding • Complications
- Reoperations

KEY POINTS

- Laparoscopic adjustable gastric banding (LAGB) underwent several changes over the years in both design and technique of insertion. These modifications contributed to the significant decrease of complications.
- LAGB has the lowest perioperative complications and hospital stays of the bariatric surgery options.
- Overall, the weight loss achieved with the band is lower than with other bariatric operations, such as gastric bypass and sleeve gastrectomy.
- The long-term complications and the need for reintervention have contributed to a significant decrease in the use of LAGB as a bariatric surgery option.

INTRODUCTION

The pandemic proportion of obesity disease is well known, with more than 300 million people affected worldwide. According to the most recent National Health and Nutrition Examination Survey, 140.2 million (64.5%) of United States adults are candidates for weight loss treatment.[1] This is a significant increase from 1998, when the estimated number was 116 million, or 20.9% of the population. Although up to 53.4% of these candidates are considered for pharmacologic treatment, 14.7% could be candidates for bariatric surgery. The increase in potential candidates for bariatric surgery translated

Disclosure: No external funds were used for this work. None of the authors has any disclosures pertinent to this work.
The Bariatric and Metabolic Institute, Department of General Surgery, Digestive Disease Institute, Cleveland Clinic Florida, 2950 Cleveland Clinic Boulevard, Weston, FL 33331, USA
* Corresponding author.
E-mail address: rosentr@ccf.org

Surg Clin N Am 96 (2016) 795–813
http://dx.doi.org/10.1016/j.suc.2016.03.010
0039-6109/16/$ – see front matter © 2016 Elsevier Inc. All rights reserved.

surgical.theclinics.com

to an increase of the number of bariatric operations performed annually, although on a much smaller scale. Of the potential 20 million bariatric surgery candidates, only 193,000 patients underwent bariatric operations in the United States in 2014 (**Table 1**). Also, the mix of cases has changed over the years. Noticeably, the popularity trajectories of 2 procedures are moving in opposite directions, as the rise of laparoscopic sleeve gastrectomy (LSG) numbers is closely paralleled with the fall of LAGB numbers. The factors that contributed to the steep rise in popularity of the LAGB and the reasons for its even quicker fall are analyzed.

HISTORY

After the disappointing experience with the first highly malabsorptive operations, such as the jejunoileal bypass, in the 1950s, the concept of only restricting the food reservoir began to take a stand in the bariatric arena.[2] One of the early adopters of the band, Steffen, has extensively highlighted the historic milestones of the evolution of the band.[3]

Nonadjustable Bands

The first experiments on purely restrictive operation were conducted in dogs by Wilkinson and Peloso in the 1970s.[4] These investigators then published their results of placing a nonadjustable polypropylene (Marlex) band around the top part of the esophagus (**Fig. 1**).[4] At approximately the same time, other investigators in different parts of the world performed similar procedures. One of the most well known was the gastric partition described by Molina and colleagues.[5] Although the results of both the Wilkinson and Peloso and Molina and colleagues procedures were similar, the main differences were the material of the band (polyester Dacron instead of Marlex) and the size of the resulting pouch (smaller in the Molina). It was soon obvious, however, that both materials create a significant inflammatory reaction and even ingrowth within the stomach. This is the primary reason similar gastric partitions started to be performed with more inert materials, such as silicone.[6]

Not unexpectedly, every fixed type of gastric band resulted in either short-term or long-term failures, regardless of the material of the band, size of the resulting pouch, or other technical variations. The idea of putting a fixed band on a distensible

Table 1
Estimated bariatric operations between 2011 and 2014

	2011	2012	2013	2014
Total	158,000	173,000	179,000	193,000
LRYGB	36.7%	37.5%	34.2%	26.8%
Band	35.4%	20.2%	14%	9.5%
Sleeve	17.8%	33%	42.1%	51.7%
Biliopancreatic diversion with duodenal switch	0.9%	1%	1%	0.4%
Revisions	6%	6%	6%	11.5%
Other	3.2%	2.3%	2.7%	0.1%

American Society for Bariatric and Metabolic Surgery total bariatric procedures numbers from 2011, 2012, 2013, and 2014 are based on the best estimation from available data (Bariatric Outcomes Longitudinal Database, American College of Surgeons/Metabolic and Bariatric Surgery Accreditation and Quality Improvement Program, National Inpatient Sample data, and outpatient estimations).
  Data from American Society for Bariatric and Metabolic Surgery (ASMBS). Available at: https://asmbs.org/.

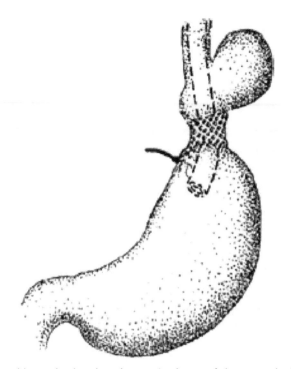

Fig. 1. Nonadjustable Marlex band at the proximal part of the stomach. (*From* Deitel M, Cowan GSM, editors. Update: Surgery for the Morbidly Obese Patient. Toronto, Ontario: FD-Communications Inc.; 2000; with permission.)

structure, such as the gastric fundus, would determine prolapse of the fundus itself and, over time, stretching of the reservoir. Both complications can lead to poor weight loss or weight regain but most importantly chronic reflux with esophageal dilatation.

Adjustable Bands

To decrease the likelihood of slippage, erosion, and chronic reflux, the idea of being able to adjust the diameter of the perigastric band started to develop. After an initial prototype was developed in the laboratory and tested on animal models by Szinicz and colleagues,[7] the first clinical application of the modern adjustable gastric band took place in Sweden by Forsell and colleauges.[8] This was the first version of the so-called Swedish band in 1985. Applying an identical concept, Kuzmak and colleagues in 1986[9] described a different design of the adjustable gastric band in the United States, initially known as the American band. Both the Swedish and American bands had an identical conceptual design of the modern bands, in which the Silastic outer ring of the band is complemented by an inner inflatable balloon. The balloon is connected to a subcutaneous port via a tube. Once accessed with a noncoring needle, the subcutaneous port allows for adjustment in the diameter of the band. Undoubtedly the ability to adjust the diameter of the band and individualize it for different patients significantly decreased the morbidity associated with the previous nonadjustable bands.[9]

Laparoscopy for Adjustable Gastric Bands

Although bands were considered safer than other more complex bariatric alternatives, the simple fact that a laparotomy was needed to implant them resulted in significant source of morbidity. It was only in 1995 that Belachew and colleagues[10] reported the first successful laparoscopic placement of an adjustable gastric band. As seen in other procedures that implemented laparoscopic techniques, the popularity of the LAGB begun to rise exponentially. This surge first started in Europe and expanded to other countries of the world, except the United States. It was only in 2001 that the Food and Drug Administration (FDA) approved the first band for use in the United States. This was the band derived from Kuzmak's prototype and commercialized as the Lap-Band (Allergan, Irvine, California; now Apollo Endosurgery, Austin, Texas) (**Figs. 2** and **3**). On the other end, the Swedish band, available in Europe since 1987, was finally marketed in the United States as the Realize band (Ethicon Endo-Surgery Cincinnati, Ohio) only 2 decades later (**Fig. 4**). Partially responsible for this late adoption of the new technology that was quickly spreading throughout the world were the disappointing results of one of the initial FDA trials in the United States.[11] These results were in definite contrast with the much more positive ones reported in both Europe and Australia.[12,13] Despite initial disappointing results, the technical simplicity and overall safety of the device contributed to the continuous expansion of the LAGB within the bariatric arena.

EVOLUTION AND TECHNICAL ADVANCEMENT OF THE LAPAROSCOPIC ADJUSTABLE GASTRIC BAND

In addition to the technical simplicity and the perioperative safety (discussed previously), several milestones contributed to the exponential rise in popularity of the LAGB.

Adoption of Laparoscopy

As previously discussed, the first major technical milestone in the history of LAGB was the adoption of the laparoscopic technique of insertion. Because, at this stage of the evolution of the band technique, the advancements were based on the previous open nonadjustable band, many of the original technical flaws were repeated in the adjustable band technique. The first laparoscopic placement was of a nonadjustable type of band done almost simultaneously by 2 investigators in different countries.[14,15] It is not surprising, then, how the early laparoscopic technique resembled the open one and consisted of placement of the band around the upper body of the stomach, also known as the perigastric technique. This resulted in 2 major consequences: the

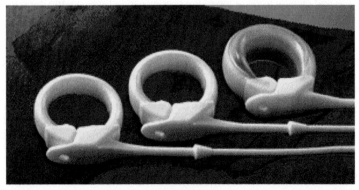

Fig. 2. First version of the Lap-Band. Note the narrow foot print, not circumferential, and the smaller volume balloon. (*Courtesy of* Apollo Endosurgery, Austin, TX; with permission.)

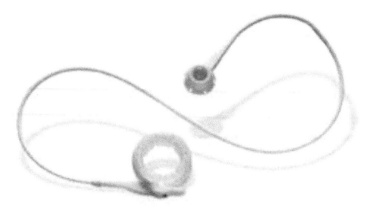

Fig. 3. Lap-Band AP. Wider footprint, larger circumferential balloon with lower volume. (*Courtesy of* Apollo Endosurgery, Austin, TX; with permission.)

inclusion of a variable portion of the distensible fundus in the pouch above the band and the violation of the lesser sac. These 2 technical points were later deemed responsible for a majority of the most common complications initially encountered with the band: prolapse and concentric pouch enlargement.[16]

The Pars Flaccida Technique

According to Belachew and colleuages'[10] original description, the band was placed around the superior portion of the stomach by creating a retrogastric tunnel from the lesser to the greater curvature across the lesser sac (perigastric technique).[10] This resulted in a generous gastric pouch of 25 cc to 30 cc, which included the gastric body and portion of the more distensible fundus. After the fundus was plicated over the band, the band was immediately filled with few milliliters of saline based on the measurements of a gastrostenometer. The high incidence of prolapse (up to 30%)

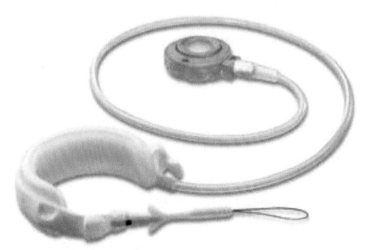

Fig. 4. Realize band equivalent to the Swedish band. (*Courtesy of* Ethicon Endo-Surgery, Cincinnati, OH; with permission.)

and of erosion (3%) was soon linked to the specific technical detail of surgical implantation. It was the recognition of those major pitfalls in the laparoscopic placement of the band that led to the second milestone in the technical evolution of the band: the adoption of the pars flaccida technique. This was the technique Forsell and colleagues[8] originally described for the placement of the Swedish band. This consists in the placement of the band higher in the stomach, preserving the lesser sac and the posterior gastric attachments. The tunnel to place the band originates from the gastrohepatic ligament above the bursa omentalis. The higher placement of the band results in the creation of a 1-cm virtual gastric pouch without any significant portion of distensible stomach. The preservation of the lesser sac attachments has been linked to the elimination of the posterior type of gastric prolapse and the significant reduction of the anterior type from 17% to 4%.[17,18] Also, the smaller gastric pouch above the band with virtually no fundus has contributed to the decrease of the concentric enlargement of the pouch, which was responsible not only for failure of weight loss and weight regain but also for chronic reflux.[16] Finally the diameter of the tunnel is kept very narrow, avoiding the disruption of the natural posterior attachments of the stomach to the diaphragmatic crura. The gastrogastric plication is made loose enough to accommodate future volume expansions of the band, and fluid is not added to the band intraoperatively but 4 weeks to 6 weeks postoperatively.

Design Changes of the Laparoscopic Adjustable Gastric Band

Additional technical advancements were made specifically to the design of the bands. The Lap-Band was originally designed with a low-volume, high-pressure inflatable balloon, not fully encircling the cardia and attached to a relatively narrow height band (footprint) (see **Fig. 2**). The superior compression on the gastric tissue was linked to higher incidence of erosion and anterior slippage.[19] Subsequent designs of the band modified the footprint of the band itself and included a 360° balloon able to accommodate higher volumes of fills and maintaining lower pressure (see **Fig. 3**). The adoption of wider bands also contributed to the decrease incidence of erosion.[19]

Increased Popularity of Laparoscopic Adjustable Gastric Band

The popularity of LAGB continued to increase exponentially. Between 2004 and 2007, the reported number of cases tripled from 7% to 23%, and between 2008 and 2010 it was the most commonly performed bariatric procedure worldwide.[20,21] The main features that determined the rapid increase of LAGB adoption were the technical simplicity; the early recovery with minimal, if any, in hospital stay; the gradual patient adjustment to the dietary modifications; the belief of total reversibility of the procedure; and the relative lower cost. These characteristics were consolidated by multiple reports of low morbidity and mortality of LAGB (11% and 0.05%, respectively) compared with the rates of the procedure more popular at the time, laparoscopic Roux-en-Y gastric bypass (LRYGB) (23.6% and 0.5%, respectively).[20] When longer-term data began to surface, the complications rate of LAGB increased to 31% to 60%, and the reoperation rates went up to 60%.[20,22] Even the concept of total reversibility began to be challenged and after removal some of the anatomic alteration of the gastroesophageal anatomy were more permanent than previously believed. A new concept of removability, instead of reversibility, started to gain ground.[20] Also the idea of lower costs started to be re-evaluated. Although true that the initial cost of the device and the quick operation with no in-hospital stay was lower, when the more intense follow-up and costs of complications and reoperations was factored in, the gap between LAGB and other operations was noticeably smaller than initially reported.[23] The continuing popularity of the band, along with the promising short-term and midterm results, resulted in a push for the application of the band in lower body mass index (BMI) ranges. This movement culminated in 2011 with the FDA approval in the United States of the LAGB for BMI between 30 kg/m^2 and 35 kg/m^2 with associated comorbid conditions.

COMPLICATIONS

To understand the reasons for the decline of the band, an in-depth analysis of its potential complications and their relative probability has to be done. Although the initial studies reported low rates of early complications, and certainly lower mortality rates of other bariatric operations,[24,25] several complications remain a substantial problems related to the LAGB.

The complications of LAGB can be divided as band related and port related (**Box 1**).

If the port-related complications are generally minor and require only minor surgery, often done under local anesthesia, the band-related complications can be the source of severe morbidity and potentially mortality.[26]

Acute Slippage

Slippage, also known as prolapse or eccentric pouch dilatation, is a herniation of portion of the stomach in a cephalad direction through the band. Based on the portion of herniated stomach, the slippage is divided in anterior or posterior. The herniation of the stomach changes the orientation of the axis of the band in a characteristic and diagnostic way. The posterior prolapse determines a counterclockwise rotation of the band with the axis of the band becoming almost parallel to the vertebral column (**Fig. 5**). On the other hand, in the anterior prolapse, the gastric tissue displaces the band clockwise, resulting in a horizontal appearance of the band (**Fig. 6**). Similarly

---

Box 1
Potential complications of laparoscopic adjustable gastric banding

Band related

- Slippage
- Erosion
- Pouch dilatation
- Esophageal dilatation
- System leak
- Infection
- Dysphagia
- GERD

Port tubing related

- Port displacement
- Tube disconnection
- System leak
- Infection

From Lo Menzo E, Szomstein S, Rosenthal R. Reoperative bariatric surgery. In: Nguyen N, Balckstone R, Morton J, et al, editors. The ASMBS textbook of bariatric surgery. New York: Springer; 2015. p. 276; with permission.

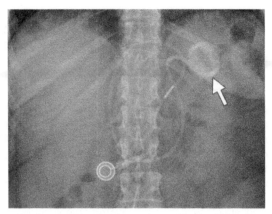

Fig. 5. Plain x-ray study showing a posterior prolapse. The band is oriented vertically almost parallel to the spine. The *arrow* denotes the typical O sign of the prolapsed band. (*From* Sonavane SK, Menias CO, Kantawala KP, et al. Laparoscopic adjustable gastric banding: what radiologists need to know. Radiographics 2012;32(4):1171; with permission.)

to other types of herniations, the prolapsed gastric tissue is at risk for ischemia and perforation. As discussed previously, the adoption of the pars flaccida technique and the band design modifications to lower pressure and higher volume balloons has eliminated the posterior prolapse.

Chronic Pouch Dilatation

Chronic pouch dilatation is one of the most common chronic findings of LAGB. Although the creation of a virtual pouch of the pars flaccida technique has decreased the incidence of pouch dilatation, this remains a significant cause of morbidity and

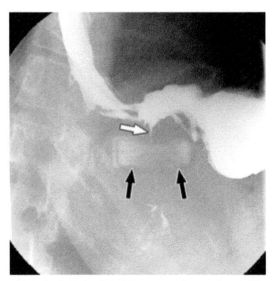

Fig. 6. Upper gastrointestinal study showing an anterior prolapse. The white arrow indicates severely narrowed outlet of the stomach. Black arrows show the horizontal position of the band.

indication for band revision, conversion, or removal. The functional stenosis at the level of the band determines a progressive dilatation of the gastric pouch. Because there is no prolapse of gastric tissue across the band, there is no risk of ischemia. The radiographic appearance is different from the prolapse (**Fig. 7**). The main contributing factor for the stenosis is an over-adjustment of the band. Dietary habits, however, are believed to play a role as well.[27] Because the loss of restriction is often interpreted as a loose band, the subsequent adjustments done without the aid of fluoroscopy create perpetuation of the outlet obstruction and worsening of the concentric dilatation.

Esophageal Dilatation

The persistent gastroesophageal obstruction with or without gastric concentric dilatation can determine insufficiency of the lower esophageal sphincter and stasis of food in the lower esophagus. Similar to primary achalasia, over time the esophageal muscle weakens and the esophageal lumen begins to dilate. If unrecognized, this process can cause permanent esophageal damage even after band removal (**Fig. 8**).

Band Erosion

Also known as band migration, the band erosion complication consists of the partial or complete penetration of the band in the gastric lumen (**Fig. 9**). The most helpful diagnostic tool is the esophagogastroduodenoscopy. Upper gastrointestinal contrast

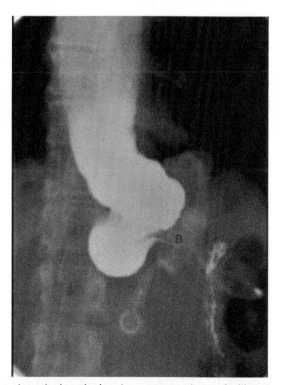

Fig. 7. Upper gastrointestinal study showing a concentric pouch dilatation. B indicates the band. (*From* Behr S, Campos G, Westphalen A. Applied radiology imaging and bariatric surgery. Appl Radiol 2012;41(6):18; with permission.)

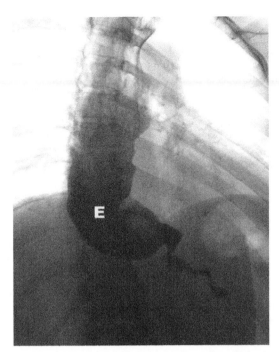

Fig. 8. Megaesophagus from chronic gastric outlet obstruction at the level of the band. E, esophagus.

study or CT scan can identify the presence of contrast media between the outside of the band and the inside of the gastric wall (**Fig. 10**). Early erosion is usually secondary to a technical error during the band placement, that is, gastric perforation. Another less common possibility is an early infection of the implant. Erosions presenting in more chronic form are mostly due to band overfilling, tight gastric plication, and,

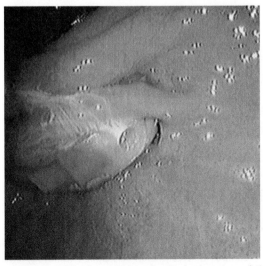

Fig. 9. Esophagogastroscopy study showing intraluminal migration of the band.

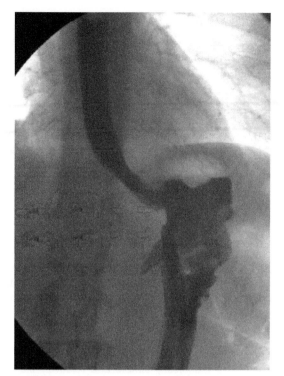

Fig. 10. Upper gastrointestinal study showing an intragastric band migration.

possibly, maladaptive eating behaviors. The development of a subcutaneous port site infection could be the first manifesting sign of band erosion.

Port-related Complications

Port-related complications account for approximately 12% of LAGB revisions.[20] The suspicion of a port tube complication should be raised when the port cannot be accessed, the band does not hold the fluid injected, or for abdominal pain of unclear origin. A fluoroscopic study with injection of contrast is the test of choice to identify the complication.

Although most of the port-related complications can be approached with minor surgery under local anesthesia, occasionally a diagnostic laparoscopy might be necessary to address problems, such as bowel obstructions and intra-abdominal dislodgement of the end of the tube.

Gastroesophageal Reflux Disease

The placement of an artificial prosthesis around the esophagogastric junction for the purpose of recreating the lower esophageal sphincter was in clinical use at the time of the description of the fixed band for weight loss. The first results of the so-called Angelchik prosthesis were reported in 1979.[28] Although initially effective, the long-term results of the device did not live up to its expectations because of the long-term outcomes and complications, in particular dysphagia, migration, and erosion.[29] According to the 2-year results on 122 patients of the APEX study, gastroesophageal reflux disease (GERD) symptoms resolved completely in 98 patients (80%), improved in 13 (11%), were unchanged in 9 (7%), and worsened in 2 (2%), leading to an overall improvement or resolution rate of 91%.[30] These impressive rates did not seem dependent on the extent of weight loss. Even objective data based on pH studies before and after the LAGB revealed short-term improvements after of LAGB.[31,32] Long-term significant worsening of both the symptoms and the pH positive reflux, however, has been demonstrated by the same investigators.[32]

Gastric Perforation

Gastric performation is a rare complication, reported in 0.1% to 0.4% of the band placements.[33] In acute settings, this is considered a technical error at the time of band insertion. Aggressive retrogastric tunnel creation can cause perforations at or near the posterior esophagogastric junction. Some of the smaller perforations can remain silent and manifest in a delayed fashion with subcutaneous port infection. The perforations that occur more chronically are due to band erosions, as previously described.

Failure of Weight Loss

Although several definitions are available, failure of weight loss is usually defined as less than 50% excess body weight loss.[34] According to these parameters, 10.5% of the patients who underwent LAGB present with inadequate weight loss at 5 years and 14% at 10 years.[35] Failure of weight loss remains the most prevalent reason for conversion surgery after LAGB (up to 62%).[36]

RESULTS

LAGB is still regarded as a technically simple and relatively inexpensive bariatric surgical option. Also, its safety is known in short-term and medium-term follow-ups. According to early studies, LAGB offered significantly lower morbidities and mortalities compared with the standard of care laparoscopic gastric bypass (mortality 0.05% vs 0.5%).[37] Even the weight loss outcomes of the LAGB were more than satisfactory compared with the potentially more morbid LRYGB. If the initial weight loss was lower compared with the LRYGB, multiple studies reported up to 65% EWL after 2 or 3 years.[37,38] The reports showed, however, a great degree of variability. Some of the variability was likely due to the lack of standardization of the postoperative band adjustments. Also it was evident how more-intense follow-ups and adjustments resulted in better weight loss outcomes, as shown by Shen and Ren.[39] Several long-term studies on LAGB are available. O'Brien and colleagues[19] reported the 15-year follow-up data on more than 3000 patients. They reported no mortality for either the primary LAGB procedure or for any subsequent revisional procedures. The EWL was 47% at 10 years and 15 years, although only 22% and 1.6% of the patients respectively were available for follow-up. They also reported a significant decrease in the need of reoperations and revisional surgeries after the introduction of the pars flaccida techniques as well as the new bad design.[19] They identified 3 separate periods in the evolution of the band and technique: the first period of the perigastric technique, the second of the pars flaccida, and the third of the newer and current designs of the band (Lap-Band AP, Apollo Endosurgery, Austin, Texas). Besides the prolapse (discussed previously), even the incidence of erosions significantly decreased with the in technique and band design. According to the investigators, the erosion rates went from 8.5%, to 2.25, and to 0.8% in the 3 evolution periods (groups 1, 2, and 3, respectively). Most of the revisions occurred for proximal pouch enlargement (26%) in the first 10 years of the investigators' experience. Port and tubing complications accounted for 21% of the revisions. Band removal occurred in 5.6% of the patients, mostly because of patients' request for reflux type symptoms. In the pooled analysis of studies reporting the results of LAGB and LRYGB with more than 10-year follow-up, they concluded that LAGB offers similar long-term weight loss, lower perioperative mortality, and similar need for revisional surgery (median of 22% for LRYGB and 26% for the LAGB).[19]

Along with the weight loss, comorbidity resolution was evident in many studies. Most of the typical manifestations of the metabolic syndrome were deeply improved by the band-related weight loss. Hypertension, for instance, has been reported improving in up to 92% of the patients.[37] Even the randomization of diabetic patient between LAGB and conventional medical treatment favor the former.[40] Also the initial concerns of creating a surgical achalasia were proved inaccurate by multiple reports showing improvement of the GERD after LAGB. Dixon and O'Brien[41] reported an 89% resolution of GERD after LAGB, 5% improvement, and only 2.5% worsening of the symptoms.

Longevity of Laparoscopic Adjustable Gastric Band

Despite a multitude of positive reports on the short-term and midterm results of LAGB, subsequent studies began to question the efficacy and durability of the LAGB long term. These results and the availability of more effective and equally safe options, such as the LSG, contributed to the significant decline in popularity of the LAGB.

One of the main concerns about the longevity of results after LAGB is attributed to the need for long-term follow-up, more so than in other bariatric operations. It is often the misconception of the need for such intense follow-up that has given the band the reputation of an easy and quick fix and is the reason it has been offered to a large nonselected cohort of patients.

Large-scale studies on LAGB have been reported; however, they tend to be single-institution and nonrandomized. Among these, Favretti and colleagues[42] reported on more than 1700 patients with an excellent 91% follow-up at 12 years. The mean weight loss was 40% at 1 year, 37% at 6 years, and 49% at 12 years. They also reported a 5.9% incidence of complication related to reoperation and 2.3% conversion for failure of weight loss or weight regain. Similar good weight loss results and resolution of comorbidities were reported in Australia by O'Brien and colleagues[38] on 709 patients. They reported an excessive weight loss (EWL) of 57% at 72 months. They also noted, however, a higher incidence of slippage (12.5%), band erosion of 2.8%, and port-related complications (3.6%). Other positive reports included the one from Switzerland of Steffen,[3] in which 824 patients were followed for 7 years. A respectable 61% EWL was reported, with, however, a 5.6% annual reoperation rate.

Concerning Results

If many positive studies on LAGB exist in the literature, more negative ones are reported, especially when longer follow-up data are available. Suter and colleagues[35] reported on 317 patients at 8 years. The overall complication rate they reported was 33%, mostly due to erosion (9.5%), port-related complications (7.6%), and slippage or pouch dilatation (6.3%). Also, the same investigators describe a worrisome 21.7% rate of major reoperations. Patel and colleagues reported a reoperation rate of 17.5% in band placed over an 8 year period.[20] In the author experience the majority of the reoperations were due to band removals alone (44%), conversion to Roux-en-Y gastric bypass (14.8%), conversion to sleeve gastrectomy (13.6%), band repositioning (10.2%), and band replacements (2.3%). Himpens and colleagues[22] also reported high rates of removal (60%). More interestingly is the failure of weight loss (EWL <25%) or need for reoperation rates, reaching 36.9% at 7 years. Similar high long-term complication rates requiring reoperations for explantation and conversions were reported by other investigators.[43] These investigators reported a 17.6% incidence of reoperation in their 448 patients followed for an average of 3.2 ± 2.2 years. Only 36% of the reoperations were considered minor. The main reasons for reoperation were again pouch dilatation (37%), erosion (20%), and insufficient weight loss (20%). They estimated the need for major reoperation after LAGB to be 4.1 interventions per 100 person-years. It is noticeable how only 19% of the patients were available for greater than 5-year follow-up.

Morino and colleagues[44] in their prospective randomized trial comparing LAGB to laparoscopic vertical banded gastroplasty found that early morbidities were similar between the 2 procedures, but the late complications were more common after LAGB (32.7% vs 14%, $P<.05$). LAGB was also more likely to require additional operations compared with laparoscopic vertical banded gastroplasty (24.5% vs 0, $P<.001$). Some of the complications of the LAGB were related to the technique (perigastric placement) used and the experience of the surgeon. Weiner and colleagues[17] reported that the rate of slippage decreased from 17% during the first 100 operations to 0 in the last 300 cases. Additional reports continued to appear on the high rate on complications (19% to 44%), reinterventions (25% or higher), and conversion for failure of weight loss.[45,46] Finally the most recent of the reports analyzed more than 19,000 LAGB patients in the state of New York over a 6-year period.[47] According to these investigators, the rate of revision after LAGB is more than 22%, 20% of which required multiple operations. Furthermore, the complication rates at the time of revisions were significantly higher (30%). The higher complication rates after revisional surgery have been well described by other investigators.[48]

Laparoscopic Adjustable Gastric Banding in Adolescents

LAGB has been selectively used in the treatment of morbid obesity in adolescents. After the first report in this patient population in 2003, multiple other studies have shown the medium-term safety and efficacy of the LAGB in the adolescent population.[49,50] Even in a randomized trial between intense medical management and LAGB in adolescents, the latter group compared favorably for weight loss and comorbidity resolution. Similarly to the adult studies, however, the overall weight loss seems inferior to the LRYGB.[51] Although solid long-term results are still lacking, there is more evidence that LAGB in adolescents presents similar long-term complication as in the adults.[51]

Laparoscopic Adjustable Gastric Banding for Lower Body Mass Indices

The other category of patients worth mentioning is those with lower BMIs (30 kg/m^2–35 kg/m^2). In a review of 6 studies encompassing 515 patients, the mean EWL% ranged from 52.5 to 78.6 at 1 year and from 57.6 to 87.2 at 2 years. The weight loss is maintained over time, as shown by the 3-year EWL of 68%. The complication rates were overall low (6.6%).[52] Again, the long-term data are missing, so only partial conclusions can be drawn from this study.

FUTURE OF LAPAROSCOPIC ADJUSTABLE GASTRIC BANDING

The rapid decline of the utilization of LAGB and the proportional steep increase in LSG popularity have put the future of LAGB in question. Even the companies producing the different bands have significantly scaled down their marketing strategies, once targeting patients directly. So the question is, Would the LAGB disappear from the bariatric arena just like the vertical banded gastroplasty did, or there are still some potential indications for it?

To attempt an answer to this question, the results of LAGB are compared with the other bariatric options.

When the authors analyze randomized trials comparing LAGB to other bariatric procedures, the conclusions are overall consistent. The LAGB is not the most effective bariatric procedure in terms of weight loss, but it is associated with lower early complications and shorter operative time and length of stay.[53] LAGB it is also effective in reducing obesity-related comorbidities, but its efficacy varies depending on the degree of success in weight loss.[53] LAGB presents, however, a higher potential for long-term of complications and reoperations.

It is well known how quality of life and self-image improve with increasing weight loss.[54] But postoperative complications, lengthy hospital admissions, and postoperative complications may reduce the general well-being of patients. In this setting, LAGB with minimal early complications and in-hospital stay might have a potential advantage over other, more complex bariatric operations. The only prospective randomized trial comparing quality of life after LRYGB and LAGB showed no significant difference between the 2 arms at 12 months.[23] Other more recent studies have confirmed the improvement of quality of life after LAGB, both short term and up to 3 years.[55] According to the same randomized study, the mean operative time and blood loss were higher, but as expected, the length of stay was also longer in the LRYGB gastric bypass group. The 30-day complication rate was higher after gastric bypass (21.6% vs 7.0% for gastric band), although the only statistically significant difference was in the minor complications. The late complications were once again higher in the LRYGB group (29% vs 10%, $P = .01$), with the most common ones anastomotic stricture (15%) and band slippage and erosion (5.8%), respectively. Treatment failure (EWL <20%), however, was only observed in the LAGB group (16.7%).

Despite the reported variability of weight loss results, it seems a consistent finding that the ability to reach adequate weight loss is greater with the LRYGB, followed by the LSG, and finally by the LAGB. The incidence of patients reaching EWL% less than 50% has been reported higher after LAGB (50%) than after LSG and LRYGB (33% and 23%, respectively).[56]

If the other potential field of application of LAGB is analyzed, the adolescent population, the results remain consistent. Even the most recent of the reviews for bariatric surgery and adolescents focuses on EWL results.[57] In this review, the investigators, reporting on the results of 37 studies, found a maximum weight loss of the LRYGB (BMI loss of 16.6 kg/m²), followed by the LSG (BMI loss of 14 kg/m²), and lastly the LAGB (BMI loss of 11.6 kg/m²). Complications of the LAGB were reported in 10.5%, and reoperation was necessary in 14% of the cases (including replacement or repositioning, removal, and port revision).

Finally, as previously reported by other investigators, the revision rate after LAGB in large studies could be as high as 34.17%.[47] Although a majority of these patients (80%) require only 1 procedure, up to 20% of them require multiple revisional and conversional operations. According to Altieri and colleagues,[47] patients particularly at risk for needing reinterventions were younger patients, female patients, and those with chronic pulmonary disease, hypothyroidism, psychoses, or rheumatoid arthritis. Despite the authors' best efforts, more than 3500 patients could not be followed up, so it is reasonable to believe that the percentages of complications could be even higher.

SUMMARY

LAGB presents fewer short-term complications and shorter hospital stays than other bariatric operations. Although its efficacy in terms of comorbidity resolution seems adequate in many studies, the variability of results is such that without robust level 1 data, final conclusions are difficult to draw. The main concern regarding LAGB remains with the long-term complications and durability of the procedure. Overall it is fair to conclude that the role of the band seems limited at the moment. The availability of more effective procedures with acceptable short-term and long-term complication rates, such as LSG, has eclipsed the role of the formally popular LAGB.

REFERENCES

1. Stevens J, Oakkar EE, Cui Z, et al. US adults recommended for weight reduction by 1998 and 2013 obesity guidelines, NHANES 2007-2012. Obesity (Silver Spring) 2015;23(3):527-31.

2. Payne JH, Dewind LT, Commons RR. Metabolic observations in patients with jejunocolic shunts. Am J Surg 1963;106:273-89. Available at: http://www.ncbi.nlm.nih.gov/pubmed/14042557. Accessed January 6, 2016.

3. Steffen R. The history and role of gastric banding. Surg Obes Relat Dis 2008; 4(3 Suppl):S7-13.

4. Wilkinson LH, Peloso OA. Gastric (reservoir) reduction for morbid obesity. Arch Surg 1981;116(5):602-5. Available at: http://www.ncbi.nlm.nih.gov/pubmed/7235951. Accessed January 6, 2016.

5. Molina M, Oria HE. Gastric segmentation: a new, safe, effective, simple, readily revised and fully reversible surgical procedure for the correction of morbid obesity. [abstract 15]. 6th Bariatric Surgery Colloquium. Iowa City (IA), June 2-3, 1983.

6. Frydenberg HB. Modification of gastric banding, using a fundal suture. Obes Surg 1991;1(3):315-7.

7. Szinicz G, Müller L, Erhart W, et al. "Reversible gastric banding" in surgical treatment of morbid obesity–results of animal experiments. Res Exp Med (Berl) 1989;189(1): 55-60. Available at: http://www.ncbi.nlm.nih.gov/pubmed/2711037. Accessed January 6, 2016.

8. Forsell P, Hallberg D, Hellers G. Gastric banding for morbid obesity: initial experience with a new adjustable band. Obes Surg 1993;3(4):369-74.

9. Kuzmak LI, Yap IS, McGuire L, et al. Surgery for morbid obesity. Using an inflatable gastric band. AORN J 1990;51(5):1307-24. Available at: http://www.ncbi.nlm.nih.gov/pubmed/2344182. Accessed January 6, 2016.

10. Belachew M, Legrand M, Vincenti V, et al. Laparoscopic placement of adjustable silicone gastric band in the treatment of morbid obesity: how to do it. Obes Surg 1995;5(1):66-70. Available at: http://www.ncbi.nlm.nih.gov/pubmed/10733796. Accessed January 6, 2016.

11. DeMaria EJ, Sugerman HJ, Meador JG, et al. High failure rate after laparoscopic adjustable silicone gastric banding for treatment of morbid obesity. Ann Surg 2001;233(6):809-18. Available at: http://www.pubmedcentral.nih.gov/articlerender.fcgi?artid=1421324&tool=pmcentrez&rendertype=abstract. Accessed December 10, 2015.

12. Fielding GA, Rhodes M, Nathanson LK. Laparoscopic gastric banding for morbid obesity. Surgical outcome in 335 cases. Surg Endosc 1999;13(6):550-4. Available at: http://www.ncbi.nlm.nih.gov/pubmed/10347288. Accessed January 6, 2016.

13. Weiner R, Wagner D, Bockhorn H. Laparoscopic gastric banding for morbid obesity. J Laparoendosc Adv Surg Tech A 1999;9(1):23-30. Available at: http://www.ncbi.nlm.nih.gov/pubmed/10194689. Accessed January 6, 2016.

14. Broadbent R, Tracey M, Harrington P. Laparoscopic Gastric Banding: a preliminary report. Obes Surg 1993;3(1):63–7.
15. Catona A, Gossenberg M, La Manna A, et al. Laparoscopic Gastric Banding: preliminary series. Obes Surg 1993;3(2):207–9. Available at: http://www.ncbi.nlm.nih.gov/pubmed/10757923. Accessed January 6, 2016.
16. Fielding GA, Ren CJ. Laparoscopic adjustable gastric band. Surg Clin North Am 2005;85(1):129–40, x.
17. Weiner R, Blanco-Engert R, Weiner S, et al. Outcome after laparoscopic adjustable gastric banding - 8 years experience. Obes Surg 2003;13(3):427–34.
18. Dargent J. Pouch dilatation and slippage after adjustable gastric banding: is it still an issue? Obes Surg 2003;13(1):111–5.
19. O'Brien PE, MacDonald L, Anderson M, et al. Long-term outcomes after bariatric surgery: fifteen-year follow-up of adjustable gastric banding and a systematic review of the bariatric surgical literature. Ann Surg 2013;257(1):87–94.
20. Patel S, Eckstein J, Acholonu E, et al. Reasons and outcomes of laparoscopic revisional surgery after laparoscopic adjustable gastric banding for morbid obesity. Surg Obes Relat Dis 2010;6(4):391–8.
21. Nguyen NT, Nguyen B, Gebhart A, et al. Changes in the makeup of bariatric surgery: a national increase in use of laparoscopic sleeve gastrectomy. J Am Coll Surg 2013;216(2):252–7.
22. Himpens J, Cadière G-B, Bazi M, et al. Long-term outcomes of laparoscopic adjustable gastric banding. Arch Surg 2011;146(7):802–7.
23. Nguyen NT, Slone JA, Nguyen XM, et al. A prospective randomized trial of laparoscopic gastric bypass versus laparoscopic adjustable gastric banding for the treatment of morbid obesity: outcomes, quality of life, and costs. Ann Surg 2009; 250(4):631–41.
24. van Dielen FMH, Soeters PB, de Brauw LM, et al. Laparoscopic adjustable gastric banding versus open vertical banded gastroplasty: a prospective randomized trial. Obes Surg 2005;15(9):1292–8.
25. Kim TH, Daud A, Ude AO, et al. Early U.S. outcomes of laparoscopic gastric bypass versus laparoscopic adjustable silicone gastric banding for morbid obesity. Surg Endosc 2006;20(2):202–9.
26. Tucker O, Sucandy I, Szomstein S, et al. Revisional surgery after failed laparoscopic adjustable gastric banding. Surg Obes Relat Dis 2008;4(6):740–7.
27. Wiesner W, Hauser M, Schöb O, et al. Spontaneous volume changes in gastric banding devices: complications of a semipermeable membrane. Eur Radiol 2001;11(3):417–21.
28. Angelchik JP, Cohen R. A new surgical procedure for the treatment of gastroesophageal reflux and hiatal hernia. Surg Gynecol Obstet 1979;148(2):246–8. Available at: http://www.ncbi.nlm.nih.gov/pubmed/154176. Accessed January 6, 2016.
29. Maxwell-Armstrong CA, Steele RJ, Amar SS, et al. Long-term results of the Angelchik prosthesis for gastro-oesophageal reflux. Br J Surg 1997;84(6):862–4. Available at: http://www.ncbi.nlm.nih.gov/pubmed/9189111. Accessed January 6, 2016.
30. Woodman G, Cywes R, Billy H, et al. Effect of adjustable gastric banding on changes in gastroesophageal reflux disease (GERD) and quality of life. Curr Med Res Opin 2012;28(4):581–9.
31. de Jong JR, van Ramshorst B, Timmer R, et al. Effect of laparoscopic gastric banding on esophageal motility. Obes Surg 2006;16(1):52–8.
32. de Jong JR, van Ramshorst B, Timmer R, et al. The influence of laparoscopic adjustable gastric banding on gastroesophageal reflux. Obes Surg 2004;14(3): 399–406.

33. Eid I, Birch DW, Sharma AM, et al. Complications associated with adjustable gastric banding for morbid obesity: a surgeon's guides. Can J Surg 2011; 54(1):61–6. Available at: http://www.pubmedcentral.nih.gov/articlerender.fcgi?artid=3038361&tool=pmcentrez&rendertype=abstract. Accessed January 6, 2016.

34. Reinhold RB. Critical analysis of long term weight loss following gastric bypass. Surg Gynecol Obstet 1982;155(3):385–94. Available at: http://www.ncbi.nlm.nih.gov/pubmed/7051382. Accessed January 6, 2016.

35. Suter M, Calmes JM, Paroz A, et al. 10-year experience with laparoscopic gastric banding for morbid obesity: high long-term complication and failure rates. Obes Surg 2006;16(7):829–35.

36. van Wageningen B, Berends FJ, Van Ramshorst B, et al. Revision of failed laparoscopic adjustable gastric banding to Roux-en-Y gastric bypass. Obes Surg 2006;16(2):137–41.

37. O'Brien PE, Dixon JB. Lap-band: outcomes and results. J Laparoendosc Adv Surg Tech A 2003;13(4):265–70.

38. O'Brien PE, Dixon JB, Brown W, et al. The laparoscopic adjustable gastric band (Lap-Band): a prospective study of medium-term effects on weight, health and quality of life. Obes Surg 2002;12(5):652–60. Available at: http://www.ncbi.nlm.nih.gov/pubmed/12448387. Accessed January 6, 2016.

39. Shen R, Ren CJ. Removal of peri-gastric fat prevents acute obstruction after Lap-Band surgery. Obes Surg 2004;14(2):224–9. Available at: http://www.ncbi.nlm.nih.gov/pubmed/15027437. Accessed January 6, 2016.

40. Dixon JB, O'Brien PE, Playfair J, et al. Adjustable gastric banding and conventional therapy for type 2 diabetes: a randomized controlled trial. JAMA 2008; 299(3):316–23.

41. Dixon JB, O'Brien PE. Selecting the optimal patient for LAP-BAND placement. Am J Surg 2002;184(6B):17S–20S. Available at: http://www.ncbi.nlm.nih.gov/pubmed/12527345. Accessed January 7, 2016.

42. Favretti F, Segato G, Ashton D, et al. Laparoscopic adjustable gastric banding in 1,791 consecutive obese patients: 12-year results. Obes Surg 2007;17(2): 168–75.

43. Silecchia G, Bacci V, Bacci S, et al. Reoperation after laparoscopic adjustable gastric banding: analysis of a cohort of 500 patients with long-term follow-up. Surg Obes Relat Dis 2008;4(3):430–6.

44. Morino M, Toppino M, Bonnet G, et al. Laparoscopic adjustable silicone gastric banding versus vertical banded gastroplasty in morbidly obese patients: a prospective randomized controlled clinical trial. Ann Surg 2003;238(6):835–41 [discussion: 841–2].

45. Weber M, Müller MK, Bucher T, et al. Laparoscopic gastric bypass is superior to laparoscopic gastric banding for treatment of morbid obesity. Ann Surg 2004; 240(6):975–82 [discussion: 982–3]. Available at: http://www.pubmedcentral.nih.gov/articlerender.fcgi?artid=1356513&tool=pmcentrez&rendertype=abstract. Accessed January 7, 2016.

46. Chevallier J-M, Zinzindohoué F, Douard R, et al. Complications after laparoscopic adjustable gastric banding for morbid obesity: experience with 1,000 patients over 7 years. Obes Surg 2004;14(3):407–14.

47. Altieri MS, Yang J, Telem DA, et al. Lap band outcomes from 19,221 patients across centers and over a decade within the state of New York. Surg Endosc 2015. http://dx.doi.org/10.1007/s00464-015-4402-8.

48. Acholonu E, McBean E, Court I, et al. Safety and short-term outcomes of laparoscopic sleeve gastrectomy as a revisional approach for failed laparoscopic adjustable gastric banding in the treatment of morbid obesity. Obes Surg 2009;19(12):1612–6.
49. Dolan K, Creighton L, Hopkins G, et al. Laparoscopic gastric banding in morbidly obese adolescents. Obes Surg 2003;13(1):101–4.
50. Holterman AX, Browne A, Tussing L, et al. A prospective trial for laparoscopic adjustable gastric banding in morbidly obese adolescents: an interim report of weight loss, metabolic and quality of life outcomes. J Pediatr Surg 2010;45(1): 74–8 [discussion: 78–9].
51. Lennerz BS, Wabitsch M, Lippert H, et al. Bariatric surgery in adolescents and young adults–safety and effectiveness in a cohort of 345 patients. Int J Obes (Lond) 2014;38(3):334–40.
52. Adegbola S, Tayeh S, Agrawal S. Systematic review of laparoscopic adjustable gastric banding in patients with body mass index $\leq$35 kg/m^2. Surg Obes Relat Dis 2014;10(1):155–60.
53. Chakravarty PD, McLaughlin E, Whittaker D, et al. Comparison of laparoscopic adjustable gastric banding (LAGB) with other bariatric procedures; a systematic review of the randomised controlled trials. Surgeon 2012;10(3):172–82.
54. Mathus-Vliegen EMH, de Wit LT. Health-related quality of life after gastric banding. Br J Surg 2007;94(4):457–65.
55. Billy HT, Sarwer DB, Ponce J, et al. Quality of life after laparoscopic adjustable gastric banding (LAP-BAND): APEX interim 3-year analysis. Postgrad Med 2014;126(4):131–40.
56. Caiazzo R, Arnalsteen L, Pigeyre M, et al. Long-term metabolic outcome and quality of life after laparoscopic adjustable gastric banding in obese patients with type 2 diabetes mellitus or impaired fasting glucose. Br J Surg 2010;97(6):884–91.
57. Paulus GF, De Vaan LEG, Verdam FJ, et al. Bariatric surgery in morbidly obese adolescents: a systematic review and meta-analysis. Obes Surg 2015;25(5): 860–78.

Biliopancreatic Diversion with Duodenal Switch

Surgical Technique and Perioperative Care

Laurent Biertho, MD*, Stéfane Lebel, MD, Simon Marceau, MD,
Frédéric-Simon Hould, MD, François Julien, MD, Simon Biron, MD, MSc

KEYWORDS

- Biliopancreatic diversion • Duodenal switch • Surgical technique
- Malabsorptive surgery • Management

KEY POINTS

- Patient selection is key to obtaining good clinical outcomes.
- Sleeve gastrectomy (SG) alone can be used as a staged approach in selected cases or to assess patient compliance with follow-up and supplementation.
- Long-term nutritional follow-up with vitamins and minerals supplements is mandatory.

 Video content accompanies this article at http://www.surgical.theclinics.com

INTRODUCTION

The duodenal switch technique, without gastric resection, was originally described for the treatment of bile gastritis, by DeMeester and colleagues in 1987.[1] In addition, Dr Scopinaro and colleagues[2] described in 1979 a technique of biliopancreatic diversion. This procedure combined a distal gastrectomy, a gastrojejunostomy, and a jejunojejunostomy to create a 50-cm common channel and a 250-cm alimentary channel. This technique resulted in excellent outcomes, but the resection of the pyloric valve and the short, 50-cm, common channel resulted in postgastrectomy syndrome, significant risks of marginal ulcer, and increased gastrointestinal side effects.[3] The technique was thus modified in the late 1980s, to perform a longitudinal gastrectomy instead of a distal gastrectomy and to increase the common channel to 100 cm.[4,5] By preserving the pyloric valve and first duodenum, the normal emptying of the stomach is preserved, the risk of marginal ulcer is decreased, and gastrointestinal side effects are reduced.[3] In short, biliopancreatic diversion with duodenal switch (BPD-DS) includes

---

Department of Metabolic and Bariatric Surgery, Institut Universitaire de cardiologie et pneumologie de Québec – Université Laval, 2725 Chemin Sainte Foy, Quebec City, Quebec G1V 4G5, Canada
* Corresponding author.
E-mail address: laurent.biertho@criucpq.ulaval.ca

Surg Clin N Am 96 (2016) 815–826
http://dx.doi.org/10.1016/j.suc.2016.03.012
0039-6109/16/$ – see front matter © 2016 Elsevier Inc. All rights reserved.
surgical.theclinics.com

3 specific components: (1) a longitudinal gastrectomy (SG) to provide some caloric restriction while decreasing acid production and maintaining a normal gastric emptying; (2) a 250-cm total alimentary limb whose role is to decrease caloric absorption; and (3) a 100-cm common channel where food bolus mixes with biliopancreatic juices, resulting in decreased protein and fat absorption (**Fig. 1**). The malabsorptive and hormonal effects of BPD-DS result from separating the flow of food from the flow of bile and pancreatic juices. This results in a reduction of caloric and food absorption, in particular lipids, and metabolic changes through modifications in incretin levels.

In 2001, Dr Gagner[6] performed the first BPD-DS by laparoscopy, but the procedure has long been long been considered the most challenging bariatric procedure. Improvements in patient selection and preparation, surgical instrumentation, and 2-stage surgery, however, have now made laparoscopic approach standard, even for patients with very high body mass index (BMI).

SURGICAL TECHNIQUE
Preoperative Planning

The goal in modern bariatric surgery should be to select the right procedure for the right patient. This can significantly improve patient compliance with vitamin

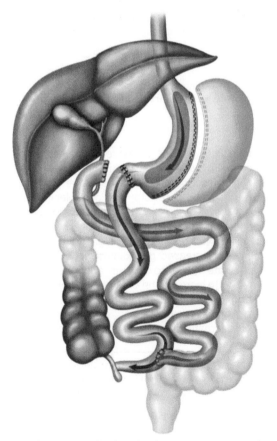

Fig. 1. BPD-DS. SG is performed and the first duodenum is anastomosed to the last 250 cm of small bowel. A 100-cm common channel is created.

supplementations, decrease dissatisfaction with side effects, and set reasonable goal expectations. The selection criteria for BPD-DS follows the standard recommendations for bariatric surgery, described in 1991 by the National Institutes of Health.[7] In addition, with the increased popularity of SG, it has become of increasing importance to be knowledgeable of laparoscopic BPD-DS for the management of weight regain. A duodenal switch allows staying away from scarred tissue at the level of the stomach, which can potentially reduce the risk of leak at the level of a gastrojejunostomy. Also, the safety and effectiveness of redo SG or conversion to Roux-en-Y gastric bypass for patients who have failed an SG can be questionable. On the other hand, adding a malabsorptive component (duodenal switch) represents an effective way to offer a successful weight loss to those patients.[8]

Contraindications for malabsorptive surgery follow the standard recommendations for bariatric surgery. In addition, the presence of Barrett esophagus is usually seen as a relative contraindication to an SG. Compliance with long-term follow-up, regular blood work, and lifelong vitamin and mineral supplementation are also of utmost importance to obtaining successful outcomes. A history of substance abuse in the prior 6 months, poorly controlled mental disease, and questionable long-term compliance represent the authors' main reasons to refuse patients for BPD-DS. Patients should quit smoking before any bariatric surgery. Slow-release medications should be converted to normal release, due to the unknown absorption after malabsorptive surgery (ie, long-acting antidepressants).

Preoperative Work-up

All bariatric patients are assessed by a multidisciplinary team, including a bariatric surgeon, specialized bariatric nurse, and dietician. Consultation with a dietician experienced with BPD-DS is of utmost importance, to correct eating disorders before surgery and for patient education of the recommended diet after BPD-DS (high-protein and low-fat diet). A psychiatric evaluation is requested for patients with a history of mental disease or when clinically indicated. Patients are screened for sleep apnea and, if needed, noninvasive positive pressure ventilation is initiated by a pneumologist before surgery. Preoperative blood work consists of a complete blood cell count, liver enzymes, albumin, calcium, parathyroid hormone, vitamin D, vitamin A, vitamin B_{12}, and folic acid. Patients also have a lipid panel and are screened for diabetes. All patients receive a multivitamin complex (Centrum Forte) before surgery (usually 3 months in advance) and vitamin D supplementation (10,000U for 1 month followed by 1000 U until surgery). Other vitamins and minerals deficiencies are corrected before surgery.

Preparation and Patient Positioning

Patients are placed under general anesthesia in a bariatric operating room table. Intravenous antibiotics (cefazolin, 2 g) and thromboprophylaxis (heparin, 5000 U, subcutaneously 2 hours before surgery, or low-molecular-weight heparin at a prophylactic dose, 12 hours before surgery) are given before the procedure starts. Pneumatic compression devices are used during the procedure and until patients are ambulatory.

The following laparoscopic instruments set is used during the surgery:

- A 5-mm or 10-mm 30° endoscope
- Nontraumatic bowel graspers, including extralong (45-cm) instruments
- Articulating linear stapler-cutter, 60 mm in length, with cartridges ranging from white to black loads (Echelon Flex long 60, Ethicon, Cincinnati, OH)
- Ace ultrasonic device (Ethicon)

- Laparoscopic curved needle holder with DeBakey forceps, with a bariatric needle holder
- 5-mm and 10-mm disposable trocars, 10 cm in length (Endopath Xcel, Ethicon), with 15-cm length trocars available
- 15-cm Veress needle
- V-Loc absorbable 3-0 suture (Covidien, Mansfield, Massachusetts)
- Long clip applier
- Fascia closure device

The basic principles of a BPD-DS are to start with the gastric mobilization and SG. The duodenum is transected 3 cm to 4 cm distal to the pylorus. The small bowel is then transected 250 cm from the ileocecal valve. A handsewn duodenoileostomy is then created. The biliary limb is anastomosed side to side to the alimentary limb, 100 cm from the ileocecal valve.

Positioning

Patients are placed in a split-legs position, with both arms open. The surgeon stands between a patient's legs, a camera operator to the right, and an assistant to the left. A 15-cm Veress needle is introduced in the left subcostal area to create a 15-mm Hg pneumoperitoneum. A 5-mm or 10-mm optical trocar is placed under direct vision, 2 handbreadths under the xyphoid, for the camera. A 12-mm port is placed at the same level in the left and right flanks. A 5-mm port is placed in the epigastrium for the liver retractor, in the left upper quadrant for the assistant, and in the left flank for the submesocolic part of the procedure (**Fig. 2**).

Surgical Approach

Step 1: gastric mobilization
The first step of the procedure is similar to a standard SG (Video 1). The gastrocolic ligament is opened starting at the level of the gastric body, using an ultrasonic scalpel (**Fig. 3**). The greater curvature of the stomach is fully mobilized from the antrum to the

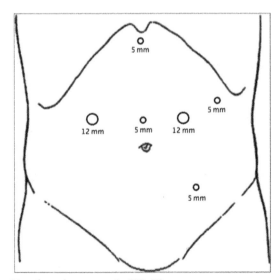

Fig. 2. Trocars position for a laparoscopic BPD-DS.

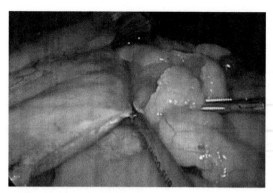

Fig. 3. Transection of the gastrocolic ligament.

angle of His. The feasibility of the duodenal switch is appraised at that point. In certain cases (ie, super-super obese man with a short mesentery, dense adhesions at the level of the duodenum or pelvis, or patients with high intra-abdominal pressure with limited working space), the surgery can be converted to SG alone, as a first-stage surgery.

Step 2: duodenal dissection

The duodenal dissection represents the main specificity of a duodenal switch and the learning curve with this dissection should be done under supervision, due to the proximity of several major anatomic structures, such as the pancreatic head, the common bile duct, and the gastroduodenal artery (Videos 2 and 3). The pylorus is identified and the peritoneum is opened at the inferior and superior edges of the duodenum. Pulling the antrum to the patient's left, from the left upper quadrant trocar, provides a good retraction of the duodenum. The common bile duct is often visualized at the superior aspect of the duodenum and can be used as a landmark for the duodenal dissection. Two different techniques exist for the mobilization of the first duodenum: a complete mobilization of the inferior and posterior attachments of the duodenum (inferior approach) and a direct approach of the duodenum to create a tunnel under the posterior aspect of the duodenum (posterior approach).

Inferior approach The gastrocolic ligament is transected using ultrasonic energy (see Video 2). The pyloric artery is controlled and dissection is continued on the first duodenum. A posterior dissection is performed to mobilize the first 3 cm to 4 cm of duodenum. The gastroduodenal artery is often used as the limit for the posterior dissection of the first duodenum. A window is then created on the upper aspect of the duodenum, and a 15-cm Penrose drain is used for retraction. The window is slightly enlarged to accommodate the anvil of a 60-mm linear stapler. An Echelon Flex with a blue cartridge is introduced through the 12-mm port in the left flank. The duodenum is then transected.

Posterior approach A window is created at the inferior part of the duodenum, 3 cm to 4 cm distal to the pylorus (see Video 3). Blunt dissection is used to identify the plane between the posterior duodenal wall and the pancreas. That dissection has to be done carefully, to avoid bleedings from the small venous branches draining the duodenum to the pancreatic head, from the gastroduodenal artery, and to prevent an injury to the back wall of the duodenum. If any difficulties are encountered, the dissection can be converted to an Inferior approach to better identify the anatomy. When the window below the duodenum is created, a 15-cm Penrose drain is used to retract the duodenum (**Fig. 4**). The window is slightly enlarged to accommodate the anvil of a 60-mm linear stapler and the duodenum is transected (**Fig. 5**).

Step 3: sleeve gastrectomy

Gastric transection is started 5 cm to 7 cm from the pylorus (**Fig. 6**, Video 4). A 60-mm Echelon Flex is used with black or green cartridges for the first 2 to 3 firings. The length of the staples is decreased (from green to blue cartridges) as the gastric transection progresses towards the fundus. A 34-French esophagogastric bougie is usually placed for guidance. Care is taken not to create the sleeve too tight along that bougie. The goal of gastric resection in BPD-DS patients is to reduce acid production and to be mildly restrictive. This is in stark contrast with SG as a stand-alone procedure, in which the sleeve has to be much more restrictive due to the absence of associated small bowel bypass. The hemostasis on the staple line must be controlled, either with clips, oversewing with a 3-0 absorbable suture or with buttressing materials. The gastrectomy specimen is then placed in a plastic bag and removed through the 12-mm trocar in the right flank.

Step 4: small bowel transection

Patients are placed in a head-down position with the left side down (Video 5). The surgeon moves to the left side of the patient and uses the 2 lower trocars in the left flank. The ileocecal junction is first identified and adhesions between the ascending colon and the omentum are released. The authors use the length of the metallic part of our bowel graspers (5 cm) to measure the alimentary limb. The small bowel is first marked at 100 cm from the ileocecal junction, using a large clip on each side of the mesentery. The small bowel is then run another 150 cm and transected at that level (250 cm from the ileocecal valve), using a 60-mm linear stapler with a white cartridge. The alimentary limb should be on the patient's right side and is directly marked using a metallic clip on the mesentery. The small bowel mesentery is usually opened a few centimeters to decrease tension on the duodenal anastomosis. Resection of the last few centimeters of small bowel can be done if there is any ischemia detected at that time.

Step 5: duodenoileal anastomosis

The duodenoileal anastomosis is usually performed first, to decrease tension on that anastomosis as much as possible (Videos 6 and 7). In smaller patients, however, the distal anastomosis (see step 6) can be performed before the duodenoileal

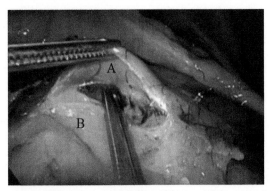

Fig. 4. (A) The duodenum is lifted up with a Penrose drain and the retroduodenal window is enlarged (B) pancreatic head and (C) pylorus.

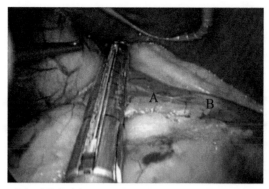

Fig. 5. Transection of the (A) duodenum using a 60-mm stapler with a blue load, 3 cm from (B) the pylorus.

anastomosis, to avoid one position change. For the duodenal anastomosis, the patient is placed in a slight head-up position and the surgeon goes between the patient's legs. The alimentary limb is brought to the right upper quadrant in an antecolic fashion and approximated to the transected duodenum. The omentum can be mobilized from its attachments to the ascending colon if there is any tension on the anastomosis. A handsewn end-to-side anastomosis is then created. A 23-cm 3-0 absorbable V-Loc suture is used for the first anastomotic layer (see Video 6). The antimesenteric side of the small bowel is anastomosed to the duodenum (**Fig. 7**). The intestinal lumens are opened and another 23-cm 3-0 V-Loc suture is used to create the back wall of the anastomosis, starting from the top of the intestinal opening. A 15-cm V-Loc suture is then used to create the anterior wall of the anastomosis, starting from the top of the anastomosis (**Fig. 8**, see Video 7). The 2 running sutures are crossed or attached together on the inferior aspect of the anastomosis. The anastomosis can be tested by insufflating air through a nasogastric tube. This also allows testing the patency of the anastomosis. The authors do not routinely test the anastomosis but rather perform an intraoperative gastroscopy in selected cases.

Step 5: ileoileal anastomosis
The ileoileal anastomosis is then created at 100 cm from the ileocecal valve (see Video 5). The patient is place head-down and the surgeon moves back to the patient's

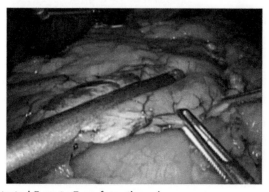

Fig. 6. The SG is started 5 cm to 7 cm from the pylorus.

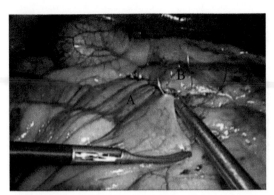

Fig. 7. The first posterior layer is created using 3-0 absorbable suture, to approximate (A) the alimentary limb to (B) the duodenum.

left side. The biliary limb is attached to the ileon using a 2-0 Vicryl in an antiperistaltic technique **(Fig. 9)**. This stitch is used to provide an adequate exposure for the anastomosis. A side-to-side anastomosis is then created using another white load of a 60-mm linear stapler-cutter. The intestinal opening is closed using a single layer of 3-0 V-Loc suture, starting from the mesenteric side **(Fig. 10)**. The small bowel is then retracted to the right upper quadrant using the 2-0 Vicryl stay suture. The mesenteric window is closed using a nonabsorbable 2-0 Prolene suture. The Petersen window is also closed as much as possible. The transverse colon is lifted up through the left upper quadrant trocar. A 2-0 Prolene suture is then used to close the Petersen defect.

A routine cholecystectomy and liver biopsy are usually performed at the end of the surgery; 12-mm trocars are closed with 2-0 Vicryl using a fascia closure device and the pneumoperitoneum is exsufflated under direct vision.

Postoperative Period

Regular or low-molecular-weight subcutaneous heparin is given the day of surgery. All patients are switched to a low-molecular-weight heparin on postoperative day 1. Patients are allowed to drink water the day of surgery. A liquid diet is started on postoperative day 1 and a soft diet on postoperative day 2. Patients are usually discharged on

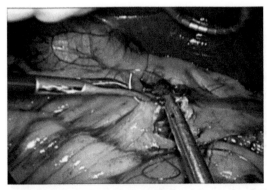

Fig. 8. The anterior wall of the anastomosis is created, using an absorbable 3-0 running suture, starting from the top of the anastomosis.

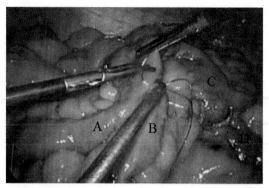

Fig. 9. A 2-0 Vicryl suture is placed to approximate (A) the common channel and (B) the biliary limb. (C) The alimentary limb is located in the patient's right flank and (D) proximal Ileon.

postoperative day 3, when tolerating a soft diet. Patients who still have their gall-bladder are placed on ursodiol (Actigall, Ciba-Geigy, Summit, New Jersey), 250 mg orally, twice a day, for 6 months. A nutritionist monitors patient intakes before discharge and instructs patients to progress to a minced diet after 2 weeks and to a regular diet after 1 month. Daily vitamins and mineral supplementations are started within the first month after surgery (ferrous sulfate, 300 mg; vitamin D, 50,000 IU; vitamin A, 20,000 IU; calcium carbonate, 1000 mg; and a multivitamin complex). These supplements are adjusted over the years, and education in consuming a high-protein diet is reinforced. The patient is followed with a blood work (similar to the blood work done in the preoperative period) after 4, 8, and 12 months and annually thereafter.

SUMMARY OF CLINICAL OUTCOMES

A recent survey of the International Federation for the Surgery of Obesity and Meta-bolic Disorders member national societies reported that the proportions of BPD-DS were 4.9% in 2008, 2.1% in 2011, and 1.5% in 2013.[9] Even though the absolute num-ber of BPD-DS procedures increased from 2008 to 2013, this suggests that other sur-geries are performed preferentially (ie, SG, which has now become the predominant surgery in North America). This decrease in the percentage of duodenal switch can

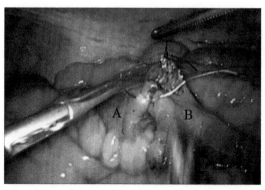

Fig. 10. The intestinal opening of the anastomosis is closed with a 3-0 absorbable suture. (A) The common channel is on the left and (B) the biliary limb is on the right.

be related to the lack of exposure of many surgical teams to the BPD-DS technique, its greater complexity, and greater concerns about gastrointestinal side effects and vitamins and protein deficiencies. In addition, BPD-DS can only be offered to super–morbidly obese patients (BMI above 50 kg/m^2) in some countries.

Long-Term Outcomes After Biliopancreatic Diversion with Duodenal Switch

Even though an exhaustive discussion of BPD-DS outcomes is beyond the goal of this article, the authors want to place long-term outcomes of BPD-DS in perspective. Only a few investigators[10–13] reported their outcomes beyond 5 years in a significant number of patients (>100 patients). These studies are summarized in **Table 1**. Overall, long-term outcomes are excellent and BPD-DS has a marked effect on obesity-related diseases, specifically type 2 diabetes mellitus (T2DM) (remission in >90% for T2D on oral medications). Similarly, Buchwald and colleagues,[14] in a meta-analysis of 32 studies with 4035 patients who underwent a biliopancreatic diversion or BPD-DS, reported a mean excess weight loss (EWL) of 70%, improvement or remission of T2DM in 98%, resolution of hypertension in 81%, resolution of sleep apnea in 95%, and improvement of hyperlipidemia in 99%.

Perioperative Morbidity and Mortality

In a meta-analysis of 361 studies, including 85,048 patients published in 2007, the mean 30-day mortality after bariatric surgery was 0.28%.[15] Perioperative mortality for BPD-DS was the highest, with a rate between 0% and 2.7% for laparoscopic procedures. More recently, global mortality after bariatric surgery has been consistently reported to be approximately 0.1%. The authors reported a complication rate in a series of 1000 consecutive BPD-DS, including the initial experience with laparoscopic BPD-DS[16]; the 90-day mortality rate was 1/1000, from pulmonary embolism. In that series, major complications occurred in 7.2%, including 1.5% leak from the SG and 1.5% leak from the duodenal anastomosis. The complication rate after BPD-DS is usually higher compared with restrictive or mixed procedure, such as gastric bypass.[17] This is partly due to the complexity of the technique but also to BPD-DS being specifically offered in superobese patients with a higher rate of metabolic

Table 1
Clinical outcomes in large series of biliopancreatic diversion with duodenal switch (>100 cases) with a minimal follow-up of 5 years

Authors	Follow-up (y)	n	Weight Loss (%)	Type 2 Diabetes Mellitus (Remission)	Hypertension	Dyslipidemia
Bolckmans & Himpens,[10] 2016	10.8 ± 4.6	153	Total body weight loss: 40.7 ± 10	87.5%	81% Improved	>90%
Marceau et al,[11] 2015	8 (5–20)	2615	EWL: 71 (55.3 kg)	93.4%	60% Cured 91% Improved	80%
Biertho et al,[12] 2010	8.6 ± 4	810	EWL: 76 ± 22	92%	60% Cured	—
Pata et al,[13] 2013	11.9 ± 3.1	874	21 points of BMI lost	67% to 97%[a]	>96%	>96%

[a] Remission was 67% for patients initially on Insulin and 97% when initially on oral medications.
Data from Refs.[10–13]

complications. Even though there has been a significant decrease in both major and minor complications with laparoscopic approach in recent years, this rate is likely to remain slightly higher compared with other surgeries with shorter operative times or lower complexity.

SUMMARY

Malabsorptive bariatric procedures, such as BPD-DS, offer sustained weight loss and marked effect on comorbidities. Offering these procedures laparoscopically can improve the complication rate and accelerate patients' return to normal activities. This should be the approach of choice in this high-risk population. Intraoperative strategies can be used to minimize surgical complications, including the use of SG as a bridge to BPD-DS. Postoperative management involves active patient participation with follow-up and adherence to dietary recommendations, including lifelong vitamin supplements. The excellent long-term medical benefits and improvement in quality of life come at the expense of some gastrointestinal side effects and vitamin supplementation.

SUPPLEMENTARY DATA

Supplementary data related to this article can be found at http://dx.doi.org/10.1016/j. suc.2016.03.012.

REFERENCES

1. DeMeester TR, Fuchs K, Ball C, et al. Experimental and clinical results with proximal end-to-end duodenojejunostomy for pathologic duodenogastric reflux. Ann Surg 1987;206(4):414–26.
2. Scopinaro N, Gianetta E, Civalleri D, et al. Bilio-pancreatic bypass for obesity: II. Initial experience in man. Br J Surg 1979;66(9):618–20.
3. Marceau P, Biron S, Hould FS, et al. Duodenal switch improved standard biliopancreatic diversion: a retrospective study. Surg Obes Relat Dis 2009;5(1):43–7.
4. Hess DS, Hess DW. Biliopancreatic diversion with a duodenal switch. Obes Surg 1998;8:267–82.
5. Marceau P, Biron S, Bourque RA, et al. Biliopancreatic diversion with a new type of gastrectomy. Obes Surg 1993;3(1):29–35.
6. Ren CJ, Patterson E, Gagner M. Laparoscopic biliopancreatic diversion with duodenal switch: a case series of 40 consecutive patients. Obes Surg 2000; 10:514–23.
7. Brolin RE. Update: NIH consensus conference. Gastrointestinal surgery for severe obesity. Nutrition 1996;12(6):403–4.
8. Dapri G, Cadière GB, Himpens J. Laparoscopic repeat sleeve gastrectomy versus duodenal switch after isolated sleeve gastrectomy for obesity. Surg Obes Relat Dis 2011;7:38–43.
9. Angrisani L, Santonicola A, Iovino P, et al. Bariatric Surgery Worldwide 2013. Obes Surg 2015;25(10):1822–32.
10. Bolckmans R, Himpens J. Long-term (>10 Yrs) outcome of the laparoscopic biliopancreatic diversion with duodenal switch. Ann Surg 2016. [Epub ahead of print].
11. Marceau P, Biron S, Marceau S, et al. Long-term metabolic outcomes 5 to 20 years after biliopancreatic diversion. Obes Surg 2015;25(9):1584–93.

12. Biertho L, Biron S, Hould FS, et al. Is biliopancreatic diversion with duodenal switch indicated for patients with body mass index <50 kg/m2? Surg Obes Relat Dis 2010;6:508–14.

13. Pata G, Crea N, Di Betta E, et al. Biliopancreatic diversion with transient gastroplasty and duodenal switch: long-term results of a multicentric study. Surgery 2013;153(3):413–22.

14. Buchwald H, Avidor Y, Braunwald E, et al. Bariatric surgery: a systematic review and meta-analysis. JAMA 2004;292:1724–8.

15. Buchwald H, Estok R, Fahrbach K, et al. Trends in mortality in bariatric surgery: a systematic review and meta-analysis. Surgery 2007;142(4):621–32 [discussion: 632–5].

16. Biertho L, Lebel S, Marceau S, et al. Perioperative complications in a consecutive series of 1000 duodenal switches. Surg Obes Relat Dis 2013;9(1):63–8.

17. Prachand VN, Davee RT, Alverdy JC. Duodenal switch provides superior weight loss in the super-obese (BMI > or = 50 kg/m2) compared with gastric bypass. Ann Surg 2006;244(4):611–9.

Revisional Bariatric Surgery

Noah J. Switzer, MD[a], Shahzeer Karmali, BSc, MD, MPH, FRCSC[b],
Richdeep S. Gill, MD, PhD, FRCSC[c], Vadim Sherman, MD, FRCSC[d],*

KEYWORDS

- Revisional surgery • Failed gastric band • Failed gastric bypass
- Failed sleeve gastrectomy • Conversion • Weight recividism

KEY POINTS

- Revisional bariatric procedures are becoming increasingly common. Inevitably 5–8% of primary bariatric procedures will fail requiring a revisional operation.
- The main reasons for revisional bariatric surgery are either primary inadequate weight loss, weight recidivism, or inherit specific complications related to the procedure itself.
- The most successful conversion strategy relies on selecting the most appropriate revisional procedure, including one-stage versus two-staged and laparoscopic versus open, and involving a multidisciplinary team approach to the patient.
- The gold standard revisional option is usually to laparoscopically convert a restrictive operation to a Roux-en-Y gastric bypass in order to have the best balance of long term weight loss, resolution of complications related to the primary procedure and acceptable rate of perioperative complications.

ADJUSTABLE GASTRIC BAND/LAPAROSCOPIC ADJUSTABLE GASTRIC BANDING
History

Initially introduced in the early 1990s, adjustable gastric banding (AGB) is the most commonly performed bariatric operation in many places in the world, including Europe, Australia, and South America, and is the second most commonly performed bariatric procedure in the United States.[1–5] Largely based on its acceptable weight loss, technical simplicity, low morbidity profile, and reversibility, more than 300,000 laparoscopic adjustable gastric banding (LAGB) procedures have been performed

Disclosure: The authors have no financial or commercial interests that conflict with the topic of this paper.
[a] Department of Surgery, University of Alberta, Room 405 CSC, 10240 Kingsway Avenue, Edmonton, Alberta T5H 3V9, Canada; [b] Department of Surgery, Minimally Invasive Gastrointestinal and Bariatric Surgery, University of Alberta, Room 405 CSC, 10240 Kingsway Avenue, Edmonton, Alberta T5H 3V9, Canada; [c] Department of Surgery, Peter Lougheed Hospital, University of Calgary, 3rd Floor West Wing, Room 3656, 3500 26th Avenue Northeast, Calgary, Alberta, T1Y 6J4, Canada; [d] Weill Cornell Medical College, Bariatric and Metabolic Surgery Center, Houston Methodist Hospital, 6550 Fannin Street, SM 1661, Houston, TX 77030, USA
* Corresponding author.
E-mail address: vsherman@houstonmethodist.org

Surg Clin N Am 96 (2016) 827–842
http://dx.doi.org/10.1016/j.suc.2016.03.004
surgical.theclinics.com

worldwide since US Food and Drug Administration approval in 2001.[3] However, as is common in primarily restrictive bariatric operations, the failure rate is quite high. Failure rates have been reported ranging between 40% and 50%, with 20% to 30% of patients requiring a revisional operation.[3]

Brief description of the surgical procedure

Using minimally invasive techniques for gaining entry, a gastric band is placed just below the gastroesophageal junction and fixed with 3 or 4 nonabsorbable sutures on the anterior aspect.[6] The approximate size of the gastric pouch should be between 50 and 80 mL.[7]

Indications for Revision

Although primary inadequate weight loss and secondary weight regain are common indications for revision after banding, other complications, including hardware malfunctions with the band, tubing, or access port; esophageal motility issues; and psychological intolerance to the band, are common causes that lead to revision (**Table 1**).[8]

Inadequate weight loss and secondary weight recividism

There are many considerations, often overlapping, when evaluating a patient for either inadequate weight loss or weight regain. These considerations include technical factors from suboptimal band adjustments, adverse gastrointestinal symptoms such as reflux, and maladaptive eating behaviors. It is important to evaluate all these factors in a multidisciplinary bariatric care clinic before considering revisional surgery of any kind.[4]

Hardware problems

Band slippage is a common postoperative issue following LAGB. With an incidence ranging between 1% and 22%, it is the primary reason for reoperation in 2% to 69% of revisional cases.[7,9,10] It is defined as either the downward migration of the band with the anterior wall of the stomach migrating through the band (anterior slip) or the herniation of the posterior wall of the stomach through the band (posterior slip).[7]

Table 1
Indications for revision following adjustable gastric band/laparoscopic adjustable gastric banding

Issues	Incidence (%)
Insufficient weight loss	13.7–62.5
Weight recidivism	33.3–40
Hardware problems	
Slippage	2–76
Band erosion	0–11
Band intolerance	0.6–6.2
Early band obstruction	0.5–11
Port and tubing problems	4.3–24
Motility problems	
Esophageal dilation	37.5
Gastric pouch dilation	0.4–40
Miscellaneous	
GERD	33
Band intolerance	0.6–6.2

Data from Refs.[4–14]

Band erosion is seen when the band gradually erodes into the gastric lumen. It has a prevalence of 3% to 11%.[7] It may result from stomach wall injury during the initial surgery but more commonly results from chronic pressure imposed by the band.

Band intolerance, defined as symptoms such as vomiting, esophageal spasm, and gastrointestinal reflux disease (GERD) in the absence of clinical obstruction, has an incidence of 0.6% to 6.2%.[11]

Port and tubing problems, as a composite complication, have an incidence of 4% to 24% and consist of band erosion or displacement and tubing leakage, breakage, or disconnection.[11]

Motility problems

Pouch enlargement is defined as dilation of the proximal gastric pouch without overt evidence of a band slip. Radiologically, there may or may not be a change in the angle of the band.[7] It is usually a consequence of chronic outlet obstruction imposed by the band, leading to proximal dilatation. Some evidence suggests it may also be related to overeating.[7]

Conversion Strategies

Key principles

1. *Appropriate revisional operation selection.* Choosing the most appropriate revisional surgery following failed LAGB depends largely on the indications for revision themselves. If the primary cause was inadequate weight loss, reflux, or band erosion/intolerance/obstruction, then conversion to a malabsorptive procedure such as Roux-en-Y gastric bypass (RYGB) or duodenal switch (DS) is most appropriate.[3] Several investigators advocate the key principle in conversion surgery is that a failed restrictive bariatric surgery due to poor weight loss should include a revisional option with a malabsorptive component. Others suggest that if the gastric band failed due to either band slippage or pouch dilatation, yet independent of weight outcomes, then potential revisional options include rebanding or conversion to a laparoscopic sleeve gastrectomy (LSG).[3] Decision-making should include the presence of symptoms related to GERD, because this should sway patients and surgeons away from another restrictive operation. Educating patients with regards to all possible options as well as their risks and benefits is of paramount importance because studies have shown that 96% of patients felt that they were unaware of all their bariatric surgical options before agreeing to an operation.[15]

2. *One-staged versus 2-staged revisional operations.* Traditional opinion was that a 2-step operation, consisting of band removal and then at a later date a conversion operation, would allow chronic inflammatory changes induced by the gastric band to settle and would therefore reduce gastric staple line leak and anastomotic stricture rates.[16,17] However, opponents of this strategy would argue that the disadvantage of 2-step operations is the potential for weight regain in the waiting period, in addition to the risks of undergoing an additional general anesthesic.[18] The literature remains divided in this recommendation. An interesting study by Tan and colleagues[19] revealed that inflammatory changes following band removal might be irreversible; therefore, the speculation might be that leak rates, regardless of timing, would be higher compared with a primary operation.

3. *Open versus laparoscopic.* Laparoscopic bariatric surgery is associated with fewer postoperative complications and decreased hospital length of stay, and therefore, should be considered the standard of treatment.[20,21]

Adjustable gastric band/laparoscopic adjustable gastric banding removal
Although there have been scattered reports of maintaining the band during conversions to LSG or RYGB, band removal is the standard of care when performing a revisional operation.[3,14] Band removal, without a subsequent conversion to another bariatric operation, will often solve many the adverse gastrointestinal symptoms; however, weight regain or inadequate weight loss will not be addressed.[3]

Common indications for band removal alone include acute slippage with necrosis or perforation, erosion, intractable nausea and vomiting, intractable dysphagia, band infection, and patient desire.[9,11]

It is important to note that conservative management consisting of band volume adjustment is indicated for initial, first-line treatment of minimal anterior slippage and esophageal dilation.[9]

*Adjustable gastric band/laparoscopic adjustable gastric banding replacement/
refixation*
Rebanding for failed gastric bands is a heavily debated topic. Successful laparoscopic refixation and rebanding have been reported in the literature, with a reduction in band slippage rates and improved excess weight loss (EWL).[6,10] In comparing rebanding with repositioning, rebanding was associated with a nonsignificant reduction in the rate of future operations (5.3% vs 22.6%).[13] Most investigators would argue that for failed weight loss, the gastric band should be converted to a malabsorptive procedure; however, for hardware failures such as band slippage or band defect such as a punctured balloon, there is a role for laparoscopic band replacement or re-fixation.[6]

*Adjustable gastric band/laparoscopic adjustable gastric banding to Roux-en-Y gastric
bypass*
Revision from the LAGB to laparoscopic Roux-en-Y gastric bypass (LRYGB) is generally considered the gold standard.[22] Conversion to RYGB is associated with excellent long-term weight loss outcomes, with a quoted decrease in body mass index (BMI) of approximately 10 kg/m^2 at 1-, 2-, and 4-year follow-ups.[3] Quoted %EWL based on prebanding weight ranges between 50% and 57%.[4,23,24] The main indications for conversion to an RYGB include inadequate weight loss, weight recidivism, reflux, and esophageal dysmotility.[8,13] Conversion to RYGB is associated with longer operative times and higher complication rates compared with primary RYGB.[4] Literature-cited complication rates following revisional RYGB range between 3% and 29.3%, with an overall complication rate of 8.5%. Anastomotic leak and bleeding rates were reported at a combined rate of approximately 3%.[25]

*Adjustable gastric band/laparoscopic adjustable gastric banding to laparoscopic
sleeve gastrectomy*
A recent review of conversion of the LAGB to LSG reported a drop in BMI at 1 and 2 years of approximately 8.8 kg/m^2 and 10.8 kg/m^2, respectively. Quoted %EWL based on prebanding weight was roughly 40%.[26,27] However, there was significant weight regain greater than 2 years after LSG of approximately 8 kg/m^2.[3] As well, increased overall complication rates following LSG were reported by Coblijn and colleagues[25] in a recent systematic review (LSG 12.2% vs RYGB 8.5%). Specifically, the quoted incidence of anastomotic leak rates following LSG was 5.6%.[25]

The advantages of the LSG over the RYGB are the technical ease of the operation, reduced mean hospital stay, and decreased operating room (OR) time.[25] However, the LSG lacks a malabsorptive component and involves the transection of the band's fibrous capsule, which could potentially lead to tissue ischemia and therefore might explain the observed higher postoperative leak rates.[12] The fibrous capsule must be removed in order to increase the chances of creating a uniformly tubular stomach with conversion to LSG.

Reflux disease leading to AGB failure should be a contraindication for conversion to an LSG.[11]

Adjustable gastric band/laparoscopic adjustable gastric banding to biliopancreatic diversion with duodenal switch

Successful conversion to the BPD-DS leads to considerable %EWL compared with RYGB, but has marked perioperative morbidities.[22] Topart and colleagues[22] reported 73% EWL for their series of 21 patients following DS from their initial weight, but had significantly higher complication rates (62 vs 12.5%) compared with RYGB. Limited evidence exists, only small case series or case reports, in the literature as to the efficacy and safety of the DS in revisional surgery from the LAGB.[22,28]

LEGACY PROCEDURE
The Nonadjustable Gastric Band

History

The nonadjustable gastric band (NAGB) was first performed in the late 1970s by Wilkinson and Peloso.[29] Based on the concept of restricting oral intake by reducing gastric volume, an implanted band material was placed around the upper part of the stomach in a process called gastric segmentation. The band material itself was variable, including polypropylene mesh, Dacron graft, silastic tubing, and Gore-Tex mesh.[29–31]

Indications for revision

Although long-term weight-loss outcomes were underwhelming, long-term complications after NAGB were significant. Band slippage, band erosion, and esophagitis were all morbid and common complications.[31,32] Naslund and colleagues[33] published one of the longest follow-up studies following NAGB in the literature, consisting of 80 patients. They found that during their almost 10-year follow-up, not only was weight regain very common, but also only 31% of patients actually had an intact band in follow-up investigations. Their conclusion was quite bold, stating that they could not recommend the NAGB as a general treatment for morbid obesity.[33]

Nonadjustable gastric band to Roux-en-Y gastric bypass The literature is sparse about revisional operations after the NAGB, but the limited case series point to the efficacy of conversion to RYGB.[31,34]

Conversion to RYGB is heavily favored over LSG, because the site of band erosion or stricturing can be avoided.[34] Because of the desmoplastic reaction caused by the NAGB, a fibrous and thickened stomach wall results. Therefore, the gastric pouch must be created proximal to the site of the capsule.[31] Band removal can be performed laparoscopically, with care taken to remove as much of the fibrous capsule as possible. Should the band erode, it can be removed either endoscopically, laparoscopically, or combined laparoendoscopically.[34]

Vertical Banded Gastroplasty

History

Vertical banded gastroplasty (VBG) was first described by Mason[35] in 1982 and quickly became the most commonly performed primary bariatric surgery in the late 1980s. Although reported short-term weight loss outcomes, roughly 50% EWL, and low perioperative morbidity rates made this procedure promising initially, high long-term failure rates in the range of 20% to 65% made the VBG less appealing.[11,36] Observed reoperative rates after VBG are between 10% and 56%.[11] VBG is associated with the highest operation failure rates compared with any other primary bariatric surgery option.[37]

Brief description of the surgical procedure As originally described by Mason and colleagues, the operator places a 32-French Ewald tube per oral into the stomach, flush to the lesser curvature. Then, a site 8 to 9 cm below the angle of His is selected for the 2.5-cm gastric window to be created with an Anvil stapler. Through this window, a noncutting stapler was then applied in the cephalad direction toward the angle of His along the Ewald tube to create a 50-cc tubularized gastric pouch. This technique was later altered by MacLean and colleagues[38] to attempt to reduce the high rates of gastrogastric fistulas by completely dividing the staple line. In addition, the outlet to the pouch was banded with either Marlex mesh, polypropylene, or silastic ring to maintain a constant stomal circumference.[11,35]

Indications for revision
Inadequate weight loss and weight recidivism are the primary indications, ranging between 5% and 61%, for patients seeking a revisional bariatric surgery.[11] However, other common indications are related to proximal gastric outlet obstruction, leading to reflux, food intolerance, band erosion, and staple line disruption (**Table 2**).

Inadequate weight loss and secondary weight recividism Poor weight outcome patients can be divided into 2 separate groups after VBG: patients with intact anatomy versus patients with abnormal anatomy. Patients with intact VBG anatomy usually fail due to maladaptive eating behaviors. Because of obstructive-like symptoms imposed by the band, patients will exhibit maladaptive eating behaviors by consuming soft or liquid foods, which tend to be calorie dense. Patients with abnormal anatomy due to staple line breakdown or band erosion may be regaining their weight due to lack of a restrictive component. Regardless, a multidisciplinary approach with counseling and nutritional education is essential in addition to the surgical therapy.

Conversion strategies
Key principles
1. *Revisional surgery is complex.* Revisional surgeries are associated with increased morbidity compared with primaries.[42] Increased adhesions and distorted anatomy

Table 2
Indications for revision following vertical banded gastroplasty

Issues	Incidence (%)
Insufficient weight loss	10–100
Weight recidivism	26–74
Technical reasons	
Wide outlet	14–17.1
Pouch dilation	3–15.8
Staple line erosion	2.7–47.6
Stoma stenosis	9.9–100
Band erosion	6.3–11
Band dehiscence	0.7
Miscellaneous	
GERD	16.6–65

Data from Refs.[26,27,38–42]

lead to longer OR times and increased rates of bleeding.[40] Consideration should be given for the placement of a gastrostomy tube during conversion to an RYGB for immediate decompression, and in the event of a leak, for long-term enteral feeding.[40] Because of technical complexity and potential for morbid perioperative complications, reoperative bariatric surgeries should be performed in tertiary care hospitals by experienced, high-volume bariatric surgeons.[11]

2. *Anastomotic strictures are common following failed VBG.* The proximal stomach is often chronically inflamed, with the presence of thickened mucosa, which together can lead to stricturing.[40] Transection of the stomach to create the gastric pouch may also disrupt the vascular supply, therefore further increasing the risk of anastomotic stricture.[42]

Vertical banded gastroplasty reversal Reversal is an option in patients not desiring conversion to RYGB or are otherwise higher-risk surgical candidates.[11] Thoreson and Cullen[39] published a series of VBG reversals in 28 patients. A gastrotomy was performed and, using a linear stapler, an intraluminal side-to-side gastrogastrostomy was created. Following surgery, presenting symptoms of gastric outlet obstruction including nausea and vomiting, reflux, and food intolerance improved in 89% of patients, with minor perioperative complications. Patients, on average, gained 8 kg at 32 months follow-up after reversal.[39]

Vertical banded gastroplasty revision Revision surgery to a re-VBG has been associated with poor surgical outcomes in the literature and is generally not performed. van Gemert and colleagues[41] compared revision re-VBG to conversion to RYGB and found that 68% of re-VBG patients will require another surgery over a 5-year time period compared with 0% of conversion RYGB patients.

In a study by Hunter and colleagues,[43] poor long-term outcomes were found in their 69 revision patients, with only 23% of patients having successful revisional surgeries. Stomal dilation and stomal stenosis, in particular, as primary indications for revision were associated with higher failure rates of 55% and 83%, respectively. The investigators concluded that although re-VBG revision surgery, in general, has poor response rates, stomal dilation or stenosis patients, in particular, should be converted to the bypass.[43] From a safety point of view, high gastric leak rates have been reported in the re-VBG perioperative period, necessitating eventual conversion to a gastric bypass.[44,45]

Vertical banded gastroplasty to Roux-en-Y gastric bypass Conversion to RYGB is the gold standard and resolves complications related to proximal gastric outlet obstruction while assisting with weight loss.[45] Gagne and colleagues,[40] in their series of 94 patients undergoing conversion for poor weight-loss outcomes, described an EWL of 47% at 26 months following conversion to LRYGB. Complications were divided between early and late, but 38% of patients reported a complication. Notable early complications (<30 days) were anastomotic leaks (4.8%) and marginal ulcers (2.9%), with reoperations (diagnostic laparoscopy) required in 9.5% of patients.[40] Notable late complications (>30 days) included anastomotic structuring (11.4%), internal herniation (1.9%), and jejunojejunostomy site perforation (1.0%), with reoperation required in 9 patients and endoscopic dilation in 10 patients.

Iannelli and colleagues[42] performed a smaller case series in 2008 on 18 patients undergoing revision from VBG to RYGB with similar results. They reported no perioperative mortalities and low conversion-to-open rates (5.5%), with similar anastomotic leak (5.5%) and stricture (11.1%) rates to Gagne and colleagues.[40] The investigators concluded that conversion of failed VBG to RYGB is the "ideal" solution.

Vertical banded gastroplasty to laparoscopic sleeve gastrectomy The specific surgical steps in conversion of VBG to LSG, as described by Iannelli and colleagues,[26] varies slightly depending on whether the original VBG was a true Mason or modified MacLean technique. For the MacLean VBG, only the distal stomach is divided, and for the Mason VBG, the stomach is divided medially to the vertical staple line.

Foletto and colleagues[27] observed high leak rates in their series of 5 VBG patients converted to an LSG, because 40% of these patients had leaks that were conservatively managed. The explanation behind the observed higher leak rates following conversion to LSG compared with RYGB may be due to proximity of the new staple line to the previous vertical staple line. More likely, though, when the site of the band or mesh is transected, the tissue is most at risk for vascular compromise leading to the high risk for leaks.[46]

Vertical banded gastroplasty to biliopancreatic diversion with duodenal switch The data are limited on the conversion of VBG to DS. Dapri and colleagues[46] converted a series of 12 patients from VBG to DS. Although the mean EWL was quite impressive at 85.1% at a mean follow-up time of 43 months, the outcomes from this case series were quite poor. Six patients suffered major complications (4 leaks) with 3 patients suffering mortality within 8 months of their surgery.[46] The average length of stay was 35 days. They concluded that laparoscopic conversion of VBG to DS has an unacceptable rate of complications and death.[46]

Laparoscopic Sleeve Gastrectomy

History
The sleeve gastrectomy was first introduced by Hess and Hess[47] in 1988 as a component of their newly introduced open hybrid operation, the biliopancreatic diversion with duodenal switch (BPD-DS). As the BPD-DS evolved, it became a laparoscopic operation[48] and subsequently LSG was performed as a first stage in a 2-staged operation in high-risk and severely obese patients.[49] After short-term weight loss was shown to be promising from the first-stage LSG, the second stage was increasingly abandoned until LSG became a stand-alone primary bariatric procedure around 2005.[49]

Brief description of the surgical procedure The lesser sac is entered via ligation of the gastroepiploic vessels along the greater curvature of the stomach using an energy device.[49] Dissection then proceeds in the cephalad direction to the left pillar of the hiatus.[49] A linear cutting stapler is then introduced along with a per-oral 32 to 40 French bougie. The stapler then fires along the length of the bougie, approximately 6 cm proximal to the pyloric valve, until the greater curvature of the stomach is completely transected.[49,50] The stomach is transformed into a "banana-shaped" gastric pouch of approximately 20% of the original stomach volume and total capacity of 100 to 150 mL.[5,49]

Indications for revision
Not surprisingly, inadequate weight loss and weight recidivism are the primary indications for patients seeking a revisional bariatric surgery.[51] However, other indications include development of GERD, staple-line stricture, pouch dilatation, and anastomotic leak (**Box 1**).

Inadequate weight loss/weight regain Although LSG is associated with good long-term weight loss, with 48% to 53% EWL, approximately 5% to 10% of patients will have poor weight loss outcomes and require a revisional procedure.[51,52]

Technical reasons Sleeve strictures leading to obstruction most commonly occur at the angularis incisura, as a result either of technical factors or from creation of an inappropriately small luminal diameter.[11] First-line treatment is usually endoscopic

---

Box 1
Indications for revision following laparoscopic sleeve gastrectomy

Issues

Insufficient weight loss

Weight recidivism

Technical reasons
  Anastomotic leaks
  Sleeve stricture
  Sleeve dilation

Miscellaneous
  GERD

Data from Brethauer SA, Kothari S, Sudan R, et al. Systematic review on reoperative bariatric surgery: American Society for Metabolic and Bariatric Surgery Revision Task Force. Surg Obes Relat Dis 2014;10(5):952–72.

---

dilatation; however, this is usually followed by definitive surgical therapy such as conversion to RYGB.[11]

Anastomotic leaks are very challenging because they are difficult to control with drainage or stenting. Acute or chronic leaks may lead to fistulous disease. Conversion to RYGB is usually the mainstay of treatment for difficult to control leaks.[11]

Miscellaneous The effect of LSG on reflux is debateable.[53,54] However, long-term studies have commented that approximately 1 in 5 patients will develop new GERD following LSG and that preoperative presence of reflux will be maintained following LSG.[55]

Conversion strategies
Key principles

1. *Sleeve dilation or not?* As a distensible organ, the stomach may stretch over time. Patients presenting with weight regain will often be found to have a dilated tubular stomach on upper endoscopy or upper gastrointestinal series. Nonetheless, a re-sleeve is not the standard of care and should not be considered as a long-term viable option for weight control.[56] Rather, a conversion to a malabsorptive operation is the mainstay of treatment.
2. *BMI ≥50 kg/m²?* Although RYGB is the gold-standard conversion procedure, surgeons must consider DS for patients with BMI of 50 kg/m² or greater.[57,58] DS has been shown to be superior in weight-loss outcomes and comorbidity resolution in the superobese patient.[57,58]
3. *GERD or not?* Resleeve should not be considered in LSG failures associated with GERD. Instead, patients should be converted to RYGB, which is the ultimate anti-reflux operation, because acid and bile will be diverted away from the esophagus.[54]
4. *Preoperative assessment is crucial.* Assessing whether the patient has significant risk factors for perioperative complications is of utmost importance. Patients with prior thromboembolic disease and nutritional deficiencies would benefit more with conversion to RYGB rather than DS because of a shorter procedural length and decreased long-term nutritional complications.[56]

Resleeve gastrectomy The RLSG involves a refashioning of the dilated gastric pouch.[59] A recent 2014 systematic review of failed LSG found that there is no difference in efficacy between the RLSG and RYGB at 24-month follow-up, with both procedures having approximately 45% EWL.[60] The advantages of the RLSG are that it is not associated with profound nutritional deficiencies; it is associated with less dumping syndrome, and it is technically a simpler operation.[59]

Conversion to a malabsorptive procedure Choosing the appropriate malabsorptive conversion procedure for failed LSG is difficult. Although conversion to RYGB is most widely accepted in the literature and there is a paucity of data on conversion to DS, the LSG was originally described as the first step in a staged BPD-DS 2-step procedure.[60] At the latest International Consensus summit on Sleeve Gastrectomy, most surgeons converted to the RYGB (46%) followed by DS (24%) for weight regain.[54] The only systematic review by Cheung and colleagues[60] on revisional LSG found that after conversion to RYGB, patients had 68% and 44% EWL at 1 year and 2 years or more, respectively. DS was not analyzed individually because of the lack of primary studies available.

Carmeli and colleagues[56] retrospectively compared BDP-DS and RYGB in 19 patients. At the last follow-up, patients had more significant weight loss following DS versus RYGB, 80.3% versus 66.6% of EWL, respectively.[56] Importantly, DS also had improved rates of comorbidity resolution, 84% versus 67%. However, DS was associated with more long-term complications, mainly nutritional.[56]

Roux-en-Y Gastric Bypass

History
Developed in 1967 by Mason, RYGB has become the gold standard in primary and revisional bariatric surgery.

Indications for revision
Around 10% to 20% of patients following RYGB, as a primary procedure, will have inadequate weight loss or weight regain at 2 years, with a subset of these individuals requiring a revisional surgery.[61–63] Other RYGB-specific complications can also be primary indications for revision, including gastric pouch dilatation, gastrogastric fistulas, anastomotic strictures or ulcers, and metabolic derangements (**Box 2**).

Metabolic/endocrine derangements Severe malnutrition, vitamin deficiency, refractory hypoglycemia, and recalcitrant hypocalcemia have all been reported as revisional indications following RYGB.[11]

Conversion strategies
Reversal of Roux-en-Y gastric bypass Reversal to normal intestinal continuity is only indicated in extreme circumstances of intractable nausea/vomiting, extreme weight loss and malnutrition, metabolic abnormalities, nonhealing ulcerations or leaks, and patient choice.[11] Case reports in the literature report successful resolution of endocrine, metabolic, and nutritional abnormalities following reversal, with improved metabolic parameters.[64,65] Refeeding syndrome is a concern for these patients, especially patients with extremely low BMI.[65] Fifty percent to 88% of patients will regain weight following reversal.[64]

Banding Roux-en-Y gastric bypass The placement of AGBs/NAGBs on the gastric pouch following failed RYGB is termed "salvage" banding. Indications for banding after RYGB failure include pouch dilation and gastrojejunostomy dilation.[63] A recent review of banding following failed RYGB included only 7 studies.[61,63] Excess BMI loss ranged between 28.3% and 64.9%.[63] The less invasive nature of banding when compared with conversion to DS makes it an appealing revisional option.[63] However,

> **Box 2**
> **Indications for revision following Roux-en-Y gastric bypass**
>
> *Issues*
>
> Insufficient weight loss
>
> Weight recidivism
>
> Extreme weight loss
>
> Technical reasons
>   Gastrogastric fistula
>   Gastric pouch dilation/stricture
>   Gastrojejunostomy dilation/stricture
>   Marginal ulcers
>   Bowel loss: internal hernia/small bowel volvulus
>   Roux stasis syndrome
>   Dumping syndrome
>
> Miscellaneous
>   Metabolic/endocrine derangements
>   Bypass intolerance
>
> *Data from* Refs.[11,62,64]

it is not without its complications, because 18% of patients developed long-term complications, which included band erosion and band slippage, with 17% of patients requiring a re-revision.[63]

Roux-en-Y gastric bypass limb lengthening The concept of Roux limb lengthening is based on increasing the malabsorption component of the gastric bypass and thereby increasing weight loss. Systematic reviews examining the efficacy of Roux limb length on weight loss found that limb length makes no difference on weight loss outcomes for non-superobese patients, but there might be a small benefit in the patients with BMI of 50 kg/m^2 or more.[66,67] Christou and colleagues[68] found that at 10-year follow-up, the length of the Roux limb (40 cm vs 100 cm) was not associated with differing weight loss outcomes. Therefore, lengthening the Roux limb as a revisional procedure seems to have little utility.

Gastric pouch revisions Revision of the gastric pouch for poor weight loss can be performed in several ways: either complete takedown of the gastrojejunostomy, trimming the gastric pouch, placing a gastric band (as mentioned previously), or endoluminal reduction.[69,70] Pouch reduction with neo-gastrojejunostomy will address an enlarged pouch and stoma; however, if there is isolated pouch enlargement on the greater curvature side, then reduction of the pouch alone may be an option.[71] Muller and colleagues[71] laparoscopically revised 5 patients for pouch dilatation by a complete reconstruction of the pouch and reported a mean change in BMI of 3.9 kg/m^2 at 23-month follow-up. Nguyen and colleagues[72] performed revisional trimming of the pouch with or without redo gastrojejunostomy anastomosis in 44 patients and reported 38% EWL.bib72 Endoluminal techniques achieve gastric pouch and stomal reduction via tissue plication. Mild short-term weight loss is reported but long-term weight-loss outcomes are poor because restriction is immediately lost once the plication sutures fail.[70,73]

Revisional options for marginal ulcer complications involve gastrojejunostomy resection with primary anastomosis with or without a truncal vagotomy. Case reports and series in the literature have shown the efficacy of this approach for patients with persistently symptomatic marginal ulcers who have failed appropriate medical management.[74,75]

Roux-en-Y gastric bypass to duodenal switch Perhaps the best indication for conversion to DS in revisional surgery is for failed RYGB.[76] Parikh and colleagues[77] converted 12 patients to DS and reported 62.7% EWL equating to a mean BMI reduction of 10.5 kg/m^2 at 11-month follow-up. Surprisingly, there were no leaks in the series, only 4 strictures that were managed with endoscopic dilation and reoperative revision. Other small case series and case reports have reported the efficacy of conversion for indications including poor weight loss outcomes, hypoproteinemia, and dumping syndrome.[76,78] A few specific technical considerations must be taken into account by the operator. The preservation or sacrifice of the Roux limb in the restoration of continuity and the preservation of the lesser curve gastric vessels that feed the new gastrogastrostomy and the sleeve gastrectomy should both be given significant consideration during conversion.[78]

SUMMARY

All bariatric surgical procedures, especially restrictive ones, are at risk for failure, from either poor weight loss outcomes or procedural-specific complications. An experienced bariatric surgeon within a multidisciplinary team should make the ultimate determination to convert. The gold standard is to laparoscopically convert a restrictive operation to an RYGB in order to have the best balance of long-term weight loss, resolution of complications related to the primary procedure, and acceptable rate of perioperative complications.

REFERENCES

1. Mann JP, Jakes AD, Hayden JD, et al. Systematic review of definitions of failure in revisional bariatric surgery. Obes Surg 2015;25(3):571–4.
2. Shimizu H, Annaberdyev S, Motamarry I, et al. Revisional bariatric surgery for unsuccessful weight loss and complications. Obes Surg 2013;23(11):1766–73.
3. Elnahas A, Graybiel K, Farrokhyar F, et al. Revisional surgery after failed laparoscopic adjustable gastric banding: a systematic review. Surg Endosc 2013;27(3):740–5.
4. Langer FB, Bohdjalian A, Shakeri-Manesch S, et al. Inadequate weight loss vs secondary weight regain: laparoscopic conversion from gastric banding to Roux-en-Y gastric bypass. Obes Surg 2008;18(11):1381–6.
5. Acholonu E, McBean E, Court I, et al. Safety and short-term outcomes of laparoscopic sleeve gastrectomy as a revisional approach for failed laparoscopic adjustable gastric banding in the treatment of morbid obesity. Obes Surg 2009;19(12):1612–6.
6. Schouten R, van Dielen FM, Greve JW. Re-operation after laparoscopic adjustable gastric banding leads to a further decrease in BMI and obesity-related co-morbidities: results in 33 patients. Obes Surg 2006;16(7):821–8.
7. Eid I, Birch DW, Sharma AM, et al. Complications associated with adjustable gastric banding for morbid obesity: a surgeon's guides. Can J Surg 2011;54(1):61–6.
8. Gagner M, Gumbs AA. Gastric banding: conversion to sleeve, bypass, or DS. Surg Endosc 2007;21(11):1931–5.

9. Dargent J. Surgical treatment of morbid obesity by adjustable gastric band: the case for a conservative strategy in the case of failure—a 9-year series. Obes Surg 2004;14(7):986–90.

10. Peterli R, Donadini A, Peters T, et al. Re-operations following laparoscopic adjustable gastric banding. Obes Surg 2002;12(6):851–6.

11. Brethauer SA, Kothari S, Sudan R, et al. Systematic review on reoperative bariatric surgery: American Society for Metabolic and Bariatric Surgery Revision Task Force. Surg Obes Relat Dis 2014;10(5):952–72.

12. Bernante P, Foletto M, Busetto L, et al. Feasibility of laparoscopic sleeve gastrectomy as a revision procedure for prior laparoscopic gastric banding. Obes Surg 2006;16(10):1327–30.

13. Ardestani A, Lautz DB, Tavakkolizadeh A. Band revision versus Roux-en-Y gastric bypass conversion as salvage operation after laparoscopic adjustable gastric banding. Surg Obes Relat Dis 2011;7(1):33–7.

14. O'Brien PE, MacDonald L, Anderson M, et al. Long-term outcomes after bariatric surgery: fifteen-year follow-up of adjustable gastric banding and a systematic review of the bariatric surgical literature. Ann Surg 2013;257(1):87–94.

15. Keshishian A, Zahriya K, Hartoonian T, et al. Duodenal switch is a safe operation for patients who have failed other bariatric operations. Obes Surg 2004;14(9):1187–92.

16. Obeid NR, Schwack BF, Kurian MS, et al. Single-stage versus 2-stage sleeve gastrectomy as a conversion after failed adjustable gastric banding: 30-day outcomes. Surg Endosc 2014;28(11):3186–92.

17. Van Nieuwenhove Y, Ceelen W, Van Renterghem K, et al. Conversion from band to bypass in two steps reduces the risk for anastomotic strictures. Obes Surg 2011;21(4):501–5.

18. Lanthaler M, Strasser S, Aigner F, et al. Weight loss and quality of life after gastric band removal or deflation. Obes Surg 2009;19(10):1401–8.

19. Tan MH, Yee GY, Jorgensen JO, et al. A histologic evaluation of the laparoscopic adjustable gastric band capsule by tissue sampling during sleeve gastrectomy performed at different time points after band removal. Surg Obes Relat Dis 2014;10(4):620–5.

20. Weller WE, Rosati C. Comparing outcomes of laparoscopic versus open bariatric surgery. Ann Surg 2008;248(1):10–5.

21. Nguyen NT, Ho HS, Palmer LS, et al. A comparison study of laparoscopic versus open gastric bypass for morbid obesity. J Am Coll Surg 2000;191(2):149–55 [discussion: 155–7].

22. Topart P, Becouarn G, Ritz P. Biliopancreatic diversion with duodenal switch or gastric bypass for failed gastric banding: retrospective study from two institutions with preliminary results. Surg Obes Relat Dis 2007;3(5):521–5.

23. Moore R, Perugini R, Czerniach D, et al. Early results of conversion of laparoscopic adjustable gastric band to Roux-en-Y gastric bypass. Surg Obes Relat Dis 2009;5(4):439–43.

24. Weber M, Muller MK, Michel JM, et al. Laparoscopic Roux-en-Y gastric bypass, but not rebanding, should be proposed as rescue procedure for patients with failed laparoscopic gastric banding. Ann Surg 2003;238(6):827–33 [discussion: 833–4].

25. Coblijn UK, Verveld CJ, van Wagensveld BA, et al. Laparoscopic Roux-en-Y gastric bypass or laparoscopic sleeve gastrectomy as revisional procedure after adjustable gastric band–a systematic review. Obes Surg 2013;23(11):1899–914.

26. Iannelli A, Schneck AS, Ragot E, et al. Laparoscopic sleeve gastrectomy as revisional procedure for failed gastric banding and vertical banded gastroplasty. Obes Surg 2009;19(9):1216–20.

27. Foletto M, Prevedello L, Bernante P, et al. Sleeve gastrectomy as revisional procedure for failed gastric banding or gastroplasty. Surg Obes Relat Dis 2010;6(2): 146–51.

28. Trelles N, Gagner M. Laparoscopic revision of gastric banding to biliopancreatic diversion with duodenal switch. Surg Obes Relat Dis 2010;6(2):200–2.

29. Oria HE. Gastric segmentation: nonadjustable banding by minilaparotomy: historical review. Surg Obes Relat Dis 2009;5(3):365–70.

30. Karmali S, Sweeney JF, Yee K, et al. Transgastric endoscopic rendezvous technique for removal of eroded Molina gastric band. Surg Obes Relat Dis 2008; 4(4):559–62.

31. Westling A, Ohrvall M, Gustavsson S. Roux-en-Y gastric bypass after previous unsuccessful gastric restrictive surgery. J Gastrointest Surg 2002;6(2):206–11.

32. Steffen R. The history and role of gastric banding. Surg Obes Relat Dis 2008; 4(Suppl 3):S7–13.

33. Naslund E, Granstrom L, Stockeld D, et al. Marlex mesh gastric banding: a 7-12 year follow-up. Obes Surg 1994;4(3):269–73.

34. Balogh J, Vizhul A, Dunkin BJ, et al. Clinical management of patients presenting with non-adjustable gastric band (NAGB) complications. Yale J Biol Med 2014; 87(2):159–66.

35. Mason EE. Vertical banded gastroplasty for obesity. Arch Surg 1982;117(5): 701–6.

36. Berende CA, de Zoete JP, Smulders JF, et al. Laparoscopic sleeve gastrectomy feasible for bariatric revision surgery. Obes Surg 2012;22(2):330–4.

37. Greenbaum DF, Wasser SH, Riley T, et al. Duodenal switch with omentopexy and feeding jejunostomy–a safe and effective revisional operation for failed previous weight loss surgery. Surg Obes Relat Dis 2011;7(2):213–8.

38. van Wezenbeek MR, Smulders JF, de Zoete JP, et al. Long-term results of primary vertical banded gastroplasty. Obes Surg 2015;25(8):1425–30.

39. Thoreson R, Cullen JJ. Indications and results of reversal of vertical banded gastroplasty (VBG). J Gastrointest Surg 2008;12(11):2032–6.

40. Gagne DJ, Dovec E, Urbandt JE. Laparoscopic revision of vertical banded gastroplasty to Roux-en-Y gastric bypass: outcomes of 105 patients. Surg Obes Relat Dis 2011;7(4):493–9.

41. van Gemert WG, van Wersch MM, Greve JW, et al. Revisional surgery after failed vertical banded gastroplasty: restoration of vertical banded gastroplasty or conversion to gastric bypass. Obes Surg 1998;8(1):21–8.

42. Iannelli A, Amato D, Addeo P, et al. Laparoscopic conversion of vertical banded gastroplasty (Mason MacLean) into Roux-en-Y gastric bypass. Obes Surg 2008; 18(1):43–6.

43. Hunter R, Watts JM, Dunstan R, et al. Revisional surgery for failed gastric restrictive procedures for morbid obesity. Obes Surg 1992;2(3):245–52.

44. Behrns KE, Smith CD, Kelly KA, et al. Reoperative bariatric surgery. Lessons learned to improve patient selection and results. Ann Surg 1993;218(5):646–53.

45. Gonzalez R, Gallagher SF, Haines K, et al. Operative technique for converting a failed vertical banded gastroplasty to Roux-en-Y gastric bypass. J Am Coll Surg 2005;201(3):366–74.

46. Dapri G, Cadiere GB, Himpens J. Laparoscopic conversion of adjustable gastric banding and vertical banded gastroplasty to duodenal switch. Surg Obes Relat Dis 2009;5(6):678–83.

47. Hess DS, Hess DW. Biliopancreatic diversion with a duodenal switch. Obes Surg 1998;8(3):267–82.

48. Ren CJ, Patterson E, Gagner M. Early results of laparoscopic biliopancreatic diversion with duodenal switch: a case series of 40 consecutive patients. Obes Surg 2000;10(6):514–23 [discussion: 524].

49. Mognol P, Chosidow D, Marmuse JP. Laparoscopic sleeve gastrectomy as an initial bariatric operation for high-risk patients: initial results in 10 patients. Obes Surg 2005;15(7):1030–3.

50. Gumbs AA, Gagner M, Dakin G, et al. Sleeve gastrectomy for morbid obesity. Obes Surg 2007;17(7):962–9.

51. Switzer N, Karmali S. The sleeve gastrectomy and how and why it can fail? Surg Curr Res 2014;4:180.

52. Eid GM, Brethauer S, Mattar SG, et al. Laparoscopic sleeve gastrectomy for super obese patients: forty-eight percent excess weight loss after 6 to 8 years with 93% follow-up. Ann Surg 2012;256(2):262–5.

53. Gautier T, Sarcher T, Contival N, et al. Indications and mid-term results of conversion from sleeve gastrectomy to Roux-en-Y gastric bypass. Obes Surg 2013; 23(2):212–5.

54. Gagner M, Deitel M, Erickson AL, et al. Survey on laparoscopic sleeve gastrectomy (LSG) at the Fourth International Consensus Summit on Sleeve Gastrectomy. Obes Surg 2013;23(12):2013–7.

55. Himpens J, Dobbeleir J, Peeters G. Long-term results of laparoscopic sleeve gastrectomy for obesity. Ann Surg 2010;252(2):319–24.

56. Carmeli I, Golomb I, Sadot E, et al. Laparoscopic conversion of sleeve gastrectomy to a biliopancreatic diversion with duodenal switch or a Roux-en-Y gastric bypass due to weight loss failure: our algorithm. Surg Obes Relat Dis 2015; 11(1):79–85.

57. Prachand VN, Ward M, Alverdy JC. Duodenal switch provides superior resolution of metabolic comorbidities independent of weight loss in the super-obese (BMI > or = 50 kg/m2) compared with gastric bypass. J Gastrointest Surg 2010;14(2): 211–20.

58. Prachand VN, Davee RT, Alverdy JC. Duodenal switch provides superior weight loss in the super-obese (BMI > or =50 kg/m2) compared with gastric bypass. Ann Surg 2006;244(4):611–9.

59. Nedelcu M, Noel P, Iannelli A, et al. Revised sleeve gastrectomy (re-sleeve). Surg Obes Relat Dis 2015;11(6):1282–8.

60. Cheung D, Switzer NJ, Gill RS, et al. Revisional bariatric surgery following failed primary laparoscopic sleeve gastrectomy: a systematic review. Obes Surg 2014; 24(10):1757–63.

61. Aminian A, Corcelles R, Daigle CR, et al. Critical appraisal of salvage banding for weight loss failure after gastric bypass. Surg Obes Relat Dis 2015;11(3):607–11.

62. Dykstra M, Switzer N, Sherman V, et al. Roux en Y gastric bypass: how and why it fails? Surg Curr Res 2014;4:165.

63. Vijgen GH, Schouten R, Bouvy ND, et al. Salvage banding for failed Roux-en-Y gastric bypass. Surg Obes Relat Dis 2012;8(6):803–8.

64. Moon RC, Frommelt A, Teixeira AF, et al. Indications and outcomes of reversal of Roux-en-Y gastric bypass. Surg Obes Relat Dis 2015;11(4):821–6.

65. Akusoba I, Birriel TJ, El Chaar M. Management of excessive weight loss following laparoscopic Roux-en-Y gastric bypass: clinical algorithm and surgical techniques. Obes Surg 2016;26(1):5–11.

66. Orci L, Chilcott M, Huber O. Short versus long Roux-limb length in Roux-en-Y gastric bypass surgery for the treatment of morbid and super obesity: a systematic review of the literature. Obes Surg 2011;21(6):797–804.

67. Stefanidis D, Kuwada TS, Gersin KS. The importance of the length of the limbs for gastric bypass patients–an evidence-based review. Obes Surg 2011;21(1): 119–24.

68. Christou NV, Look D, Maclean LD. Weight gain after short- and long-limb gastric bypass in patients followed for longer than 10 years. Ann Surg 2006;244(5): 734–40.

69. Marks VA, de la Cruz-Munoz N. Three techniques to laparoscopically improve restriction after failed gastric bypass: revision of failed LRYGB restriction. Surg Obes Relat Dis 2011;7(5):659–60.

70. Goyal V, Holover S, Garber S. Gastric pouch reduction using StomaphyX in post Roux-en-Y gastric bypass patients does not result in sustained weight loss: a retrospective analysis. Surg Endosc 2013;27(9):3417–20.

71. Muller MK, Wildi S, Scholz T, et al. Laparoscopic pouch resizing and redo of gastro-jejunal anastomosis for pouch dilatation following gastric bypass. Obes Surg 2005;15(8):1089–95.

72. Nguyen D, Dip F, Huaco JA, et al. Outcomes of revisional treatment modalities in non-complicated Roux-en-Y gastric bypass patients with weight regain. Obes Surg 2015;25(5):928–34.

73. Horgan S, Jacobsen G, Weiss GD, et al. Incisionless revision of post-Roux-en-Y bypass stomal and pouch dilation: multicenter registry results. Surg Obes Relat Dis 2010;6(3):290–5.

74. Lo Menzo E, Stevens N, Kligman M. Laparoscopic revision of gastrojejunostomy and vagotomy for intractable marginal ulcer after revised gastric bypass. Surg Obes Relat Dis 2011;7(5):656–8.

75. Birriel TJ, El Chaar M. Laparoscopic revision of chronic marginal ulcer and bilateral truncal vagotomy. Surg Obes Relat Dis 2016;12(2):443–4.

76. Trelles N, Gagner M. Revision bariatric surgery: laparoscopic conversion of failed gastric bypass to biliopancreatic diversion with duodenal switch. Minerva Chir 2009;64(3):277–84.

77. Parikh M, Pomp A, Gagner M. Laparoscopic conversion of failed gastric bypass to duodenal switch: technical considerations and preliminary outcomes. Surg Obes Relat Dis 2007;3(6):611–8.

78. Moon C, Ghiassi S, Higa K. Laparoscopic revision of distal Roux-en-Y gastric bypass to duodenal switch for weight loss failure and symptoms. Surg Obes Relat Dis 2015;11(1):259–61.

Management and Prevention of Surgical and Nutritional Complications After Bariatric Surgery

CrossMark

Eric Marcotte, MD, MS[a],*, Bipan Chand, MD[b]

KEYWORDS

- Bariatric surgery • Complications • Nutrition

KEY POINTS

- Bariatric surgery procedures are safe and carry a low risk of complications, especially in the setting of specialized centers.
- Intraoperative complications should be recognized and their management is usually straightforward.
- Surgeons should be aware of postoperative complications and have a high index of suspicion when caring for bariatric patients.
- All patients after bariatric surgery should be on nutritional (proteins, vitamins, and minerals) supplements, for life.

Bariatric and metabolic surgery has proven health benefits, such as weight loss (and most importantly long-term weight loss maintenance) and resolution of comorbidities associated with obesity. The field has been revolutionized in the last decades with the advent and diffuse adaptation of laparoscopy as a standard of care and the development of centers of excellence.[1] Many large cohort studies demonstrated a decrease in the complication rates (most notably mortality, surgical site infections [SSI], and cardiopulmonary events) of a laparoscopic approach over an open approach.[2,3] This is reflected by the increase of bariatric procedures in the last decade.[4] This article reviews the surgical and nutritional complications of the commonly performed bariatric procedures, including Roux-en-Y gastric bypass (RYGB), laparoscopic adjustable gastric band (LAGB), laparoscopic sleeve gastrectomy (LSG), and biliopancreatic

The authors have nothing to disclose.
[a] Department of Surgery, Stritch School of Medicine, Loyola University Medical Center, 2160 South First Avenue, Maywood, IL 60153, USA; [b] Stritch School of Medicine, Loyola Center for Metabolic Surgery and Bariatric Care, Loyola University Medical Center, 2160 South First Avenue, Maywood, IL 60153, USA
* Corresponding author.
E-mail address: eric.marcotte@lumc.edu

Surg Clin N Am 96 (2016) 843–856
http://dx.doi.org/10.1016/j.suc.2016.03.006
0039-6109/16/$ – see front matter © 2016 Elsevier Inc. All rights reserved.
surgical.theclinics.com

diversion with duodenal switch (BPD-DS). An emphasis is made on ways to prevent specific complications.

An important element in prevention of complications is patient selection, preoperative investigations, and optimization. It is important to assess the patient for medical conditions that would increase the risk of complication, such as a coagulation disorder, obstructive sleep apnea, or uncontrolled diabetes (see Fouse T, Brethauer S: Resolution of Comorbidities and Impact on Longevity Following Bariatric and Metabolic Surgery; Cruz ADG, Portenier DD: Patient selection and Surgical Management of High Risk Patients with Morbid Obesit; and Genser L, Mariolo JRC, Castagneto-Gissey L, et al: Obesity, Type2 Diabetes and the Metabolic Syndrome – Pathophysiologic relationships and Guidelines for Surgical Intervention, in this issue).

PERIOPERATIVE COMPLICATIONS

The Bariatric Outcomes Longitudinal Database is a large cohort study from Bariatric Centers of Excellence across the United States.[5] Their analysis of 36,254 patients who underwent an RYGB (92% laparoscopic) demonstrated a 1.38% rate of adverse events at 30 days post-RYGB, the most common complications being anastomotic leak (0.42%), renal failure (0.31%), respiratory failure (0.27%), and death (0.12%). The Scandinavian Obesity Surgery Registry reported the 30-day complications (8.7%) of 25,038 laparoscopic RYGB in 44 accredited centers in Sweden.[6] The most common complications were bleeding (2.1%), leaks or abscesses (1.8%), and small bowel obstruction (1%). They also reported their intraoperative adverse events, such as unintentional small bowel injury (1.5%), bleeding (0.6%), and instrument failure (0.2%). The Michigan Bariatric Surgery Collaborative evaluated the 30-day operative complications that presented in 7.3% of 15,275 patients undergoing surgery, more specifically 3.1% for RYGB, 2.2% for LSG, and 0.78% for LAGB.[7] Most were minor complications (SSI, 5.9%) and the overall mortality was reported at 0.1%. The Longitudinal Assessment of Bariatric Surgery reported the outcomes of 5882 patients (73% RYGB [88% laparoscopic] and 27% LAGB).[8] Thirty-day major surgical complication rate was 4.1% and mortality is reported at 0.3%.[3] Adverse intraoperative events were associated with worse outcome and consisted of anesthesia events (0.9%), bowel injury (0.9%), instrument/equipment failure (0.8%), liver injury (0.4%), anastomosis revision (0.3%), and splenic injury (0.2%) with all events being more frequent for RYGB.

INTRAOPERATIVE SURGICAL COMPLICATIONS
Laparoscopic Entry Technique

A recent Cochrane review based on 46 randomized controlled trials that included 7389 participants demonstrated no statistical difference in the rates of major complications (vascular or visceral injury) when comparing different entry techniques.[9] All three major techniques (open-entry, Veress needle entry, and direct vision entry) have been described safely for morbidly obese patients.[10] It is important, however, to always rule out an injury after gaining access and be familiar with different techniques.

Small Bowel/Hollow Organ Injury

Although not specific to bariatric procedures, the morbidly obese patient presents with specific characteristics that might lead to a bowel injury. Torque on the trocars (caused by a thick abdominal wall) might lead to lack of control of the instrument and a thermal injury/laceration. Blind instrument insertion (especially if the trocar is very lateral) might also lead to unrecognized injury. For a higher risk trocar location or a nonexperienced assistant, it is therefore recommended to always insert instruments under direct visualization. It is recommended to use sharp dissection and not surgical energy when lysing adhesions. If an injury arises and is recognized, it can usually be repaired primarily (in a transverse fashion to prevent stricture) either laparoscopically or open, depending on the surgeon's comfort level. An unrecognized bowel injury can lead to deep SSI and peritonitis and should be suspected if a patient becomes septic in the postoperative period.

Solid Organ Injury

The left segment of the liver rests on top of the stomach and is particularly prominent in the setting of obesity and steatosis, which makes it very fragile. When using the liver retractor to lift it up, great attention should be paid to not lacerate the parenchyma. Another risk for injury is blind entry of instruments through a port in the right upper quadrant (especially if placed too cephalad). It is important to keep in mind the position of susceptible organs and entering instruments under direct visualization is recommended to prevent this avoidable complication. The spleen lays in close proximity to the gastric fundus. It is particularly at risk while dissection of the greater curve during LSG and while performing retrogastric dissection at the angle of His during LAGB and RYGB. Management of bleeding varies with the degree of laceration but common basic principles are as follows:

1. Packing compression with an opened surgical sponge passed through a 10+ mm port
2. Use of surgical energy: either electrocautery (bipolar or monopolar) or advanced energy, such as vessel-sealing bipolar devices or ultrasonic energy devices
3. Use of hemostatic agents, such as oxidized regenerated cellulose, topical thrombin, and fibrin sealants[11,12]
4. Use of argon beam coagulation
5. Resection (partial hepatectomy or splenectomy) for severe refractory cases[13]
6. Conversion to laparotomy based on surgeon's experience and judgment

Anastomosis Revision

During RYGB and BPD-DS, it is important to assess the anastomosis for two important criteria: adequate perfusion and integrity. Ischemia can be diagnosed by discoloration of either the serosa by laparoscopic view or the mucosa by endoscopic view. It can be caused by the following factors:

1. Tension (commonly gastrojejunal [GJ] anastomosis of RYGB) on the mesentery, which can be reduced by using a retrocolic-retrogastric technique, achieving a complete omental split and, for a patient with a short mesentery, creating a slightly longer gastric pouch.
2. Twisting of the mesentery, always important to rule out. A standardized technique can avoid this problem.
3. Undercutting the mesentery of the biliopancreatic limb of the Roux limb, which is important to rule out before performing the anastomosis, at which point the compromised portion of bowel (tip of the limb) can easily be resected as needed.

Integrity of the anastomosis is evaluated through a leak test, by insufflating at the anastomosis (either with the use of an endoscope or an orogastric tube connected to air flow), clamping the distal bowel, and immersing the anastomosis under water to look for bubbles. It can also be done by injecting methylene blue dye and looking for extravasation. In the case of a positive leak test, it is important to examine all sides of the anastomosis and look for a defect (the site of leak is guided by the origin of extravasation of either air or dye). The defect can be repaired primarily and an omental patch reinforces the repair. It is afterward important to repeat the leak test to confirm adequate repair of the leak.

Staple Line Bleeding

During LSG, the long staple line is often a source of bleeding. It is often caused by superior staple height of tissue (selected for thick gastric tissue) that does not compress vessels, especially when the staple line is close to the larger vessels of the lesser curve. Management of bleeding is compression with opened surgical sponge or application of clips or hemostatic agents. For diffuse bleeding, the staple line can be oversewn, but great care should be taken to prevent obstruction, especially in critical areas, such as the angle of His and the incisura angularis. Using staple line reinforcement can prevent bleeding.[14–16]

Bleeding from Trocar Site

Trocars compress injured abdominal wall vessels (most importantly the inferior epigastric vessels) during the case and tamponade off the bleeding. It is important to take trocars out under direct visualization. If hemorrhage is noted, a figure-of-eight stitch using a suture passer can be placed and tied after the trocar is removed. If not recognized during the case, it leads to a hematoma of the abdominal wall. If the hematoma is expanding or large, anticoagulants (thromboprophylaxis) should be suspended. Surgical intervention is rarely required but is warranted in cases of hemodynamic instability, hemoperitoneum, and superinfection of the hematoma.[17]

POSTOPERATIVE SURGICAL COMPLICATIONS
Bleeding

Although rare, a postoperative hemorrhage is life-threatening. For RYGB or BPD-DS, the incidence in the early postoperative period (less than 30 days) has been reported to be less than 5% and can arise from many sources and vary in clinical presentation.[18–20] Intraluminal bleeding (GJ or duodenoileal anastomosis and jejunojejunal [JJ] or ileoileal [II] anastomosis) presents with either hematemesis (GJ/duodenoileal) or melena/hematochezia (JJ/II). It can also present as a small bowel obstruction caused by a clot (discussed later). Late (more than 30 days postoperative) intraluminal bleed is classically caused by a marginal ulcer.[21,22] Extraluminal bleeding can appear through an incision site or a drain or be diagnosed by findings of hemoperitoneum on imaging or a drop in hemoglobin. It can arise from a staple line, a trocar site, mesentery, omentum, or solid organ injury, unrecognized during surgery.[23] Management of patients depends on hemodynamic stability and failure of self-resolution after suspending anticoagulants and transfusions as needed (more than 2 units of packed red blood cells).[18] Endoscopic management of intraluminal bleeding by adrenaline injection, electrocoagulation, or hemostatic endoclips is successful and safe, with low failure rates. This therapy can be repeated.[24,25] Management of extraluminal bleeding refractory to conservative management is return to the operating room for exploratory laparoscopy and hemostasis, as previously described.

Postoperative bleeding after LSG has been reported as below 5%.[26,27] The main source of bleeding is the staple line and can present as intraluminal or extraluminal hemorrhage. Management is as previously described.

Postoperative bleeding after LAGB is even rarer. Early bleeding is usually caused by solid organ injury and is managed as previously described. Delayed hemorrhage can be secondary to erosion and is life-threatening.[28]

Obstruction

A common complication of gastrointestinal (GI) surgery, small bowel obstruction has been reported in 1% to 5% of RYGB and BPD-DS patients who underwent an open procedure.[29] Although less frequent with the laparoscopic approach, it has been described in up to 3.6% of patients.[29–31] Adhesive disease represents a common cause when performing open surgery but should not be considered as the default cause for patients who have undergone laparoscopy. Internal hernias are common causes of small bowel obstruction and can occur through well-recognized spaces: Petersen space (between the mesentery of the Roux limb and the transverse colon), the JJ, or II mesenteric defect for both RYGB and BPD-DS and the transverse mesocolon defect created to perform a retrocolic approach for the GJ anastomosis of RYGB.[30] Internal hernias are prevented by closing mesenteric defects.[30,32,33] For RYGB, an antecolic configuration of the Roux limb for the GJ anastomosis was demonstrated to lead to fewer internal hernias and small bowel obstruction than a retrocolic approach.[34] Another common cause of small bowel obstruction postbariatric surgery is abdominal wall hernia, including trocar site hernias.[31] Great care should be applied when closing the trocar site fascial defect to prevent those from occurring.

The patient presenting with small bowel obstruction should be evaluated and managed while keeping that differential diagnosis in mind. Routine investigations usually consist of abdominal series, upper GI studies ± computed tomography scan (with oral and intravenous contrast). Diagnostic laparoscopy is often warranted to rule out closed loop obstruction or bowel ischemia. The cure of obstruction can also be performed laparoscopically or open, depending on the surgeon's abilities and comfort. Bowel distention is too important to perform the laparoscopic approach safely and conversion to laparotomy should be perceived as a good judgement for patient safety instead of a technical failure.

For patients with a history of LAGB who present with pain and obstructive symptoms (nausea, vomiting, dysphagia), it is important to rule out a gastric slip, which has been reported to occur in up to 24% of the patients after undergoing LAGB.[35] Suspicion of slippage arises when the band lies in a horizontal orientation and is confirmed by upper GI series showing the obstructed passage of contrast through the band with dilation proximal to the band.[36] A band that is too tight appears in a correct position but shows the same pattern on the upper GI series. Immediate management should be to access the system and remove all fluid.[37]

For patients that underwent LSG, stenosis of the tabularized stomach has been reported to occur in up to 4% of cases.[38] The gastroesophageal junction and the incisura angularis are well-recognized critical zones to protect from narrowing when performing the sleeve gastrectomy. It is important to always use a Bougie as a guide.[39] When a stenosis is suspected, it should be investigated by upper GI series and upper GI endoscopy. The initial management is endoscopic and consists of balloon dilation and may require stent placement.[38,40] Refractory cases are managed by either laparoscopic surgical correction (seromyotomy) or conversion to RYGB.[41]

Infections

SSI are minor complications but can lead to pain and undesired discomfort from wound care and consequences on the health care system, such as increased visits in the emergency department and increased readmission rates.[42] Bariatric surgery patients have multiple risk factors for the development of SSI, such as obesity and diabetes. Great efforts should be conducted to limit the prevalence of SSI. Apart from prophylactic antibiotics, many changes in operative techniques have been linked to a decrease in SSI rates.[43,44] A laparoscopic approach over open leads to a decrease in the incidence of SSI, for both RYGB[2] and BPD-DS.[29]

Leaks are life-threatening complications of bariatric surgery. Although they remain rare, at a reported frequency of usually less than 5%, they can happen after RYGB, BPD-DS, and LSG.[2,18,27,45] Leaks can happen at staple lines (sleeve, gastric pouch, or duodenal stump) or anastomoses.[29] It is important to perform a leak test on proximal anastomoses, as previously reported. Leaks for LSG happen most commonly proximal, close to the gastroesophageal junction and great care should be applied to prevent the superior staple line to be on esophagus, because the tissue is thinner and more fragile.[46] It is also believed that a tighter sleeve leads to increased pressure and would lead to increased risk of leak. Leaks should be suspected in all postbariatric surgery patients presenting with sepsis (tachycardia, pain, fever, hypotension). A leak can be confirmed radiographically with an upper GI series or computed tomography scan with water-soluble contrast, but even if the test is negative, it is important to explore laparoscopically when clinically suspected. Imaging should never delay intervention in an unstable patient. Goals of surgical management of a leak are peritoneal washout and wide drainage, identification (leak test) and repair of the defect as previously described, enteral access for postoperative nutritional support (feeding jejunostomy for LSG and BPD-DS; gastrostomy in the bypassed gastric remnant for RYGB), and cultures and wide-spectrum antibiotics.

NUTRITIONAL COMPLICATIONS

Although the goals of bariatric surgery are weight-loss and resolution of comorbidities, it is important to realize that those operations affect either intake or absorption of nutritional elements, or both at the same time.[47] The benefits of reduced intake of fat and carbohydrate are obvious, but great care needs to be taken to make sure patients after their surgeries do not suffer malnutrition or micronutrient deficiencies (**Table 1**).

Postoperative Diet

Before discharge, the patients are placed on a clear liquid diet to ensure tolerance.[47] While in the hospital, intravenous fluids are given to compensate for a limited oral intake. Nausea is frequent and can impede oral intake, therefore it should be

Table 1
Vitamin supplement recommendations

	Procedure			
Vitamins	LAGB	LSG	RYGB	BPD-DS
Multivitamin with minerals	✔	✔	✔	✔
Vitamin B_{12}	—	✔	✔	—
Calcium with vitamin D	✔	✔	✔	✔
Iron	—	—	✔	✔
Vitamin C	—	—	✔	—
Vitamin A	—	—	—	✔
Vitamin K	—	—	—	✔

controlled. We routinely use a scopolamine patch to prevent and antinausea medications to treat this complication as needed. Once the patients demonstrate adequate oral intake, they are discharged home.

The diet progression is staged, with the goal of tolerating a solid diet 1 month after surgery.[48] Although the duration of each of the phases varies from different programs, the concept is progression in consistencies (to minimize early satiety and reflux) and selection of foods to maximize weight loss and preservation of lean body mass. It goes from clear liquid diet (inpatient), to full liquid diet (10–14 days), to puree (10–14 days), to mechanical soft (14 days), to regular. Emphasis is put on maintaining proper hydration status by drinking at least 60 oz of fluids daily. Protein intake should be 60 to 80 g per day after LAGB, LSG, and RYGB and 80 to 120 g per day after BPD-DS.[49]

Nutrient Metabolism

It is important to understand basic concepts of macronutrient and micronutrient metabolism to understand the need for supplementation for these patients, and the potential for deficiencies. The American Society for Metabolic and Bariatric Surgery nutritional guidelines review all of them in detail.[47]

Vitamin B_{12} needs the intrinsic factor as a cofactor to be absorbed in the distal ileum. Intrinsic factor is produced by parietal cells of the stomach. LSG and RYGB limit the production of intrinsic factor, therefore leading to deficiency, although the level of deficiency is more than 3 times more for RYGB than for LSG.[50–52]

Iron is primarily absorbed in the duodenum and proximal jejunum. The bypassing of these parts of the GI tract after RYGB and BPD-DS therefore puts patients at an increased risk for iron deficiency, which leads to anemia.[53] Iron deficiency has also been reported after LSG, frequencies of which were similar to RYGB.[52] This is believed to be caused by the reduced levels of gastric acid, an important element to cleave dietary iron. Vitamin C deficiency is rare after bariatric surgery and leads to scurvy. Consuming fruits, especially citrus, can prevent it. However, vitamin C has been demonstrated to increase the absorption of iron after RYGB and is therefore recommended as a supplement.[54]

Calcium is absorbed preferentially in the duodenum and proximal jejunum. Its absorption is facilitated by vitamin D, which is itself absorbed in the jejunum and ileum. It is therefore limited after RYGB and BPD-DS. Because calcium is better absorbed in an acidic environment, LSG patients are also at an increased risk for deficiency.[55] A vitamin D deficiency would not lead to hypocalcemia right away because of the parathyroid hormone (PTH) pathway. As calcium stores deplete, PTH levels rise, leading to bone resorption and preservation of calcium by the kidneys. Therefore, hypocalcemia occurs only in the setting of osteoporosis, which is to be avoided.

An important mechanism of action of BPD-DS is the reduction in absorption of fat caused by the delay to mix pancreatic and gastric enzymes with nutrients until the last 50 to 100 cm of ileum (common channel).[56] Fat-soluble vitamins A, D, E, and K are mainly absorbed in the distal jejunum and ileum and are therefore at a very high risk to become deficient after BPD-DS.[49] Deficiencies have, however, also been described after RYGB, LAGB, and LSG, albeit at a lesser extent as for BPD-DS.[57,58]

Thiamine (vitamin B_1) has many important roles that regulate the heart, the GI tract, and the peripheral and central nervous system. Thiamine deficiency can lead to devastating consequences, such as Wernicke encephalopathy (WE) and Korsakoff psychoses. WE presents with peripheral neuropathies and the classic triad of confusion, ataxia with unsteadiness of gait, and nystagmus with diplopia.[59] Because thiamine is primarily absorbed in the duodenum and proximal jejunum, RYGB and BPD-DS are at an increased risk for deficiency but thiamine deficiency has been associated with all bariatric procedures. The main cause is limited intake and the classical presentation of WE is following a period of nausea and vomiting while not taking vitamin supplements, or a patient maintained on a prolonged clear liquid diet without vitamin supplementation, typically in the first 4 to 12 weeks after bariatric surgery.[60] Thiamine deficiency is treated by supplements and needs to be recognized as soon as possible to increase the chances of recovery. Infusing bariatric surgery patients with a solution of dextrose without giving vitamins and thiamine first can deplete thiamine stores and can precipitate WE and aggravate neurologic damage.[61]

Deficiencies (Macronutrients and Micronutrients)

Protein deficiency usually arises from intolerance to protein-rich foods and failure to take protein supplements.[47,62] Common symptoms of protein deficiency are edema, weakness, decreased muscle mass, and thinning hair. Dosage of serum albumin, prealbumin, and creatinine can confirm the deficiency. The first line of treatment is increasing oral protein supplements. Refractory cases may need enteral or parenteral nutritional support and might require reversal of the procedure in extreme cases.

Vitamin B_{12} deficiency can present with fatigue (pernicious anemia) and neurologic symptoms, such as tingling or numbness in fingers and toes, ataxia, mood changes, memory loss, and dementia. It is confirmed by drawing a complete blood count (CBC) and serum B_{12} levels. Repletion with oral or sublingual B_{12} (500 μg/d) for 1 month is recommended as the first phase. Refractory cases should be treated with intramuscular injections of B_{12} (1000–2000 μg/month) for 2 to 3 months.

Iron deficiency also leads to anemia (fatigue, pale skin, palpitations, cold hands and feet). It is confirmed with CBC, serum iron, iron-binding capacity, and ferritin. It is treated with ferrous sulfate, 300 mg two to three times per day with vitamin C. Refractory cases should get intravenous iron infusions.

Hypocalcemia rarely gets severe enough to be symptomatic but can present with tetany and cramping. Dosage of total and ionized serum calcium levels and PTH are necessary to pose the diagnosis. Treatment is with oral supplements of calcium citrate, 1200 to 200 mg/d.

Vitamin D deficiency can lead to hypocalcemia. A low 25-hydroxy vitamin D level confirms the diagnosis. First-line repletion therapy is oral vitamin D, 50,000 IU once weekly for 3 months, which is increased to 50,000 IU twice a week for another 3 months if still deficient. Refractory cases should get oral calcitriol vitamin D, 1000 IU/d.

Folate deficiency leads to the development of macrocytic anemia and neural tube defects in pregnant postbariatric surgery patients. Measuring CBC, serum folate levels, and homocysteine levels leads to the diagnosis. Oral repletion with 400 μg/d (included in multivitamin) for 1 month is recommended. Refractory cases should have the dosage increased to 1000 μg/d.

Zinc deficiency leads to poor wound healing, hair loss, diarrhea, and alteration in taste. It is diagnosed when low levels of serum zinc are found. Repletion is with oral zinc, 220 mg/d for 1 month. Refractory cases can have the dosage increased to 220 mg two or three times a day for another month.

Copper deficiency leads to weakness, fatigue, skin sores, and hair and skin discoloration. These patients should be repleted with oral copper, 2 to 4 mg/d for 1 month.

Vitamin A deficiency leads to night blindness, dry eyes, dry skin, and dry hair. It is diagnosed with a low serum vitamin A level. Treatment is initially with oral vitamin A, 5000 to 10,000 IU/d for 1 month. Refractory cases should then have the dosage increased to 50,000 IU/d for 1 month.

Box 1
Nutritional follow-up laboratory studies
LAGB: 6 months, 12 months, and annual
CBC
Comprehensive Metabolic Panel
Folate
PTH
Iron and transferrin
Vitamin B_{12}
Vitamin D, 25-OH
LSG: 6 months, 12 months, and annual
CBC
CMP
Folate
PTH
Iron and transferrin
Vitamin B_{12}
Vitamin D, 25-OH
RYGB: 6 months
CBC
CMP
Folate
PTH
Iron and transferrin
Magnesium
Phosphorus
Zinc
Copper
Vitamin B_{12}
Vitamin D, 25-OH
RYGB: 12 months and annual
Bone density: dual photon study
CBC
CMP
Folate
PTH
Iron and transferrin
Magnesium
Phosphorus
Zinc

Copper

Vitamin B_{12}

Vitamin D, 25-OH

BPD-DS: 6 months

CBC

CMP

Folate

PTH

Iron and transferrin

Magnesium

Phosphorus

Zinc

Copper

Vitamin A

Vitamin B_1

Vitamin B_{12}

Vitamin D, 25-OH

Vitamin E

BPD-DS: 12 months and annual

Bone density: dual photon study

CBC

CMP

Folate

PTH

Iron and transferrin

Magnesium

Phosphorus

Zinc

Copper

Vitamin A

Vitamin B_1

Vitamin B_{12}

Vitamin D, 25-OH

Vitamin E

Vitamin E deficiency leads to hair loss, leg cramps, and pain/tingling in the extremities. It is diagnosed with finding of low serum vitamin E levels and is repleted with oral vitamin E (initially 400 IU/d for 1 month, then 800 IU/d for another month for refractory cases).

Vitamin K deficiency leads to coagulopathy and can present with bruising, hematuria, or menorrhagia. It is diagnosed with low serum vitamin K levels (more commonly used for research purposes) but can also be suspected with an international normalized ratio greater than 1.4. Repletion is with oral vitamin K, 5 to 10 mg/d, or it can also be treated with a single dose of 10 mg intramuscular.

Follow-Up of Laboratory Studies for Monitoring

It is important to always emphasize at every encounter with the patient the importance of observance in taking supplements after bariatric surgery. It is also very important to monitor nutritional status of the patient to catch a deficiency or more importantly prevent a deficiency from arising. In our centers, laboratory studies are performed routinely at 6 months and 12 months postoperative and more frequently should a suspicion arise (either by symptoms suspicious of deficiency or by behaviors that would lead to a deficiency, such as poor observance, food aversion, or nausea/vomiting). **Box 1** lists the laboratory studies drawn per our actual protocol, dependent on procedure and timing postoperatively.

SUMMARY

Although major complications after bariatric surgeries remain rare, it is important to recognize their presentation and understand their management. Prevention is key and a few of these complications are avoided by simple actions in the operating room. Observance of nutritional supplements after bariatric surgery is a crucial determinant of whether or not complications will occur. Counseling on supplements and nutritional monitoring is important. "Are you taking your vitamins and supplements?" should be part of every encounter with patients after a bariatric procedure, for the rest of their life.

REFERENCES

1. Pratt GM, Learn CA, Hughes GD, et al. Demographics and outcomes at American Society for Metabolic and Bariatric Surgery Centers of Excellence. Surg Endosc 2009;23:795.
2. Lancaster RT, Hutter MM. Bands and bypasses: 30-day morbidity and mortality of bariatric surgical procedures as assessed by prospective, multi-center, risk-adjusted ACS-NSQIP data. Surg Endosc 2008;22:2554.
3. Flum DR, Belle SH, King WC, et al. Perioperative safety in the longitudinal assessment of bariatric surgery. N Engl J Med 2009;361:445.
4. Nguyen NT, Masoomi H, Magno CP, et al. Trends in use of bariatric surgery, 2003-2008. J Am Coll Surg 2011;213:261.
5. DeMaria EJ, Pate V, Warthen M, et al. Baseline data from American Society for Metabolic and Bariatric Surgery-designated Bariatric Surgery Centers of Excellence using the Bariatric Outcomes Longitudinal Database. Surg Obes Relat Dis 2010;6:347.
6. Stenberg E, Szabo E, Agren G, et al. Early complications after laparoscopic gastric bypass surgery: results from the Scandinavian Obesity Surgery Registry. Ann Surg 2014;260:1040.
7. Maciejewski ML, Winegar DA, Farley JF, et al. Risk stratification of serious adverse events after gastric bypass in the Bariatric Outcomes Longitudinal Database. Surg Obes Relat Dis 2012;8:671.
8. Greenstein AJ, Wahed AS, Adeniji A, et al. Prevalence of adverse intraoperative events during obesity surgery and their sequelae. J Am Coll Surg 2012;215:271.
9. Ahmad G, Gent D, Henderson D, et al. Laparoscopic entry techniques. Cochrane Database Syst Rev 2015;(8):CD006583.

10. Kassir R, Blanc P, Lointier P, et al. Laparoscopic entry techniques in obese patient: Veress needle, direct trocar insertion or open entry technique? Obes Surg 2014;24:2193.

11. Chung BI, Desai MM, Gill IS. Management of intraoperative splenic injury during laparoscopic urological surgery. BJU Int 2010;108:572.

12. Cui H, Luckeroth P, Peralta R. Laparoscopic management of penetrating liver trauma: a safe intervention for hemostasis. J Laparoendosc Adv Surg Tech A 2007;17:219.

13. Peters TG, Steinmetz SR, Cowan GS Jr. Splenic injury and repair during bariatric surgical procedures. South Med J 1990;83:166.

14. Consten EC, Gagner M, Pomp A, et al. Decreased bleeding after laparoscopic sleeve gastrectomy with or without duodenal switch for morbid obesity using a stapled buttressed absorbable polymer membrane. Obes Surg 2004;14:1360.

15. D'Ugo S, Gentileschi P, Benavoli D, et al. Comparative use of different techniques for leak and bleeding prevention during laparoscopic sleeve gastrectomy: a multicenter study. Surg Obes Relat Dis 2014;10:450.

16. Shikora SA, Mahoney CB. Clinical benefit of gastric staple line reinforcement (SLR) in gastrointestinal surgery: a meta-analysis. Obes Surg 2015;25:1133.

17. Fernandez EM, Malagon AM, Arteaga I, et al. Conservative treatment of a huge abdominal wall hematoma after laparoscopic appendectomy. J Laparoendosc Adv Surg Tech A 2005;15:634.

18. Schauer PR, Ikramuddin S, Gourash W, et al. Outcomes after laparoscopic Roux-en-Y gastric bypass for morbid obesity. Ann Surg 2000;232:515.

19. Dick A, Byrne TK, Baker M, et al. Gastrointestinal bleeding after gastric bypass surgery: nuisance or catastrophe? Surg Obes Relat Dis 2010;6:643.

20. Heneghan HM, Meron-Eldar S, Yenumula P, et al. Incidence and management of bleeding complications after gastric bypass surgery in the morbidly obese. Surg Obes Relat Dis 2012;8:729.

21. El-Hayek K, Timratana P, Shimizu H, et al. Marginal ulcer after Roux-en-Y gastric bypass: what have we really learned? Surg Endosc 2012;26:2789.

22. Braley SC, Nguyen NT, Wolfe BM. Late gastrointestinal hemorrhage after gastric bypass. Obes Surg 2002;12:404.

23. Chand B, Prathanvanich P. Critical care management of bariatric surgery complications. J Intensive Care Med 2015. [Epub ahead of print].

24. Fernandez-Esparrach G, Bordas JM, Pellise M, et al. Endoscopic management of early GI hemorrhage after laparoscopic gastric bypass. Gastrointest Endosc 2008;67:552.

25. Jamil LH, Krause KR, Chengelis DL, et al. Endoscopic management of early upper gastrointestinal hemorrhage following laparoscopic Roux-en-Y gastric bypass. Am J Gastroenterol 2008;103:86.

26. Csendes A, Braghetto I, Leon P, et al. Management of leaks after laparoscopic sleeve gastrectomy in patients with obesity. J Gastrointest Surg 2010;14:1343.

27. Alvarenga ES, Lo Menzo E, Szomstein S, et al. Safety and efficacy of 1020 consecutive laparoscopic sleeve gastrectomies performed as a primary treatment modality for morbid obesity. A single-center experience from the metabolic and bariatric surgical accreditation quality and improvement program. Surg Endosc 2015. [Epub ahead of print].

28. Rao AD, Ramalingam G. Exsanguinating hemorrhage following gastric erosion after laparoscopic adjustable gastric banding. Obes Surg 2006;16:1675.

29. Biertho L, Lebel S, Marceau S, et al. Perioperative complications in a consecutive series of 1000 duodenal switches. Surg Obes Relat Dis 2013;9:63.

30. Comeau E, Gagner M, Inabnet WB, et al. Symptomatic internal hernias after laparoscopic bariatric surgery. Surg Endosc 2005;19:34.
31. Martin MJ, Beekley AC, Sebesta JA. Bowel obstruction in bariatric and nonbariatric patients: major differences in management strategies and outcome. Surg Obes Relat Dis 2011;7:263.
32. Ren CJ, Patterson E, Gagner M. Early results of laparoscopic biliopancreatic diversion with duodenal switch: a case series of 40 consecutive patients. Obes Surg 2000;10:514.
33. Schweitzer MA, DeMaria EJ, Broderick TJ, et al. Laparoscopic closure of mesenteric defects after Roux-en-Y gastric bypass. J Laparoendosc Adv Surg Tech A 2000;10:173.
34. Champion JK, Williams M. Small bowel obstruction and internal hernias after laparoscopic Roux-en-Y gastric bypass. Obes Surg 2003;13:596.
35. Egan RJ, Monkhouse SJ, Meredith HE, et al. The reporting of gastric band slip and related complications; a review of the literature. Obes Surg 2011;21:1280.
36. Sonavane SK, Menias CO, Kantawala KP, et al. Laparoscopic adjustable gastric banding: what radiologists need to know. Radiographics 2012;32:1161.
37. Freeman L, Brown WA, Korin A, et al. An approach to the assessment and management of the laparoscopic adjustable gastric band patient in the emergency department. Emerg Med Australas 2011;23:186.
38. Parikh A, Alley JB, Peterson RM, et al. Management options for symptomatic stenosis after laparoscopic vertical sleeve gastrectomy in the morbidly obese. Surg Endosc 2012;26:738.
39. Gagner M, Deitel M, Erickson AL, et al. Survey on laparoscopic sleeve gastrectomy (LSG) at the Fourth International Consensus Summit on Sleeve Gastrectomy. Obes Surg 2013;23:2013.
40. Eubanks S, Edwards CA, Fearing NM, et al. Use of endoscopic stents to treat anastomotic complications after bariatric surgery. J Am Coll Surg 2008;206:935.
41. Dapri G, Cadiere GB, Himpens J. Laparoscopic seromyotomy for long stenosis after sleeve gastrectomy with or without duodenal switch. Obes Surg 2009; 19:495.
42. Chopra T, Marchaim D, Lynch Y, et al. Epidemiology and outcomes associated with surgical site infection following bariatric surgery. Am J Infect Control 2012; 40:815.
43. Alasfar F, Sabnis A, Liu R, et al. Reduction of circular stapler-related wound infection in patients undergoing laparoscopic Roux-en-Y gastric bypass, Cleveland Clinic technique. Obes Surg 2010;20:168.
44. Beitner M, Luo Y, Kurian M. Procedural changes to decrease complications in laparoscopic gastric bypass. JSLS 2015;19. e2014.00256.
45. Aurora AR, Khaitan L, Saber AA. Sleeve gastrectomy and the risk of leak: a systematic analysis of 4,888 patients. Surg Endosc 2012;26:1509.
46. Elariny H, Gonzalez H, Wang B. Tissue thickness of human stomach measured on excised gastric specimens from obese patients. Surg Technol Int 2005;14:119.
47. Aills L, Blankenship J, Buffington C, et al. ASMBS allied health nutritional guidelines for the surgical weight loss patient. Surg Obes Relat Dis 2008;4:S73.
48. Bosnic G. Nutritional requirements after bariatric surgery. Crit Care Nurs Clin North Am 2014;26:255.
49. Slater GH, Ren CJ, Siegel N, et al. Serum fat-soluble vitamin deficiency and abnormal calcium metabolism after malabsorptive bariatric surgery. J Gastrointest Surg 2004;8:48.

50. Smith CD, Herkes SB, Behrns KE, et al. Gastric acid secretion and vitamin B12 absorption after vertical Roux-en-Y gastric bypass for morbid obesity. Ann Surg 1993;218:91.
51. Marcuard SP, Sinar DR, Swanson MS, et al. Absence of luminal intrinsic factor after gastric bypass surgery for morbid obesity. Dig Dis Sci 1989;34:1238.
52. Kwon Y, Kim HJ, Lo Menzo E, et al. Anemia, iron and vitamin B12 deficiencies after sleeve gastrectomy compared to Roux-en-Y gastric bypass: a meta-analysis. Surg Obes Relat Dis 2014;10:589.
53. Skroubis G, Sakellaropoulos G, Pouggouras K, et al. Comparison of nutritional deficiencies after Roux-en-Y gastric bypass and after biliopancreatic diversion with Roux-en-Y gastric bypass. Obes Surg 2002;12:551.
54. Rhode BM, Shustik C, Christou NV, et al. Iron absorption and therapy after gastric bypass. Obes Surg 1999;9:17.
55. Vix M, Liu KH, Diana M, et al. Impact of Roux-en-Y gastric bypass versus sleeve gastrectomy on vitamin D metabolism: short-term results from a prospective randomized clinical trial. Surg Endosc 2014;28:821.
56. Scopinaro N, Adami GF, Marinari GM, et al. Biliopancreatic diversion. World J Surg 1998;22:936.
57. Ledoux S, Msika S, Moussa F, et al. Comparison of nutritional consequences of conventional therapy of obesity, adjustable gastric banding, and gastric bypass. Obes Surg 2006;16:1041.
58. Belfiore A, Cataldi M, Minichini L, et al. Short-term changes in body composition and response to micronutrient supplementation after laparoscopic sleeve gastrectomy. Obes Surg 2015;25:2344.
59. Nautiyal A, Singh S, Alaimo DJ. Wernicke encephalopathy: an emerging trend after bariatric surgery. Am J Med 2004;117:804.
60. Chaves LC, Faintuch J, Kahwage S, et al. A cluster of polyneuropathy and Wernicke-Korsakoff syndrome in a bariatric unit. Obes Surg 2002;12:328.
61. Mason EE. Starvation injury after gastric reduction for obesity. World J Surg 1998;22:1002.
62. Heber D, Greenway FL, Kaplan LM, et al. Endocrine and nutritional management of the post-bariatric surgery patient: an Endocrine Society Clinical Practice Guideline. J Clin Endocrinol Metab 2010;95:4823.

Novel Endoscopic and Surgical Techniques for Treatment of Morbid Obesity
A Glimpse into the Future

Matthew Davis, MD, Matthew Kroh, MD*

KEYWORDS

- Endoluminal bariatric techniques • Metabolic surgery
- Revisional bariatric procedures • Weight regain

KEY POINTS

- New technologies involving minimally invasive endoscopic and laparoscopic procedures give patients and providers more options for treating obesity and metabolic disease.
- Primary procedures performed endoscopically include intragastric balloons, endoluminal sleeve barrier devices, sutured gastroplasty, and gastric aspiration devices.
- Novel laparoscopic surgical procedures include a modification of the duodenal switch procedure, gastric plication, and gastric electrical stimulation.
- Revisional procedures based on endoscopic platforms address mechanical aspects of existing anatomy, and use new technologies including suturing and plicating devices, and injection therapy.
- Many of these new technologies show early promise with minimally invasive approaches. Safety, efficacy, and long-term durability will determine the role that such techniques will serve in the treatment of obesity and metabolic disease.

INTRODUCTION

Obesity and weight-related comorbid diseases affect significant numbers of patients worldwide. Increasingly, data show excellent short- and longer-term outcomes for most patients undergoing bariatric surgery. The current and most accurate perspective on obesity is that of a chronic disease. Bariatric and metabolic surgery, although durable and highly effective as a treatment for obesity and its associated comorbid diseases, has potential shortcomings, including side effects, complications, and

Pertinent Disclosures: None.
Section of Surgical Endoscopy, Department of General Surgery, Digestive Disease Institute, Cleveland Clinic Lerner College of Medicine, 9500 Euclid Avenue, Cleveland, OH 44195, USA
* Corresponding author.
E-mail address: krohm@ccf.org

failures. Just as the first metabolic surgeries were performed via laparotomy, and have largely been supplanted by minimally invasive laparoscopic techniques, new and innovative technologies are rapidly advancing this field. The current pace of technologic advances in the health industry supports optimism that the future of surgery, and metabolic surgery specifically, will be even less invasive, while allowing patients access to a more diverse breadth of therapeutic options.

This trend to less-invasive procedures, with different therapeutic targets, efficacy profiles, and complication risks, has the potential to benefit more patients across a spectrum of obesity and comorbid diseases. Evaluation of metrics is important. Similar to the successes of laparoscopy including decreased length of stay, decreased postoperative recovery time, and quicker return to work, these advances may also produce newer outcomes including reversibility, incisionless advantages for endoluminal procedures, and improvements of cost and patient desirability. For patients with significant metabolic comorbid disease, the possibility of providing effective interventions with safer periprocedural outcomes seems ideal. Such effects have propelled many of the currently performed laparoscopic bariatric procedures.

This movement is at the center of novel laparoscopic procedures that target other mechanisms of the gastrointestinal tract and endoluminal procedures that may entirely circumvent any surgical procedure. Such techniques and technologies may be applied as primary bariatric procedures alongside well-established, currently performed laparoscopic surgeries, addressing similar or different patient populations. Additionally, evolving concepts of obesity as a chronic disease and recognizing that certain bariatric surgical procedures will impart complications, initial failures, or longer-term weight recidivism, indicate that there is opportunity to affect patient care and outcomes in this area.

With new strategies and technologies being introduced frequently, it is important to develop standards before offering them to patients. Each technique or improvement will invariably require new technical demands and likely have applications to different spectrums of patients. Thus, objective evaluation of new techniques through Institutional Review Board–mediated research, in addition to regimented training programs for physicians, is necessary to allow for proper evaluation of the safety and efficacy of these procedures and the technical performance of them. The American Society for Metabolic and Bariatric Surgery,[1] the Society of American Gastrointestinal and Endoscopic Surgeons,[2] and, more recently, the American Society for Gastrointestinal Endoscopy (ASGE)[3] have written position statements focused on these new procedures. In this way, proper indications, expected outcomes, and, most importantly, safety standards and contraindications can be developed and maintained.

As with all aspects of metabolic surgery, these novel procedures must be incorporated into a comprehensive bariatric management program that includes medical, psychosocial, and procedural components. This multidisciplinary approach is essential to identify who might benefit most from a given procedure. To maximize the effectiveness of an intervention, it must be the best option for the patient, taking into account all components of goals for treatment of obesity and weight-related comorbid diseases. This multidimensional approach allows for the best intervention to be selected for an individual patient, weighing the anticipated risks against expected benefits, incorporating medical therapy along with endoluminal and surgical procedures.

This article discusses novel endoscopic and surgical approaches to weight loss and treatment of weight related comorbid diseases. Additionally, new and cutting edge modifications to existing procedures are described. Unless otherwise stated, the following interventions are currently under clinical trials and are actively undergoing study to determine their appropriateness and efficacy.

NOVEL PRIMARY ENDOSCOPIC BARIATRIC PROCEDURES
Space-occupying Procedures

Although commonly used worldwide for years, the intragastric balloon has recently been approved for use in the United States. The intragastric balloon serves as an artificial bezoar and was first introduced in 1982.[4] A space-occupying device, the balloon produces a restrictive effect on the stomach based on volume, causing early satiety and thus diminishing oral intake.

Currently, there are 2 US Food and Drug Administration (FDA)-approved devices, the ORBERA (Apollo Endosurgery Inc., Austin, TX) and ReShape (ReShape Medical, San Clemente, CA) balloons. These balloons are placed deflated into the stomach via endoscopy. Once in position, they are then filled with saline, ranging in final volume from 500 to 750 mL. Methylene blue may be mixed into the saline to provide an indicator of balloon rupture, resulting in urine color change if this were to occur. This adjunctive maneuver alerts the patient to balloon deflation, and should prompt evaluation by a physician. The balloons are left in place for 6 months, after which they are then deflated and retrieved endoscopically.

The ORBERA is a single-balloon system (**Fig. 1**). The ReShape Duo balloon is a double balloon system that was developed to diminish the risk of distal migration beyond the stomach (**Fig. 2**).

The 2010 REDUCE study,[5] a prospective, randomized, multicenter trial, was the first US trial for the ReShape device. Its initial phase enrolled 30 patients in a 2:1 ratio of balloon placement or sham procedure. Tolerance of the device was excellent, with only 4 patients reporting postprocedural nausea. No major complications were encountered, and no early device removals were performed. Percentage of excess weight loss (%EWL) at device removal (6 months) was 32% in the treatment group compared with 18% in the sham group.

In 2012 to 2013, the pivotal stage of this trial was performed.[6] A total of 326 patients were randomly assigned to treatment or sham. Both groups were followed up for an

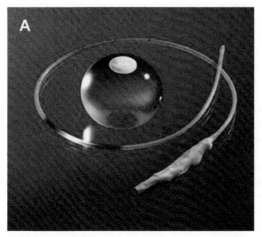
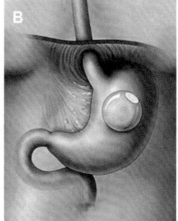

Fig. 1. (*A*) ORBERA single balloon system. (*B*) ORBERA balloon in the stomach. (*Courtesy of* Apollo Endosurgery, Inc, Austin, TX; with permission.)

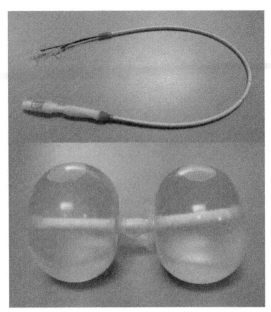

Fig. 2. ReShape® Integrated Dual Balloon duo double balloon system. (*Courtesy of* ReShape Medical, San Clemente, CA; with permission.)

additional 6 months after explantation to determine weight loss maintenance. The sham group was given the option of device placement during this second 6-month follow-up period. The primary endpoints in this study were treatment patients achieving at least 25% EWL and a significant difference in %EWL versus diet and lifestyle modification. Both of these endpoints were met, as the treatment group achieved %EWL of 25.1% and the sham group 11.3%. Statistically significant improvements of comorbid conditions were also seen in the intervention group, including decreases in HbA1c, systolic blood pressure, and serum triglycerides. One percent to 2% of treated patients experienced mild-to-moderate nausea with 9% undergoing early removal.

Both prospective and randomized, controlled trials have been performed using the ORBERA balloon. A systematic review by the ASGE reported %EWL ranging from 11% to 51% at 6 months after removal of the balloon (balloon was placed for 6 months).[7]

The pivotal US trial for ORBERA was recently completed. This trial was a multicenter, prospective, randomized, nonblinded trial involving 225 patients. All participants engaged in a 12-month behavioral modification program, while 125 patients were randomly assigned to also have the ORBERA placed for the first 6 months. The intervention group achieved a %EWL at 6 and 12 months of 38% and 29%, respectively. This percentage was significantly greater than that in the control group ($P<.001$). Additionally, 46% of ORBERA patients achieved at least 15% EWL.[8] The FDA approved the ORBERA balloon for primary treatment of obesity in August 2015.

An ASGE task force systematic review determined that the ORBERA was statistically superior to either sham procedure or lifestyle modification as both a primary and bridge bariatric therapy.[9] As well, this device was found to decrease hyperglycemia, hypertriglyceridemia, and, in some cases, hepatic steatosis.[10] These promising results have promoted further studies to determine if placement of a second balloon might further increase weight loss and metabolic effects. Also, trials are exploring the possibility of leaving the balloon in for longer duration.

Intragastric balloons have been in use outside of the United States for years with variable results. A 2008 meta-analysis pooled data from 15 studies of the BioEnterics Intragastric Balloon (BIB; BioEnterics Corp, Carpinteria, CA).[11] This systematic review comprised 3608 patients. Overall, a 32% EWL was seen at 6 months. Early device removal was required in approximately 4% of patients. Adverse events were few, with the most common being nausea and vomiting. Bowel obstruction was seen in less than 1% of patients. Gastric perforation, the most severe complication reported, occurred at a rate of 0.1% and resulted in 2 deaths.

An older study from Belgium reported on 126 patients who underwent placement of the BIB.[12] Although %EWL at 6 months was promising at 51%, most patients (77%) experienced at least 1 week of nausea. After removal at 6 months, a questionnaire was sent to patients with 40% of respondents indicating that they were "totally unsatisfied" with their degree of weight loss. The authors concluded that the BIB was best used in a carefully selected patient population and proposed that use might be helpful to select those patients who would succeed with a more permanent restrictive procedure, such as a sleeve gastrectomy.

One of the longest-term studies was performed in the Netherlands in 2005.[13] Enrolled patients in the treatment group had a BIB placed for an initial 3 months followed by replacement at 3-month intervals for 3 more occurrences (12 months total). The sham group had an initial sham procedure followed by balloon placement every 3 months for 3 occurrences. Both groups were subsequently followed up for a second year to assess weight loss maintenance. Although more than 40% of patients achieved greater than 20% weight loss in the treatment group at 1 year, this was similar to the sham group. At 2 years, both groups had a low percent weight loss, at approximately 10%.

Another device, the Obalon balloon (Obalon Therapeutics, Carlsbad, CA) is a gas-filled balloon that is initially attached to an inflation catheter. The capsule is swallowed and confirmed to be intragastric via fluoroscopy. Once in appropriate position, the catheter is used to inflate the balloon with air. Preliminary studies have yielded 36% EWL at 3 months.[14] This device is currently in use in Europe and is seeking FDA approval for US applications.

Balloon therapy may serve different roles to effect metabolic improvement in patients. As a simple intervention with few side effects, a balloon may be used in patients with lower body mass index who either do not have access to or do not qualify for more invasive procedures. Patients with no desire at all for a surgical procedure might also be interested in undergoing an endoscopic therapy. Potentially, balloons may also serve as bridges to other therapies, including surgery, by decreasing weight and improving comorbid disease for safer procedures. Finally, with the potential for subsequent placements of a balloon, this therapy may be an enduring, standalone metabolic intervention.

Endoscopic Barrier Therapy

Pure endoscopic metabolic devices have also shown promise as primary interventions and as exclusionary techniques. The EndoBarrier (GI Dynamics Inc, Lexington, MA) is a plastic sleeve 60 cm in length that is placed in the duodenal bulb and extends into the small bowel (**Fig. 3**). This placement results in passage of food through the duodenum and proximal jejunum before mixing with bile and pancreatic fluid. This technique may in some ways be similar to the duodenal-jejunal bypass created by

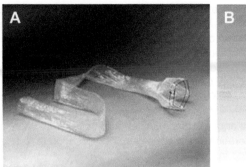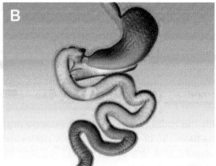

Fig. 3. (*A*) EndoBarrier plastic sleeve. (*B*) The sleeve is placed in the duodenal bulb and extends into the small bowel, resulting in the passage of food through the duodenum and proximal jejunum before mixing with bile and pancreatic fluid. (*Courtesy of* GI Dynamics Inc, Lexington, MA; with permission.)

Roux limb construction in gastric bypass. The device is placed endoscopically and left in place for 1 year before being retrieved endoscopically.

A prospective, open-label trial of 42 patients reported 39 successful initial placements.[15] Although 15 were explanted before the 1-year mark, the remaining 24 patients experienced 47% EWL. Another multicenter, randomized, controlled trial reported on 31 patients who had 32% EWL at 12 months.[16] This finding was statistically greater than that in the control group with 16% EWL. In a third study, 25 patients who had an EndoBarrier placed experienced 22% EWL at 3 months. This study reported a higher complication rate, as 5 patients (20%) were explanted earlier than 12 weeks because of upper gastrointestinal bleeding.[17] In addition to weight loss, these studies showed metabolic effects of decreasing antihyperglycemic and antihypertensive medication use with the device.

Reported complications attributable to the EndoBarrier include obstruction of the stent lumen, stent migration, and bleeding at the proximal anchor point in the duodenum. Recently, while undergoing US clinical trials, however, the FDA shut down phase 2 trials because of a higher-than-expected incidence of liver abscesses (>2%).

The ValenTx endoscopic sleeve (ValenTx, Inc, Carpinteria, CA) combines the malabsorptive component of an endoluminal sleeve with a restrictive aspect (**Fig. 4**).

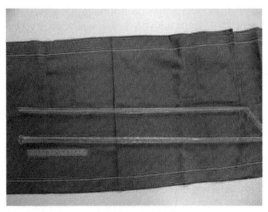

Fig. 4. ValenTx device. (ValenTx, Inc, Carpinteria, CA.)

This restriction is accomplished by using a longer device that anchors proximally in the distal esophagus and passes distally into the jejunum, effectively bypassing stomach capacity. The proximal cuff is sutured to the GE junction endoscopically. This is currently performed under direct laparoscopic vision; however, future applications will aim to secure the device endoscopically alone. This device is left in place for 1 year and then removed endoscopically after cutting the anchoring sutures.

A 2012 prospective, single-center trial reported 1-year results of 36% EWL with a 71% reduction in antihypertensives in the group studied.[18] Complications similar to those seen with the EndoBarrier have been reported in similar frequency for the ValenTx, except for liver abscesses. Also, because of its positioning at the gastroesophageal junction, dysphagia and odynophagia have been observed. This device is currently undergoing US clinical trials.

Endoscopic Sutured Gastroplasty

The Primary Obesity Surgery Endoluminal (POSE) procedure was designed to create an endoscopic bariatric procedure with long-term durability. The procedure uses the Incisionless Operating Platform (USGI Medical, San Clemente, CA), which gained FDA approval in 2006 for grasping, mobilization, and approximation of soft tissue in minimally invasive gastroenterological procedures. The device uses specialized instruments that grasp gastric tissue to create a robust fold and then deploy a suture anchor that maintains the folded tissue in a plicated position (**Fig. 5**).[19] The procedure is performed by placing approximately 8 sutures along the fundus, with 4 more in the antrum opposite the incisura (**Fig. 6**).

One-year results from a 2015 study of 147 patients with class 1 and 2 obesity showed a 44% EWL.[20] Patients reported satisfaction with weight loss results, and they were found to have a 50% decrease in hunger. Only minor complications were reported, including minor bleeding. No long-term complications have been reported.

The ESSENTIAL trial, a multicenter, randomized, double-blind trial is underway to compare the POSE procedure with a sham with an initial follow-up of 12 months.

Endoscopically Placed Aspiration Therapy Device

A novel approach to weight loss was recently devised using gastrostomy tube technology. The AspireAssist (Aspire Bariatrics, King of Prussia, PA) uses a modified gastrostomy tube as access to the stomach for evacuation of an ingested meal (**Fig. 7**). The tube is placed endoscopically using a standard "pull" type technique under sedation. At 2 weeks, the external tube is cut at the level of the skin and a port is attached. The drainage device is then attached to this site after meal ingestion and used to aspirate a portion (~30%) of ingested food in exchange for water.

Combined with lifestyle modification, aspiration yielded a 1-year 49% EWL.[21] Because of the concern for promotion of adverse eating behaviors, postaspiration psychological testing was performed. However, no binge eating events were observed. Adverse event profile was similar to that of standard percutaneous endoscopic gastrostomytube placement and included peristomal pain, bleeding, irritation, and nausea/vomiting. One patient in this series experienced persistent gastrocutaneous fistula after device removal that was managed nonoperatively. A prospective, multicenter clinical trial, the PATHWAY trial is currently ongoing.

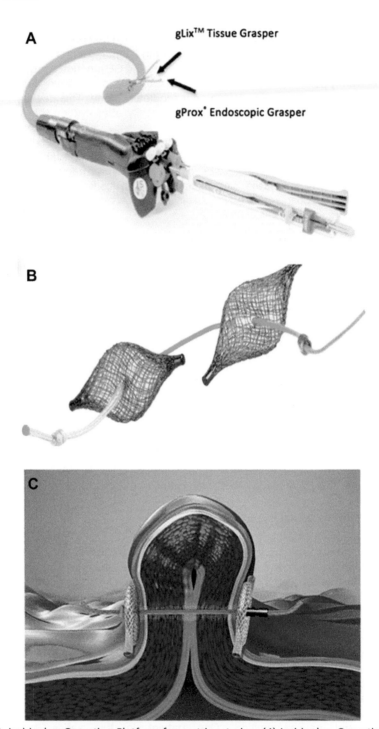

Fig. 5. Incisionless Operating Platform for gastric suturing. (*A*) Incisionless Operating Platform with TransPort Endoscopic Access Device. (*B*) g-Cath EZ Suture Anchors. (*C*) Schematic of anchors holding plicated tissue permitting serosal approximation. (*Courtesy of* USGI Medical, San Clemente, CA; with permission.)

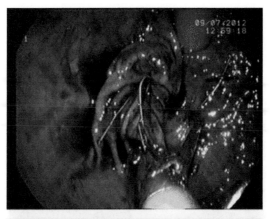

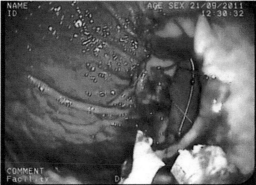

Fig. 6. Sutures placed during POSE procedure. (*From* Espinós JC, Turró R, Mata A, et al. Early experience with the Incisionless Operating Platform (IOP) for the treatment of obesity: the primary obesity surgery endoluminal (POSE) procedure. Obes Surg 2013;23:1381; with permission.)

NOVEL PRIMARY LAPAROSCOPIC SURGICAL BARIATRIC PROCEDURES
Laparoscopic Single-anastomosis Duodeno-Ileostomy with Sleeve Gastrectomy

Data and experience have emerged regarding a novel surgical weight loss procedure partly based on aspects of the duodenal switch. First described in 2007, this procedure is commonly now referred to as *single anastomosis duodeno-ileal bypass with sleeve gastrectomy*, or SADI-S. Performed laparoscopically, the initial part of the operation involves construction of a sleeve gastrectomy. After this step is completed, the duodenal bulb is divided and then anastomosed side to side with the midileum. A 300-cm common channel is measured from the ileocecal valve to find the point of for duodeno-ileostomy anastomosis formation (**Fig. 8**).[22]

A 2010 series reported %EWL at 1 and 3 years of 95% and 114%, respectively.[23] A more recent study showed %EWL of 91% at 1 year and 98% at 5 years.[24] Seventy-two percent of diabetic patients in that study had a decrease in HbA1c to less than 6% in the first year, and 52% maintained that level out to 5 years. Hypertension remission was seen in 52%. In this study, hypoalbuminemia was seen in 14% and 12% of patients in the first and third year, respectively. Vitamin and mineral deficiencies ranged from 8% to 44% of patients at 1 year and from 3% to 53% at 3 years. Of the 168 patients studied, there was one anastomotic leak and 2 reoperations.

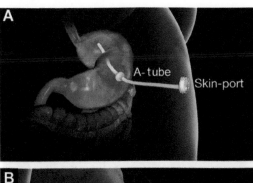

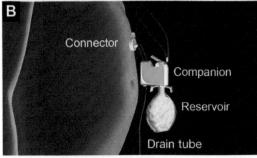

Fig. 7. AspireAssist. (*A*) The tube is placed endoscopically using a standard "pull" type technique under sedation. (*B*) At 2 weeks, the external tube is cut at the level of the skin, and a port is attached. The drainage device is then attached to this site after meal ingestion and used to aspirate a portion (~30%) of ingested food in exchange for water. (*Courtesy of Aspire Bariatrics Inc., King of Prussia, Pa; with permission.*)

Laparoscopic Greater Curvature Plication

First described in 2006, laparoscopic greater curvature plication is an attempt to produce gastric volume reduction without resection.[25] After division of the short gastric vessels, the greater curvature of the stomach is sutured in an imbricated fashion, invaginating that portion of the stomach into the lumen (**Fig. 9**). This technique is repeated for a second and sometimes third layer. This technique aims to create a diminished gastric volume, typically around 100 mL. Initial results of this procedure produced a 57% EWL at 3 years with an acceptable safety profile.

Modifications of the technique have emerged. Huang and colleagues[26] described a modification to plication with the addition of an adjustable gastric band for additional restriction. In this short-term study, 60% EWL at 1 year was shown; however, data were only available for 5 patients at this time point, and no longer-term data are reported.

Perioperative complications of plication with and without a band are reported to be as high as 15% for solitary plication[27] and 12% for banded plication.[28] However, widespread use of this technique has been limited because of poor durability. Talebpour and colleagues[29] reported 800 cases over a 12-year period. Overall, 31% of patients experienced weight regain, with 38 (5%) undergoing revisional bariatric surgery.

Laparoscopic Gastric Stimulation Therapy for Obesity

Another emerging laparoscopic restrictive operation is the gastric electrical stimulator. Different than mechanical restriction, the device imparts a functional restrictive

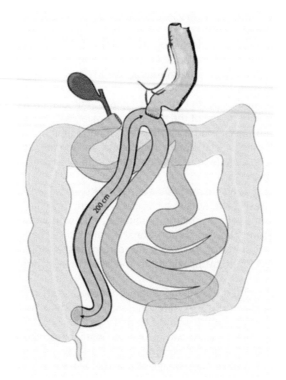

Fig. 8. SADI-S procedure. (*Courtesy of* SADI-S. Obezite Tedavi. Istanbul, Turkey.)

therapeutic effect. Initially found to be beneficial in the management of gastroparesis, the stimulator was used for weight loss soon after. Animal studies found that modulation of gastric motility affects the production and regulation of gastrointestinal hormones, including ghrelin, glucagon-like peptide-1, peptide YY, leptin, and

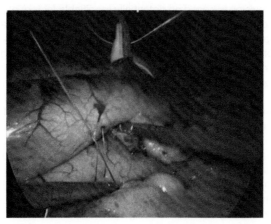

Fig. 9. Laparoscopic greater curvature plication (with proximal adjustable gastric band in place).

cholecystokinin. A decrease in the level of ghrelin, for example, leads to appetite reduction, thereby leading to decreased food intake. There are currently several stimulators undergoing evaluation, including the TANTALUS[30] (MetaCure, Atir Yeda 17 Kfar Saba, Israel), Transcend Implantable Gastric Stimulator[31] (Medtronic Transneuronix, Minneapolis, MN), Enterra (Medtronics), and RGES[32] (World Precision Instrument, Sarasota, FL).

Currently, human studies on the effects of gastric stimulation have produced heterogeneous results.[33] Because of the number of available devices and studies being in preliminary stages, there are no current recommendations on stimulation pattern (eg, long vs short pulses, stimulation frequency). In addition, some studies have looked at the effects of antegrade versus retrograde pulsation without conclusive evidence to either method.

The only FDA-approved neuromodulator, the Maestro Rechargeable System[34] (EnteroMedics, St Paul, MN), acts in a manner different than the above stimulators. Instead of having its effect on gastric peristalsis, this stimulator inhibits the vagal impulses on the stomach. The device consists of similar components, including electrodes and the generator; however, the electrodes are placed at the gastroesophageal junction, in close proximity to the anterior and posterior vagal nerve trunks.

The ReCharge trial,[35] a double-blind, sham-controlled study is currently assessing the outcomes of this device. The most recent results published are from the 18-month interval. At this time point, %EWL with the device was 24% compared with 10% in the sham group. Adverse events were mainly mild and within an acceptable safety profile. One patient did experience gastric perforation during explantation of the device after the patient's decision to discontinue in the study. This trial remains active to determine long-term effects of neurostimulation.

Revisional Endoscopic Procedures

Bariatric surgery is proven to be durable and effective. However, a certain segment of patients may have initial failures or recidivism after success. The indications for reintervention must be carefully evaluated on an individual patient basis. Weight regain and associated comorbid diseases are evaluated in the context of a multidisciplinary therapeutic approach to patients, including the surgeon, psychologist, nutritionist, and medical bariatrician. After careful evaluation including behavioral factors and diet, consideration for revision is based on potentially modifiable factors of existing anatomy.

Revisions include correction of existing operations, conversion to a different type of operation, and, rarely, reversal. Newer technologies and devices focus on particular aspects of anatomy that can be altered. Common therapeutic targets after gastric bypass include enlarged gastric pouch, gastro-gastric fistula, and dilated gastrojejunostomy. Revisional bariatric surgery can be performed safely with good results, but complication rates are consistently higher than with primary procedures.[36] As such, there is an opportunity to circumvent the previous operative field and perform procedures from an endoluminal access site.

To treat dilation of the gastric pouch, the StomaphyX device (EndoGastric Solutions, Redmond, WA) was created.[37] This endoscopic adjunct was granted FDA approval in 2007 for "approximation and ligation in the GI tract." The device is introduced transorally with a gastroscope. Using suction, gastric tissue is pulled into the device and an H-shaped suture is deployed to approximate the tissue. This method is done sequentially to form a ridge and decrease gastric pouch volume.

This procedure has not produced significant short-term weight loss or sustained long-term effects. One study showed a 12% EWL at 1 and 6 months, indicating a low level of efficacy and early plateau. Additionally, weight regain was seen at longer-term follow-up of 2 to 4 years.[38]

More recently, for treatment of an enlarged gastrojejunostomy, the Overstitch Endoscopic Suturing System (Apollo Endosurgery Inc., Austin, TX) has been used (**Fig. 10**). The system attaches to a double-channel endoscope (GIF-2T16; Olympus America, Central Valley, PA), which allows multiple suture patterns with a single pass of the scope. The device uses a helical grasper to position anastomotic tissue and deploy a full-thickness suture in a circular motion parallel to the device's axis. Then a t-tag suture anchor is released and cinched down to approximate the tissue (**Fig. 11**).

A series of 25 patients with dilated gastrojejunostomy after gastric bypass underwent endoscopic revision.[39] Mean weight regain at up to 6 years postoperatively was 24 kg. Six months after endoscopic suturing therapy, patients were able to lose up to 70% of this regained weight. This percentage decreased to 56% at 1 year, however, and longer-term data are not been reported. Complications associated with the device are low and similar to other interventional endoscopic procedures. Most commonly, complications include nausea, oropharyngeal discomfort, and, rarely, bleeding.

The PROMISE trial, in which the Overstitch device is being used to perform endoscopic sleeve gastroplasty, is currently ongoing.

The EndoCinch (C.R. Bard, Inc, Murray Hill, NJ), operates similar to the StomaphyX, but has been applied to the gastrojejunostomy rather than the pouch. The device is attached to a standard endoscope and inserted in tandem. The tip of the device suctions in tissue, and suture is passed through that tissue using a hollow needle. The suture is then tied with a knot pusher. This technique results in partial-thickness suturing only.

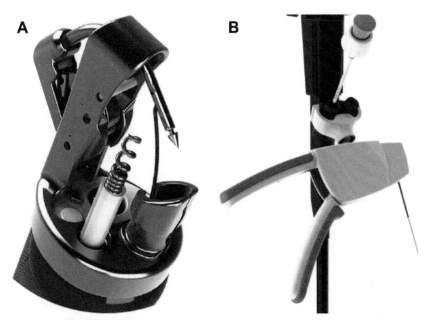

Fig. 10. Overstitch Endoscopic Suturing System. (*A*) The system attaches to a double-channel endoscope (GIF-2T16; Olympus America), which allows multiple suture patterns with a single pass of the scope. (*B*) The device uses a helical grasper to position anastomotic tissue and deploy a full-thickness suture in a circular motion parallel to the device's axis. (*Courtesy of* Apollo Endosurgery Inc, Austin, TX; with permission.)

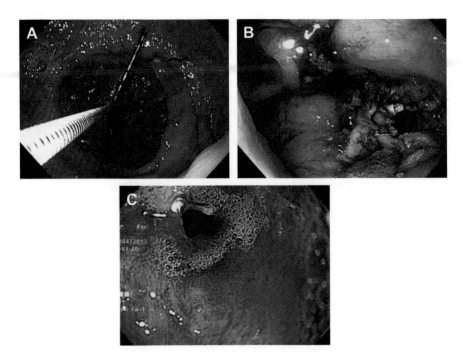

Fig. 11. Dilated gastrojejunostomy revision after Overstitch therapy. (*A*) Dilated gastrojejunal anastomosis (GJA). (*B*) GJA after transoral outlet reduction (TORe) with a full-thickness suturing device. (*C*) GJA 6 months after full-thickness TORe. (*From* Kumar N, Thompson CC. Comparison of a superficial suturing device with a full-thickness suturing device for transoral outlet reduction (with videos). Gastrointest Endosc 2014;79(6):986; with permission.)

The RESTORe trial, a multicenter, randomized, double blind, sham-controlled trial was completed in 2010.[40] The study involved 77 patients who presented with inadequate weight loss or weight regain after gastric bypass. At 6 months, patients in the EndoCinch group achieved 4.7% weight loss, compared with 1.9% in the sham group. An average of 4 stitches were placed, and successful reduction of the stoma to less than 1 cm was achieved in 89% of participants.

A 2014 matched cohort comparison study[41] compared the EndoCinch and Overstitch devices in patients with weight regain after gastric bypass. All patients had dilation of their gastrojejunostomy to greater than 2 cm. One-year %EWL was 18.9% with the Overstitch versus 9.1% using the EndoCinch. This finding was statistically significant. Both procedures were found to be safe, with only one bleeding event requiring transfusion occurring in each group.

Both the EndoCinch and the Overstitch have also been used for revision of gastrogastric fistulae, another common cause of weight regain after bariatric surgery. Although this has been shown to be technically feasible, consistent long-term durability of gastro-gastric fistula closure has yet to be demonstrated.

A novel method for treating an enlarged gastrojejunal stoma is sclerotherapy by injection of sodium morrhuate. This substance, more commonly used as a sclerosing agent to obliterate esophageal varices, is delivered via an endoscopic catheter and is injected circumferentially around the dilated stoma.

A recent study[42] with a mean follow-up of 18 months found that 64% of patients had success with this therapy, which was defined as initial reduction of stoma size

$\leq$1.2 cm and eventual loss of $\geq$75% of weight that was regained after previous gastric bypass. One instance of stoma stenosis was identified and treated successfully with endoscopic balloon dilation.

SUMMARY

Obesity is a chronic disease, and its associated metabolic diseases impact the length and quality of many patients' lives. Although current metabolic and bariatric procedures effectively address much of this burden, new minimally invasive procedures give patients and medical providers more therapeutic options. Novel endoscopic and laparoscopic procedures may provide different treatment choices for patients, both as primary and revisional procedures. Institution of any of these procedures should be performed within the context of a multidisciplinary and comprehensive bariatric treatment program to appropriately identify the best intervention. The long-term success of these exciting new approaches will be determined by evaluation of safety, efficacy, and durability, as they apply to individual patients, to treat their metabolic disease.

REFERENCES

1. Emerging Technologies and Clinical Issues Committees of the ASMBS. American Society for metabolic and bariatric surgery position statement on emerging endo-surgical interventions for the treatment of obesity. Surg Obes Relat Dis 2009;5(3): 297–8.
2. Position statement on Endoluminal Therapies for Gastrointestinal Diseases. Available at: http://www.sages.org/publications/guidelines/position-statement-on-endoluminal-therapies-for-gastrointestinal-diseases. Accessed December 1, 2015.
3. ASGE Bariatric Endoscopy Task Force, Sullivan S, Kumar N, Edmundowicz SA, et al. ASGE position statement on endoscopic bariatric therapies in clinical practice. Gastrointest Endosc 2015;82(5):767–72.
4. Nieben OG, Harboe H. Intragastric balloon as an artificial bezoar for treatment of obesity. Lancet 1982;1(8265):198–9.
5. Ponce J, Quebbemann BB, Patterson EJ. Prospective, randomized, multicenter study evaluating safety and efficacy of intragastric dual-balloon in obesity. Surg Obes Relat Dis 2013;9:290–5.
6. Ponce J, Woodman G, Swain J, et al, REDUCE Pivotal Trial Investigators. The REDUCE pivotal trial: a prospective, randomized controlled pivotal trial of a dual intragastric balloon for the treatment of obesity. Surg Obes Relat Dis 2015;11(4):874–81.
7. ASGE Bariatric Endoscopy Task Force, ASGE Technology Committee, Abu Dayyeh BK, Edmundowicz SA, Jonnalagadda S. Endoscopic bariatric therapies. Gastrointest Endosc 2015;81(5):1073–86.
8. Abu Dayyeh BK, Eaton LL, Woodman G, et al. A randomized, multi-center study to evaluate the safety and effectiveness of an intragastric balloon as an adjunct to a behavioral modification program, in comparison with a behavioral modification program alone in the weight management of obese subjects. Presented at Digestive Disease Week. Washington, DC, May 16–19, 2015.
9. Abu Dayyeh BK, Kumar N, Edmundowicz SA, et al. ASGE Bariatric Endoscopy Task Force systematic review and meta-analysis assessing the ASGE PIVIV thresholds for adopting endoscopic bariatric therapies. Gastrointest Endosc 2015;82(3):225–38.

10. Forlano R, Ippolito AM, Iacobellis A, et al. Effect of the BioEnterics intragastric balloon on weight, insulin resistance, and liver steatosis in obese patients. Gastrointest Endosc 2010;71:927–33.

11. Imaz I, Martinez-Cervell C, Garcia-Alvarez EE, et al. Safety and effectiveness of the intragastric balloon for obesity. A meta-analysis. Obes Surg 2008;18:841–6.

12. Totté E, Hendrickx L, Pauwels M, et al. Weight reduction by means of intragastric device: experience with the bioenterics intragastric balloon. Obes Surg 2001;11:519–23.

13. Mathus-Vliegen EM, Tytgat GN. Intragastric balloon for treatment-re- sistant obesity: safety, tolerance, and efficacy of 1-year balloon treat- ment followed by a 1-year balloon-free follow-up. Gastointest Endosc 2005;61:19–26.

14. Mion F, Ibrahim M, Marjoux S, et al. Swallowable Obalon gastric balloons as an aid for weight loss: a pilot feasibility study. Obes Surg 2013;23(5):730–5.

15. Escalona A, Pimentel F, Sharp A, et al. Weight loss and metabolic improvement in morbidly obese subjects implanted for 1 year with an endoscopic duodenal-jejunal bypass line. Ann Surg 2012;255:1080–5.

16. Koehestanie P, de Jonge C, Berends FJ, et al. The effect of the endoscopic duodenal-jejunal bypass liner on obesity and type 2 diabetes mellitus; a multi-center randomized controlled trial. Ann Surg 2014;260:984–92.

17. Tarnoff M, Rodriguez L, Escalona A, et al. Open label, prospective, randomized controlled trial of an endoscopic duodenal-jejunal bypass sleeve versus low cal-orie diet for pre-operative weight loss in bariatric surgery. Surg Endosc 2009;23:650–6.

18. Sandler B, Rumbaut R, Swain CP, et al. One-year human experience with a novel endoluminal, endoscopic gastric bypass sleeve for morbid obesity. Surg Endosc 2015;29:3298–303.

19. Espinós JC, Turró R, Mata A, et al. Early experience with the Incisionless Oper-ating Platform (IOP) for the treatment of obesity: the Primary Obesity Surgery Endoluminal (POSE) procedure. Obes Surg 2013;23:1375–83.

20. López-Nava G, Bautista-Castaño I, Jimenez A, et al. The Primary Obesity Surgery Endoluminal (POSE) procedure: one-year patient weight loss and safety out-comes. Surg Obes Relat Dis 2015;11(4):861–5.

21. Sullivan S, Stein R, Jonnalagadda S, et al. Aspiration therapy leads to weight loss in obese subjects: a pilot study. Gastroenterology 2013;145:1245–52.

22. Sánchez-Pernaute A, Rubio Herrera MA, Pérez-Aguirre E, et al. Proximal duodenal-ileal end-to-side bypass with sleeve gastrectomy: proposed technique. Obes Surg 2007;17:1614–8.

23. Sánchez-Pernaute A, Herrera MA, Pérez-Aguirre ME, et al. Single anastomosis duodeno-ileal bypass with sleeve gastrectomy (SADI-S). One to three-year follow-up. Obes Surg 2010;20(12):1720–6.

24. Sánchez-Pernaute A, Rubio MÁ, Cabrerizo L, et al. Single-anastomosis duode-noileal bypass with sleeve gastrectomy (SADI-S) for obese diabetic patients. Surg Obes Relat Dis 2015;11(5):1092–8.

25. Talebpour M, Amoli BS. Laparoscopic total gastric vertical plication in morbid obesity. J Laparoendosc Adv Surg Tech A 2007;17(6):793–8.

26. Huang C, Lo C, Shabbir A, et al. Novel bariatric technology: laparoscopic adjust-able gastric banded plication: technique and preliminary results. Surg Obes Re-lat Dis 2012;8:41–7.

27. Ji Y, Wang Y, Zhu J, et al. A systematic review of gastric plication for the treatment of obesity. Surg Obes Relat Dis 2014;10(6):1226–32.

28. Chaudhry UI, Osayi SN, Suzo AJ, et al. Laparoscopic adjustable gastric banded plication: case-matched study from a single U.S. center. Surg Obes Relat Dis 2015;11:119–24.

29. Talebpour M, Motamedi SM, Talebpour A, et al. Twelve year experience of laparoscopic gastric plication in morbid obesity: development of the technique and patient outcomes. Ann Surg Innov Res 2012;6(1):7.

30. Bohdjalian A, Prager G, Aviv R, et al. One-year experience with Tantalus: a new surgical approach to treat morbid obesity. Obes Surg 2006;16:627–34.

31. D'Argent J. Gastric electrical stimulation as therapy of morbid obesity: preliminary results from the French study. Obes Surg 2002;12(Suppl 1):21S–5S.

32. Zhang Y, Du S, Fang L, et al. Retrograde gastric electrical stimulation suppresses calorie intake in obese subjects. Obesity (Silver Spring) 2014;22:1447–51.

33. Cha R, Marescaux J, Diana M. Updates on gastric electrical stimulation to treat obesity: Systematic review and future perspectives. World J Gastrointest Endosc 2014;6(9):419–31.

34. Shikora S, Toouli J, Herrera MF, et al. Vagal blocking improves glycemic control and elevated blood pressure in obese subjects with type 2 diabetes mellitus. J Obes 2013;2013:245683.

35. Shikora SA, Wolfe BM, Apovian CM, et al. Sustained weight loss with vagal nerve blockade but not with sham: 18-month results of the ReCharge Trial. J Obes 2015;2015:365604.

36. Jones KB Jr. Revisional bariatric surgery—potentially safe and effective. Surg Obes Relat Dis 2005;1:599–603.

37. Mikami D, Needleman B, Narula V, et al. Natural orifice surgery: initial US experience utilizing the StomaphyX device to reduce gastric pouches after Roux-en-Y gastric bypass. Surg Endosc 2010;24:223–8.

38. Goyal V, Holover S, Garber S. Gastric pouch reduction using StomaphyX in post Roux-en-Y gastric bypass patients does not result in sustained weight loss: a retrospective analysis. Surg Endosc 2013;27:3417–20.

39. Jirapinyo P, Slattery J, Ryan MB, et al. Evaluation of an endoscopic suturing device for transoral outlet reduction in patients with weight regain following Roux-en-Y gastric bypass. Endoscopy 2013;45:532–6.

40. Thompson CC, Roslin MS, Chand B, et al. M1359 RESTORE: randomized evaluation of endoscopic suturing transorally for anastomotic outlet reduction: a double-blind, sham-controlled multicenter study for treatment of inadequate weight loss or weight regain following Roux-en-Y gastric bypass. Gastroenterology 2010;138. S–388.

41. Kumar N, Thompson CC. Comparison of a superficial suturing device with a full-thickness suturing device for transoral outlet reduction (with videos). Gastrointest Endosc 2014;79(6):984–9.

42. Catalano MF, Rudic G, Anderson AJ, et al. Weight gain after bariatric surgery as a result of a large gastric stoma: endotherapy with sodium morrhuate may prevent the need for surgical revision. Gastrointest Endosc 2007;66(2):240–5.

Body Contouring Surgery in the Massive Weight Loss Patient

Dennis J. Hurwitz, MD[a],*, Omodele Ayeni, MD, FRCSC[b]

KEYWORDS

- Body contouring surgery • Massive weight loss • Total body lift • Liposuction
- VASER

KEY POINTS

- Body contouring surgery after bariatric surgery addresses the large quantities of inelastic skin after massive weight loss.
- The author puts forth 11 surgical principles to approach body contouring in the massive weight loss patient.
- Proper patient selection, unique preoperative preparation, intraoperative planning, and resource management improve results and reduce morbidity.
- Technical advances in women include improved management of adiposity with spiral flap augmentation/suspension of the breasts and concomitant ultrasonic-assisted lipoplasty and lipoaugmentation.
- Direct oblique excision of flank bulges extending posterior to the abdominoplasty instead of the traditional lower body lift is yielding better mid/lower torso contours.

INTRODUCTION

An estimated 36.7% of the adult population in the United States is obese.[1] Defined as a body mass index of greater than 30 kg/m^2, obesity is associated with comorbidities that double mortality from cancer, cardiovascular disease, and diabetes.[2] Predictions based on a linear time trend suggest that 51% of the US population will be obese, and 9% will be morbidly obese by 2030.[3] Weight loss by dietary changes and exercise usually does not achieve the desired weight loss goals on an individual.[4] As such, bariatric surgery has become the treatment of choice for obesity and morbid obesity.[5] The Roux-En-Y gastric bypass procedure remains the gold standard surgical option for the

The authors declare no commercial or financial conflicts of interest and any funding sources in the preparation of this article.
[a] University of Pittsburgh Medical School, Suite 500, 3109 Forbes Avenue, Pittsburgh, PA 15213, USA; [b] Southlake Regional Health Centre, Newmarket, Ontario, Canada
* Corresponding author.
E-mail address: drhurwitz@hurwitzcenter.com

obese patient with gastric sleeve gaining traction. In the course of achieving massive weight loss (MWL) and alleviation of comorbidities, bariatric surgery creates quality-of-life problems for the plastic surgeon.

Minimally invasive gastrointestinal bypass surgery for morbid obesity was successfully pioneered by Phillip Schauer at the University of Pittsburgh Medical Center.[6] Despite their numerous health advantages, disgruntled patients soon complained of disturbing lax skin and subcutaneous tissue. Schauer asked the senior author to help. Addressing a hospital auditorium full of MWL patients, Hurwitz learned of the disheartening changes in body contour with repulsive hanging skin and bizarre rolls of skin and fat. They were embarrassed by flattened breasts, hanging pannus, ptotic mons pubis, and sagging inner thighs. Clothes fit poorly. Vigorous activity was difficult. Skin beneath folds becomes moist, malodorous, and inflamed.

In the late 1990s, plastic surgeons limited their treatment of skin redundancy of the torso and thigh by a circumferential abdominoplasty, a lower body lift, and a medial thighplasty.[7–13] Sagging breast were treated independently. The results often fell below expectations. Delayed wound healing was common. There was scant precedent for successfully performing body contouring surgery after MWL. The bypass patients of the 1980s usually underwent the physiologically disruptive jejunal-ileal bypass and were poor candidates for prolonged body contouring surgery. Modern minimally invasive surgery with the Roux-en-Y gastrointestinal bypass delivered a much less traumatized and healthier patient. After 4 years of innovative effort, we introduced a comprehensive single stage solution called total body lift surgery.[14]

Body contouring after MWL is now embraced as a safe and reliable option to improve self-esteem, social life, work ability, physical activity, and sexual activity.[15–21] Most often excisional, body contouring surgery can also use liopaspiration, dermal suspension techniques, and autologous fat grafting. It has been estimated that as many as one-third of MWL patients will require reconstructive surgery after their weight loss. Estimates as high as 80% purport that patients desire body contouring surgery after MWL; however, only 12% undergo the corrective surgery.

CURRENT APPROACH AND PRINCIPLES

Because of comorbidities and prolonged postoperative negative nitrogen balance (starvation), we avoid panniculectomy coincidental with gastric bypass. Moreover, the panniculectomy scar may preclude optimal subsequent surgical planning for definitive torso contour correction. After MWL, panniculectomy is simply the removal of hanging panniculus by a long anterior transverse excision of skin and fat between the umbilicus and pubis. There is no undermining of the superior flap or alteration or reconstruction of the umbilicus. Panniculectomy may be complemented with liposuction of surrounding, non-undermined bulging skin. It satisfies the medical indications by correcting the inflammatory sequelae of an overhanging pannus. This limited abdominoplasty is rarely aesthetically adequate.

Our innovative total body lift approach features comprehensive and coordinated planning in as few stages as possible.[14] Loose skin is excised and gender-specific features sculpted. Female adipose-related features of the breasts, waist, hips, and buttocks are shaped.[22] Men have restoration of upper body dominance and visibility of broad superficial muscles with aggressive treatment of gynecomastia and love handles.[22] These are extensive and complex operations over large portions of the body, requiring a team of operators, working in consort from 3 to 6 hours with the patient under general anesthesia. Minor wound healing complications were common, but major morbidity is rare.[23] Before embarking on such lengthy procedures, the surgeon and the support team and hospital should have experience working together on less extensive procedures. Two days of hospital care are essential. The larger the patient and the longer the procedure, the more likely are complications.

These multiple operations are lengthy, envelop large portions of a big body, and require position changes and high-tension closure of undermined and thinned flaps. The operative plan is based on the application of plastic surgical principles that incorporate artistry, with minimal trauma to tissues.[24] Accordingly, we have listed the 11 relevant plastic surgery principles for successful results with a low complication rate. The precise technique varies according to the deformity and surgeon preferences, but the principles are inviolate (**Box 1**).

The first principle is to analyze the patient and deformity. Consider body shape (endomorph, mesomorph, or ectomorph), extent of deformity, impact on the patient, patient priorities, lifestyle, and tolerance for risk. MWL leaves a deflated shape related to familial and gender-specific fat depositions and skin to fascia adherences. In men there is a tendency to retain adipose around the flanks, intraabdominally, and breasts. Female fullness lies in the subcutaneous fat of the abdomen, hips, and thighs. Redundant skin hangs over regions of fibrous adherence of dermis to deep fascia. Oversized people, endomorphs, cannot be transformed into ectomorphs. However, with the aid of complimentary VASERlipo, minimally traumatic debulking can be done.

Exclude from total body lift surgery candidates having unstable chronic medical and/or psychiatric illnesses and unrealistic expectations. Borderline cases may undergo limited procedures such as an abdominoplasty.

The consultation continues with a focused examination with the aid of a full-length mirror. Digital preoperative images are manipulated for the patient to understand the anticipated changes. Electronic pens draw anticipated incision lines, indicating the direction of tissue tensions and final scar placement on multiple views. Their estimated new silhouette can be morphed with no promises. During follow-up, both disappointed and pleased patients are reminded of the extent of their original deformity by having a monitor with all possible images available near the examination room. There are often extensive layered folds, wrinkling, and striae. The skin is like an oversized in elastic suit and in no dimension, vertical or horizontal, is there normal skin tension.

Box 1
Plastic surgery principles with a low complication rate

1. Analyze deformity and patient

2. Efficiency in design, organization, and execution

3. Optimal orientation of tissue excision

4. Accurate preoperative incision planning

5. Focus on contour and shape

6. Contour with autogenous tissues

7. Integration of liposuction with excisional surgery

8. Preserve dermis, subcutaneous fascia, and neurovasculature

9. Tight and secure closure

10. Anticipatory perioperative management

11. Analyze clinical experience

Efficiency in design, organization, and execution is the second principle. The surgeon should develop a consistent procedure so that the surgical assistants can anticipate. Instrument requests are made before they are needed. Wasted motion and repeated effort lengthens an already long operation, thereby increasing bleeding, medical and wound healing complications, surgeon fatigue, and costs. Slow but steady is the rule.

Reliable preoperative markings expedite team surgery. The most effective and efficient positioning and turning of the patient starts in the prone and ends in the supine positions, which includes placing the leg in abduction. The flap with the greatest movement is elevated first. The operation starts with the inferior incision of the lower body lift. Once mobilized, the buttock and thigh flap is pulled superiorly and the anticipated superior incision line is confirmed and incised. The intervening low back and flank skin is removed as an island of skin and fat from side to side. Appropriate traction and countertraction permit rapid resection through a potentially bloody and nondistinct plane of dissection. Care is taken to leave behind the ideal and symmetric adipose level along the flanks and hips. The central back closure is not too tight to better tolerate the marked flexion needed for the subsequent abdominal closure. Before the patient is turned, the posterior portion of the medial thighplasty is performed superficially along the inferior gluteal fold. Later, the patient is turned and placed in the supine position onto a second operating room table and sterile sheets for the abdominoplasty. Experienced residents assist or perform portions of the procedure with both the attending and the residents suctioning fat or suturing simultaneously.

The third principle is to excise skin in the optimal orientation. Skin redundancy is predominantly vertical, and crisscrossing with vertical excisions leaves compromised flap tips. Transverse scars are easily placed within underwear areas and are less likely to hypertrophy. Plan the trunk scar along the bikini line, which is easily covered and represents the greatest circumference of the female torso. When the relatively narrow waist level excess skin is advanced over the iliac crests, much of the transverse excess is taken in. An inverted superior anterior midline V excision is reserved for removal of widened and depressed surgical scars. A posterior V-shaped excision is limited to the midline buttock flap, to help rotate in excessively redundant lateral thigh skin. A broad vertical segment of midline back skin is invariably adherent, and therefore it is only excised as the end of a transversely oriented ellipse. A series of oblique excisions are reserved for the muscular male.[22]

Preoperative definitive incision planning, the fourth principle leaves, level scars. Most excisions are planned with the patient reclining, but checked standing. Mid and upper abdominal transverse scars are included in the excision, to avoid possible skin necrosis, whenever possible.

The fifth principle is to focus on the contour and shape of the tissue left behind, much as in a breast reduction. Do not let the removal of excess skin distract from this ultimate goal.

The sixth principle is to contour with autogenous tissue, such as regional flaps or lipoaugmentation whenever augmentation of adipose related features is needed.

The seventh principle, integration of liposuction with excisional surgery, necessitates gentle fat removal. Preliminary VASER (Solta, Valient Pharmapseudicals) ultrasound system disrupts only fat, and the not the neurovascuature allowing for minimally traumatic follow-up lipoaspiration.

The eighth principle preserves dermis and subcutaneous fascia by preliminary infiltration along the anticipated incision of 100 of mL of lactated Ringer's solution with 1 mg of epinephrine and 40 mL of 1% xylocaine per liter. This preparation minimizes bleeding and limits the use of electrocautery to pinpoint coagulation through the incision. The incision is slightly beveled along the dermis and then made perpendicular through the fat and subcutaneous fascia.

The ninth principle dictates a high-tension skin flap closure. After MWL, skin flaps are inelastic. The flap vessels are large, a remnant of the prior obesity, permitting greater undermining and closure tension on the flaps. Correction of the lateral thigh saddlebag deformity has been improved by fully abducting the leg onto a side utility table while closing with the patient in the prone position.[25] Nevertheless, the farther from the suture line, the less effective is the pull. Therefore, following a bikini line closure and upper thighplasty, residual laxity is seen in the epigastrium, midlateral trunk, and distal thighs. This upper laxity can be treated secondarily through a reverse abdominoplasty, which we have transformed into the upper body lift. Lower thigh laxity is corrected by direct excisions along the medial and posterior thighs. When high-tension closure is present, some late thinning of the subcutaneous tissues can occur, particularly in the lateral buttock region. The inclusion of a deepithelialized upper buttock flap fills out the central flattened buttocks, but not laterally. Preliminary approximation with towel clips keeps the tension during closure of the wound minimal. Optimal torso closures are achieved by flexing the trunk, approximating the wound edges with #2 PDO Quill large subcutaneous tissue bites followed by intradermal 3-0 Monoderm. These barbed sutures evenly distribute closure tension. Along with the absence of knots, the Quill device has considerably reduced our operative time and minor wound healing problems.[26]

The tenth principle is anticipatory perioperative management. A complete medical and nutritional evaluation with provision of needed supplements is essential.[27,28] The opportune time to perform body contouring is when the patient has completed the catabolism and has reduced comorbidities. In the event that a motivated patient is unable to achieve their desired weight loss goal, the author has successfully incorporated a 42-day injectable human chorionic gonadotropin/500 calories per day program.[28] Since 2004, this program has been used by the Hurwitz Centre for Plastic Surgery in Pittsburgh and has witnessed an average of nearly 1 pound lost per day per patient without complications.

Experienced anesthesiologists will be prepared for the position change and protection of the face and weight-bearing surfaces. A foam rubber mask with a cutout for the endotracheal tube has been our preferred approach (Gentle Touch 5″ headrest pillow by Orthopaedic Systems Inc, Union City, CA). Intravenous fluids are scaled down in consideration of the use of several liters of saline tumescent subcutaneous injections for liposuction. The anesthesia team controls intraoperative fluid and medical management. The need for colloid and blood replacement is discussed during the procedure. All patients are monitored continuously, which includes urine output. Hemoglobin concentration is optimized with iron and vitamin supplements, resorting to iron infusions if necessary. Erythropoietin may be taken a month before surgery, accepting an increased risk for thromboembolism. Larger patients pre donate 1 to 2 units of blood for later transfusion. Or, preferably, our anesthesiologist removes about 500 mL at the beginning of the case, replenishes the volume with saline, and then administers the donated blood at the end of the case. In that way, patients do not receive thrombogenic old banked blood. A liter of Hespan, colloids helps to restore both volume and oncotic pressure. Intermittent leg pressure pumps are activated and intravenous antibiotics are given before the induction of general anesthesia. Additional risk factors for thrombophlebitis, a history of phlebitis, thromboembolism, lower extremity swelling, age greater than 50 years, prolonged surgery and obesity prompts the use of low-molecular-weight heparin.

Patients are hospitalized for about 2 days for fluids, electrolytes, and pain management. In addition, their movements are assisted to reduce excessive tension on tight suture lines.

Edema, infections, phlebitis, and seromas are reduced by closing wounds as expeditiously as possible over suction catheters. Elasticized garments with minimal pressure over the lower abdomen are comfortable and reassuring to the patient. Aside from some periumbilical and groin flap tacking sutures, we have not closed the abdominoplasty dead space. Lower abdominal subscarpa fascia lymphatics are preserved as much as possible. Seromas are a rare. Postoperative external ultrasound (VASERshape, Solta, Valient) has speed resolution of edema.

The 11th principle is that analyzing the aesthetic results and the patient outcomes 1 year or more postoperative is very instructive. Inquire about patient satisfaction and consider measures for improvement. Review standard photography to gauge results. Our deformity and outcome grading scale is applied.[22,29] Correction of deformity may not always equate with optimal aesthetic results, but it is an improvement. The best aesthetics leave the most unobtrusive symmetric scars and gender-specific contours.

CLINICAL EXPERIENCE

Over the past 16 years, this author has performed more than 1800 procedures on more than 400 patients after MWL, pregnancy, or aging. These include singly or in

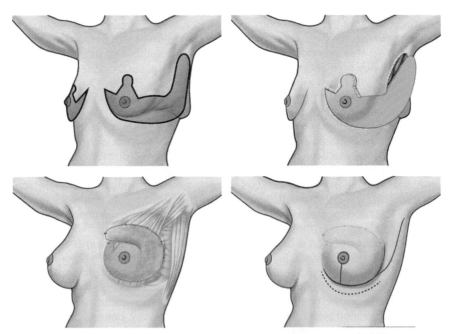

Fig. 1. Drawing of J torsoplasty upper body lift and breast reshaping with spiral flap augmentation and suspension. (*Upper left*) Outlining the Wise pattern mastopexy deepithelialization and flap incisions with J torsoplasty. (*Upper right*) The incisions and deepithelialization is completed. (*Lower left*) The lower flap has been flipped up against the breast and the J torsoplasty spiraled around the superior pole. Both flaps suspend the breast. (*Lower right*) The Wise pattern has been closed over the flaps.

combination abdominoplasty, lower body lift, upper body lift, medial thighplasty, bra-chioplasty, mastopexy, breast reduction, facelift, gynecomastia correction, liposuc-tion, and lipoaugmentation. The body mass index ranged from 24 to 42 kg/m^2. Owing to the potential for a high rate of complications,[30] we have treated few patients with morbid obesity.

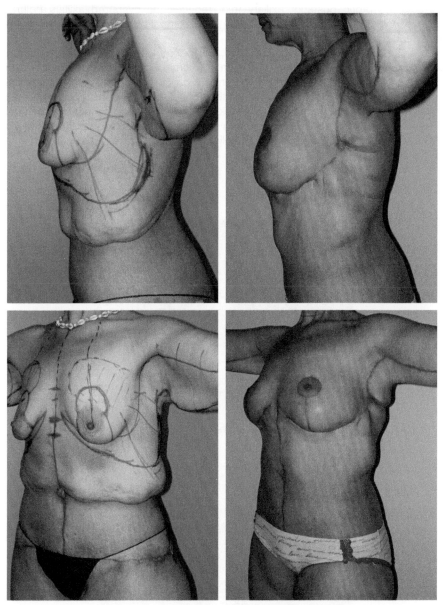

Fig. 2. J torsoplasty combined with spiral flap reshaping of the breasts and L brachioplasty in a 42-year-old massive weight loss patient. (*Left*) Before left lateral and oblique views with preoperative markings. (*Right*) Result with uncomplicated healing at 6 months.

An upper body lift treats epigastric skin, mid back folds, and flattened, distorted breasts. In males, upper body lifts treat ptotic gynecomastia in continuity with loose chest skin and back rolls. In women, the upper body lift focuses on establishing a higher and firm inframammary fold. The breasts are raised and augmented with nearby spiral flaps.[31] For all but the most severe deformity, a J-shaped lateral torsoplasty is perform to avoid back braline scars (**Figs. 1** and **2**).[22] Commonly, these operations are extended through arm reduction surgery via an L brachioplasty.[32] This method corrects the ptotic posterior axillary fold, reduces the oversized axillary hollow, removes excess subaxillary skin, and defines the lateral border of the breast seamlessly and smoothly.

When a much deeper waist is envisioned, the abdominoplasty is extended obliquely posterior over the flanks[33] (**Figs. 3** and **4**). In addition to this, we have found success in the combined lipoabdominoplasty with central high-tension closure. Defatting of the abdominal skin flap significantly increases the upper flap dispensability and preserves the perforating blood supply. Caution is taken by not suctioning the midline fat in the area of the 3-flap deepithelialized umbilical cutout.[23] Tension at the central distal end of the abdominoplasty is reduced by the plication of small epigastric skin flaps to the fascial base of the umbilicus.[34]

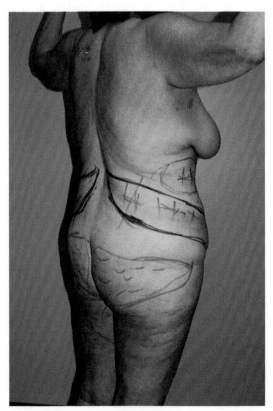

Fig. 3. Left posterior oblique view of a 59-year-old massive weight loss patient marked for abdominoplasty extending obliquely over the flanks and lipoaugmentation of the buttocks.

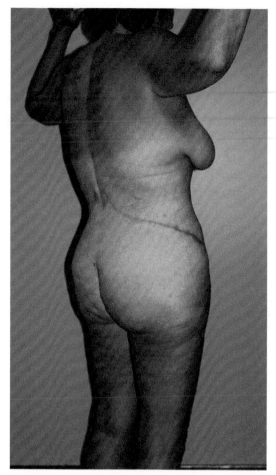

Fig. 4. Left posterior Oblique view of a 59-year-old massive weight loss patient 5 months after abdominoplasty extending obliquely over the flanks and lipoaugmentation of the buttocks.

SUMMARY

A dedicated and experience surgical team can safely and effectively offer total body lift surgery after MWL. Recent advances have improved safety and aesthetic results.

REFERENCES

1. Ogden CL, Carroll MD, Kit BK, et al. Prevalence of obesity in the United States 2009-2010. NCHS Data Brief 2012;(82):1–8.
2. Dixon J. The global burden of obesity and diabetes [Chapter 1]. In: Brethauer SA, Schauer PR, Schirmer BD, editors. Minimally invasive bariatric surgery. 2nd edition. New York: Springer; 2015. p. 1–13.
3. Finkelstein EA. Obesity and severe obesity forecasts through 2030. Am J Prev Med 2012;42:6.

4. Burguera B, Tur J. Medical management of obesity [Chapter 3]. In: Brethauer SA, Schauer PR, Schirmer BD, editors. Minimally invasive bariatric surgery. 2nd edition. New York: Springer; 2015. p. 15–38.

5. Dan AG, Lynch R. History of bariatric and metabolic surgery [Chapter 4]. In: Brethauer SA, Schauer PR, Schirmer BD, editors. Minimally invasive bariatric surgery. 2nd edition. New York: Springer; 2015. p. 39–48.

6. Schauer PR, Ikramuddin S, Gourash W, et al. Outcomes after laparoscopic Roux-en-Y gastric bypass for morbid obesity. Ann Surg 2000;4:515–29.

7. Lockwood TE. Lower body lift with superficial fascial system suspension. Plast Reconstr Surg 1993;92:1112–22.

8. Lockwood TE. Lower body lift. Aesthet Surg J 2001;21:355–60.

9. Hamra S. Circumferential body lift. Aesthet Surg J 1999;19(3):244–51.

10. Pascal JF, Le Louarn C. Remodeling body lift with high lateral tension. Aesthetic Plast Surg 2002;26:223–30.

11. Aly AS, Cram AE, Chao M, et al. Belt lipectomy for circumferential truncal excess: the University of Iowa experience. Plast Reconstr Surg 2003;111:398–413.

12. Van Geertruyden JP, Vandeweyer E, de Fontanie S, et al. Circumferential torsoplasty. Br J Plast Surg 1999;52:623–30.

13. Hunstad JP. Addressing difficult areas in body contouring with emphasis on combined tumescent and syringe techniques. Clin Plast Surg 1996;23:57–80.

14. Hurwitz DJ. Single stage total body lift after massive weight loss. Ann Plast Surg 2004;52(5):435–41.

15. Modarressi A, Balague N, Huber O, et al. Plastic surgery after gastric bypass improves long term quality of life. Obes Surg 2013;23:24–30.

16. Tremp M, Delko T, Kraljević M, et al. Outcome in body contouring surgery after massive weight loss: a prospective matched single-blind study. J Plast Reconstr Aesthet Surg 2015;68:1410–6.

17. Colwell AS. Current concepts in post bariatric body contouring. Obes Surg 2010; 20:1178–82.

18. Hasanbegovic E, Sørensen JA. Complications following body contouring surgery after massive weight loss: a meta-analysis. J Plast Reconstr Aesthet Surg 2014; 67:295–301.

19. Matarasso A, Aly A, Hurwitz DJ, et al. Aesthet Surg J 2004;24(5):452–63.

20. Klopper EM, Kroese-Deutman HC, Berends FJ. Massive weight loss after bariatric surgery and the demand (desire) for body contouring surgery. Eur J Plast Surg 2014;37(2):103–8.

21. Gusenoff JA, Messing S, O'Malley W, et al. Patterns of plastic surgical use after gastric bypass: who can afford it and who will return for more. Plast Reconstr Surg 2008;122(3):951–8.

22. Hurwitz DJ. Aesthetic refinements in body contouring in the massive weight loss patient: trunk. Plast Reconstr Surg 2014;134:1185–95.

23. Hurwitz DJ, Agha-Mohammadi S, Ota K, et al. A clinical review of total body lift. Aesthet Surg J 2008;28(3):294–304.

24. Hurwitz DJ. Principles and basic techniques in comprehensive body contouring: theory and practice [Chapter 3]. New York: Springer; 2016. p. 27–61.

25. Hurwitz DJ, Rubin JP, Risen M, et al. Correcting the saddlebag deformity in the massive weight loss patient. Plast Reconstr Surg 2004;114(5):1313–25, 22.

26. Hurwitz DJ, Reuben B. Quill™ barbed sutureIn body contouring surgery: a six year comparison study with running absorbable braided sutures. Aesthet Surg J 2013;33(Supp 3):44S–56S.

27. Agha-Mohammadi S, Hurwitz DJ. Nutritional deficiency of post- bariatric body contouring patients: what every plastic surgeon should know. Plast Reconstr Surg 2008;122(2):604–13.
28. Agha-Mohammadi S, Hurwitz DJ. Potential impacts of nutritional deficiency of post-bariatric patients on body contouring. Plast Reconstr Surg 2008;122(6): 1901–14.
29. Song AY, Jean RD, Hurwitz DJ, et al. A classification of contour deformities after massive weight loss: the Pittsburgh rating scale. Plast Reconstr Surg 2005; 116(5):1535–44.
30. Matory WE Jr, O'Sullivan J, Fudem G, et al. Abdominal surgery in patients with severe morbid obesity. Plast Reconstr Surg 1994;94:976–80.
31. Hurwitz DJ, Agha-Mohammadi S. Post bariatric surgery breast reshaping: the spiral flap. Ann Plast Surg 2006;56(5):481–6.
32. Hurwitz DJ, Holland SW. The L brachioplasty: an innovative approach to correct excess tissue of the upper arm, axilla and lateral chest. Plast Reconstr Surg 2006; 117(2):403–11, 25.
33. Hurwitz DJ, Wooten A. Plastic surgery for the obese. International Journ Adipose Tis 2007;1:5–11.
34. Hurwitz DJ. Body contouring surgery for women in comprehensive body contouring: theory and practice [Chapter 4]. New York: Springer; 2016. p. 63–179.

Index

Note: Page numbers of article titles are in **boldface** type.

Surg Clin N Am 96 (2016) 887–899
http://dx.doi.org/10.1016/S0039-6109(16)52038-6
0039-6109/16/$ – see front matter

surgical.theclinics.com

Moving?

Make sure your subscription moves with you!

To notify us of your new address, find your **Clinics Account Number** (located on your mailing label above your name), and contact customer service at:

Email: journalscustomerservice-usa@elsevier.com

800-654-2452 (subscribers in the U.S. & Canada)
314-447-8871 (subscribers outside of the U.S. & Canada)

Fax number: 314-447-8029

Elsevier Health Sciences Division
Subscription Customer Service
3251 Riverport Lane
Maryland Heights, MO 63043

*To ensure uninterrupted delivery of your subscription, please notify us at least 4 weeks in advance of move.

Printed and bound by CPI Group (UK) Ltd, Croydon, CR0 4YY

03/10/2024

01040393-0009